Nutrition
in the Childbearing Years

LEEDS BECKETT UNIVERSITY
LIBRARY
DISCARDED

Leeds Metropolitan University

17 0557787 9

DISCARDED

Nutrition in the Childbearing Years

Emma Derbyshire

BSc, PhD, RNutr

Senior Lecturer and Researcher in Human Nutrition,
Manchester Metropolitan University

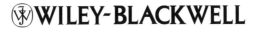

WILEY-BLACKWELL

A John Wiley & Sons, Ltd., Publication

This edition first published 2011 by Blackwell Publishing Ltd. © 2011 by Emma Derbyshire

Blackwell Publishing was acquired by John Wiley & Sons in February 2007. Blackwell's publishing program has been merged with Wiley's global Scientific, Technical and Medical business to form Wiley-Blackwell.

Registered office: John Wiley & Sons, Ltd, The Atrium, Southern Gate, Chichester, West Sussex, PO19 8SQ, UK

Editorial offices: 9600 Garsington Road, Oxford, OX4 2DQ, UK
The Atrium, Southern Gate, Chichester, West Sussex, PO19 8SQ, UK
2121 State Avenue, Ames, Iowa 50014-8300, USA

For details of our global editorial offices, for customer services and for information about how to apply for permission to reuse the copyright material in this book please see our website at www.wiley.com/wiley-blackwell.

The right of the author to be identified as the author of this work has been asserted in accordance with the UK Copyright, Designs and Patents Act 1988.

All rights reserved. No part of this publication may be reproduced, stored in a retrieval system, or transmitted, in any form or by any means, electronic, mechanical, photocopying, recording or otherwise, except as permitted by the UK Copyright, Designs and Patents Act 1988, without the prior permission of the publisher.

Designations used by companies to distinguish their products are often claimed as trademarks. All brand names and product names used in this book are trade names, service marks, trademarks or registered trademarks of their respective owners. The publisher is not associated with any product or vendor mentioned in this book. This publication is designed to provide accurate and authoritative information in regard to the subject matter covered. It is sold on the understanding that the publisher is not engaged in rendering professional services. If professional advice or other expert assistance is required, the services of a competent professional should be sought.

Library of Congress Cataloging-in-Publication Data

Derbyshire, Emma.
  Nutrition in the childbearing years / Emma Derbyshire.
      p. ; cm.
  Includes bibliographical references and index.
  ISBN 978-1-4443-3305-3 (pbk. : alk. paper)   1. Pregnancy–Nutritional aspects.   I. Title.
  [DNLM: 1. Maternal Nutritional Physiological Phenomena.   WQ 175]
  RG559.D47 2011
  618.2'42–dc22
                                                                                  2011007521

A catalogue record for this book is available from the British Library.

This book is published in the following electronic formats: ePDF 9781444344769; Wiley Online Library 9781444344790; ePub 9781444344776; Mobi 9781444344783

Set in 10/12pt Sabon by Aptara® Inc., New Delhi, India

Printed and bound in Malaysia by Vivar Printing Sdn Bhd

1   2011

LEEDS METROPOLITAN
UNIVERSITY
LIBRARY

1705577879
NF-B
CC-123634
31·10·11
618·242 DER

Contents

APPENDICES

CASE STUDIES

Foreword

Nutrition during the childbearing years plays a major role in the health of both mother and child. Poor maternal nutritional status is associated with adverse outcomes for mother and child both in the short term and in later years, and in recognition of its imperative to global public health, 'improving maternal health' is one of the United Nations Millennium Development Goals (MDG5). The link between maternal health and that of the child is critical, as stated in the WHO Global Strategy for Infant and Young Child Feeding:

> The health and nutritional status of mothers and children are intimately linked. Improved infant and young child feeding begins with ensuring the health and nutritional status of women, in their own right, throughout all stages of life and continues with women as providers for their children and families. Mothers and infants form a biological and social unit; they also share problems of malnutrition and ill-health. Whatever is done to solve these problems concerns both mothers and children together.
>
> (WHO, 2003, p. 5)

A clearer understanding of the relationship between nutrition during the childbearing years and health outcomes may provide a basis for developing nutritional interventions that will improve pregnancy outcomes and reduce maternal and child mortality and morbidity. Improving nutrition during this critical period to promote long-term health could also be a driver for future economic growth (World Bank, 2006; SACN, 2011).

One of the main challenges for practitioners working in fields allied to maternal and child nutrition is to translate intricate scientific concepts into simple advice about food and health that can be easily understood by all members of society. As our understanding advances, new controversies and challenges are introduced – this book provides a balanced view of the evidence base and will assist readers in coming to a clear understanding of these complex issues.

The first two chapters in this book set out the nutritional requirements prior to conception, both in terms of their influence on fertility and in the provision of adequate nutrient reserves for the mother and foetus during pregnancy. As illustrated in these chapters, many women of childbearing age do not meet the recommended nutrient intakes for key nutrients, particularly iron and folate. Although historically much effort has been directed at interventions to improve maternal nutritional status that are delivered during mid- or late-gestation, particularly with regard to food or micronutrient supplementation, there is a growing realisation that the mother's nutritional status at and prior to conception exerts strong effects (Williams, 2009).

There is an increasing interest in the potential that early life interventions, including those around the time of the mother's own conception (which take into account powerful intergenerational influences) could offer greater health benefits to both mother and her child.

Chapters 6 and 7 in this book clearly illustrate the wide variation in global micronutrient recommendations during pregnancy. These disparities have arisen from the use of different concepts and sometimes different data and because the expert committees who set the recommendations often base their decisions on judgments concerning the quality of the available research (Pijls et al., 2009). As national reference values are reviewed at different time points, decisions may also be based on different scientific data (Doets et al., 2008). Divergence in the terminology used to describe reference values also creates difficulties with making comparisons across countries, leading to confused messages that may have a serious impact on policy and significant health consequences (Pavlovic et al., 2007).

As nutrient recommendations form the basis of food policy and food-based dietary guidelines, and are used in nutrition labelling, the need to harmonise recommendations is clear. Chapter 7 describes the EURRECA project, which recognises the need for evidence-based policy making, transparent decision-making, stakeholder involvement and alignment of policies across Europe. The EURRECA network aims to develop a common framework that uses consistent terminology in order to develop and maintain nutrient recommendations based on the best current evidence.

The crucial role of maternal nutrition in influencing birth outcomes is discussed in Chapter 8. As a modifiable risk factor, maternal nutrition is of high public health importance with the potential to prevent adverse birth outcomes, particularly amongst developing/low-income populations. Whilst the evidence from experimental animal studies is strong, the research in humans is much less consistent, due, in part, to secondary factors that differ from study to study (e.g. baseline maternal nutritional status, socio-economic status of the study population, timing and methods of assessing or manipulating maternal nutritional variables) (Abu-Saad and Fraser, 2010). A further limitation of the usefulness of the evidence base is that most of the studies investigating maternal nutrition and birth outcomes have approached the issue by investigating single nutrients in isolation, and studies that address and bring together the broader picture of multiple nutrient intakes or deficiencies are still lacking. This work is vital as nutrient deficiencies, generally found amongst low-income populations, are more likely to involve multiple rather than single deficiencies (Abu-Saad and Fraser, 2010).

The issue of weight gain during and after pregnancy remains highly controversial. As described in Chapter 9, almost half of all women of childbearing age in England are overweight or obese, and this number is predicted to rise significantly in the coming years (NHS, 2011). This predicament is compounded by the lack of knowledge amongst mothers and health professionals about the recommended levels of weight gain and different cultural beliefs and perceptions about weight gain in pregnancy. In the United Kingdom, at present, there are no formal evidence-based guidelines from the government or professional bodies on what constitutes appropriate weight gain during pregnancy (NICE, 2010).

Chapter 10 describes some special cases that may require specific nutritional attention. One of the groups discussed includes adolescent mothers. Approximately one-fifth of all births worldwide are to adolescent mothers; this represents a significant global public health issue. Reviews have shown that the intakes and nutritional status of pregnant adolescents are suboptimal (Hall Moran, 2007a, 2007b). Of particular concern is compromised iron and folate status, which has been related to an increased incidence of small-for-gestational-age birth and preterm delivery amongst adolescents. Pregnant adolescents have also been shown to be at risk of vitamin D deficiency with inadequate vitamin D intake compounded with evidence to suggest that darker skinned adolescents may be unable to absorb sufficient ultraviolet B radiation even during the summer months (Baker *et al.*, 2009).

The final chapters in this book explore issues concerned with nutrition following birth. The reset hypothesis is discussed, which suggests that regular breastfeeding may help the mother's metabolic profile return to normal by reversing the pregnancy-related changes in triglyceride levels and insulin resistance more quickly and more completely in women who breastfeed their infants. An adequate diet during lactation is essential to replenish maternal nutrient stores, optimise the nutrition quality of breast milk and support the health of both mother and child. Lactation is a highly demanding state for the mother with a nutritive burden considerably greater than that of pregnancy. The duration and intensity of lactation may have a differential impact on a mother's nutritional status – an exclusively breastfeeding woman has much greater energy and nutrient needs (with the exception of iron attributed to the potential protective effect of lactational amenorrhoea) than a woman who is only partially breastfeeding (Dewey, 2004). Although it is well acknowledged that some of the additional nutrient requirement originates from stores accrued during pregnancy, there are recommendations for breastfeeding women to increase their intake of some nutrients. The setting of nutrient recommendations for lactation, however, is beset with methodological difficulties. As metabolic data upon which estimates of requirements are based are often lacking for physiological states such as lactation because of practical difficulties or ethical limitations in conducting research in women during these reproductive stages, differences between nutrient recommendation values can be partly ascribed to differences in methodological approaches and how these approaches are applied (Atkinson and Koletzko, 2007). Other factors associated with suboptimal maternal nutritional status during lactation, including maternal age, diet and lifestyle factors and spacing of consecutive births, should also be considered (Hall Moran *et al.*, 2010).Given the wide variation in breastfeeding practices across the world, it is crucial to first examine the cultural practices within populations to assess the relevance before making nutrient recommendations for lactating women.

Throughout this book, there is strong recognition that consumption behaviour in pregnancy is influenced by a complex range of psychological, socio-demographic and cultural factors. Low income and low maternal education have been found to be associated with poor-quality diet, and diet-related diseases, such as obesity and diabetes, are increasing amongst lower and middle-income groups (Popkin, 2003; Arkkola *et al.*, 2006). Such groups are more likely to have diets low in protein, fibre and many micronutrients, a low intake of fruit and vegetables and higher intake of processed and convenience food. Barriers to good nutritional practices of women living in conditions of material deprivation include problems with access, cost and storage of food (Reid and Adamson, 1997). Over time, such ways of 'managing' poverty can become second nature, despite the potential costs to the individual's physical and emotional well-being (Attree, 2005). Few studies which explore nutrition during this critical period of life take sufficient account of the socio-economic and living circumstances of their participants. Without a clearer understanding of the context within which women live, it is not possible to identify accurately those in need of specific nutritional intervention.

Care should be taken to avoid assumptions that providing the 'correct' information on nutritional requirements during the childbearing years will lead women to make the 'right choices' in terms of their own nutrition. This consumerist concept of decision-making ('knowledge in–behaviour out') is based on an illusion of linearity, and it ignores the complexities of decision-making. In reality, decisions will be made on the basis of macro-level (structural) factors, such as socio-economic and political contexts, gender relationships and food availability, along with micro-level factors, such as local cultural practices, norms, lifestyles, attitudes and beliefs (Bilson and Dykes, 2009; Hall Moran et al., 2010). For any given community, understanding of these variables is required while attempting to understand nutritional needs in this critical period of life (Cetin et al., 2010).

Since the ultimate goal of nutrition in the childbearing years is the optimal health and development for both mother and child, it is helpful to envisage the topic in the context of the Life Course Development framework. This is a conceptual approach to understanding the interrelating adverse and beneficial factors that influence health and development, thereby enabling an integrated implementation and assessment of related research and policy (Halfron and Hochstein, 2002). The Life Course Development framework shows:

- Health is a consequence of multiple determinants operating in a nested genetic, biological, behavioural, social and economic context that change as a person develops.
- Health development is an adaptive process composed of multiple transactions between these contexts and the bio-behavioural regulatory systems that define human functions.
- Different health trajectories are the product of accumulative risk and protective factors and other influences that are programmed into bio-behavioural regulatory systems during critical and sensitive periods.
- The timing and sequence of biological, psychological, cultural and historical events and experiences influence the health and development of both individuals and populations (Halfron and Hochstein, 2002, p. 433).

This framework, therefore, allows us to understand how nutritional risk factors, protective factors and early life experiences affect an individual's long-term well-being. With an improved understanding of health development, it may be possible to manipulate early risk factors and protective factors and help us shift our emphasis from managing the outcomes of these factors to the promotion of earlier, more effective preventative strategies and interventions focused on maximising optimal health and development. This book explores nutrition in the childbearing years within such a life course framework, highlighting the influence of complex interrelating factors and contexts upon the health of the mother and her infant.

Any pregnancy, although perhaps especially the first, is increasingly viewed by organisations at local, national and international levels as a significant 'window of opportunity' within which to promote healthier lifestyles and encourage women to take responsibility for safeguarding or improving their own health and that of their child. Thus, the consumption habits and weight gain of pregnant women, and subsequently of their infants, are of interest to maternity and related professionals seeking to optimise outcomes and address inequalities in maternal and child health.

The childbearing years are clearly a fundamental period during which family-focused public health opportunities can be maximised (Stapleton and Keenan, 2009). It is, therefore, essential that we capitalise on this opportunity and offer up-to-date, evidence-based and consistent advice on diet, weight gain, dietary supplements and food safety during the childbearing years. This book provides a valuable resource for academics and health professionals looking for the latest information on a wide range of topics in this area.

Victoria Hall Moran
Senior Editor, Maternal & Child Nutrition

References

Abu-Saad K and Fraser D (2010) Maternal nutrition and birth outcomes. *Epidemiologic Reviews* 32, 5–25.

Arkkola T, Uusitalo U, Pietikäinen M, Metsälä J, Kronberg-Kippilä M, Erkkola M (2006) Dietary intake and use of dietary supplements in relation to demographic variables among pregnant Finnish women. *British Journal of Nutrition* 96, 913–20.

Atkinson SA and Koletzko B (2007) Determining life-stage groups and extrapolating nutrient intake values (NIVs). *Food & Nutrition Bulletin* 28, 61S–76S.

Attree P (2005) Low-income mothers, nutrition and health: a systematic review of qualitative evidence. *Maternal and Child Nutrition* 1, 227–40.

Baker PN, Wheeler SJ, Sanders TA *et al.* (2009) A prospective study of micronutrient status in adolescent pregnancy. *American Journal of Clinical Nutrition* 89, 1114–24.

Bilson A and Dykes F (2009) A bio-cultural basis for protecting, promoting and supporting breast-feeding. In: *Infant and Young Child Nutrition: Challenges to Implementing a Global Strategy*, eds F Dykes and V Hall Moran, pp. 32–42. Wiley-Blackwell: Oxford.

Cetin I, Berti C and Calabrese S (2010) Role of micronutrients in the periconceptional period. *Human Reproduction Update* 16(1), 80–95.

Dewey KG (2004) Impact of breastfeeding on maternal nutritional status. *Advances in Experimental Medicine & Biology* 554, 91–100.

Doets EL, de Wit LS, Dhonukshe-Rutten RA *et al.* (2008) Current micronutrient recommendations in Europe: towards understanding their differences and similarities. *European Journal of Nutrition* 47(Suppl. 1), 17–40.

Halfron N and Hochstein M (2002) Life course health development: an integrated framework for developing health, policy, and research. *The Millbank Quarterly* 80, 433–79.

Hall Moran V (2007a) Nutritional status in pregnant adolescents: a systematic review of biochemical markers. *Maternal & Child Nutrition* 3, 74–93.

Hall Moran V (2007b) A systematic review of dietary assessments of pregnant adolescents in industrialized countries. *British Journal of Nutrition* 97, 411–25.

Hall Moran V, Lowe L, Crossland N *et al.* (2010) Nutritional requirements during lactation. Towards European alignment of reference values: the EURRECA network. *Maternal & Child Nutrition* 6(Suppl. 2), 39–54.

NHS (2011) Statistics on obesity, physical activity and diet: England, 2011 Report. Available at: http://www.ic.nhs.uk/statistics-and-data-collections/health-and-lifestyles/obesity/statistics-on-ob esity-physical-activity-and-diet-england-2011.

NICE (National Institute for Clinical Excellence) (2010) Dietary interventions and physical activity interventions for weight management before, during and after pregnancy. NICE Public Health Guidance 27. Available at: http://www.nice.org.uk/nicemedia/live/13056/49926/49926.pdf.

Pavlovic M, Prentice A, Thorsdottir I, Wolfram G and Branca F (2007) Challenges in harmonising energy and nutrient recommendations in Europe. *Annals of Nutrition and Metabolism* 51, 108–14.

Pijls L, Ashwell M and Lambert J (2009) EURRECA – A network of excellence to align European micronutrient recommendations. *Food Chemistry* **113**, 748–53.

Popkin BM (2003) The nutrition transition in developing world. *Development Policy Review* **21**, 581–97.

Reid M and Adamson H (1997) *Opportunities for and Barriers to Good Nutritional Health in Women of Childbearing Age, Pregnant Women, Infants under 1 and Children Aged 1 to 5*. Health Education Authority: London.

Scientific Advisory Committee on Nutrition (SACN) (2011) *The Influence of Maternal, Fetal and Child Nutrition on the Development of Chronic Disease in Later Life*. TSO: London.

Stapleton H and Keenan J (2009) Bodies in the making: reflections on women's consumption practices in pregnancy. In: *Infant and Young Child Nutrition: Challenges to Implementing a Global Strategy*, eds F Dykes and V Hall Moran, pp. 119–45. Wiley-Blackwell: Oxford.

WHO (2003) *Global Strategy for Infant and Young Child Feeding*. WHO: Geneva.

Williams A (2009) Lifecycle influences and opportunities for change. In: *Infant and Young Child Nutrition: Challenges to Implementing a Global Strategy*, eds F Dykes and V Hall Moran, pp. 163–80. Wiley-Blackwell: Oxford.

World Bank (2006) Repositioning nutrition as central to development: a strategy for large-scale action. Available at: http://web.worldbank.org/WBSITE/EXTERNAL/TOPICS/EXTHEALT HNUTRITIONANDPOPULATION/EXTNUTRITION/0,,contentMDK:20787550~menuPK: 282580~pagePK:64020865~piPK:149114~theSitePK:282575,00.html.

Preface

For women, a diet adequate in the right nutrients is important throughout her child-bearing years. Poor quality diets can not only affect women's health and nutrition status but can also influence the health of the next generation. Even though in the developed world we now have access to more foods than ever before, making the right food choices is no easy task. In addition, confusing and sometimes conflicting health messages can complicate this matter further.

With the help from scientists that have been dedicated to this field of work, it is now well established that women's diet not only during but also before and after pregnancy can affect the health of the next generation in the short and longer terms. Infertility, gestational diabetes, pre-eclampsia and medical complications linked to rising obesity rates are just some examples of the problems that health services are experiencing more frequently. It is also becoming increasingly apparent that children who are not well nourished when *in utero* or during the phases of breastfeeding may not reach their true potential from a health, growth or cognitive perspective. These are important issues that need to be better communicated so that the next generation is given the best start in life.

One problem that I have come across is the amount of complex and conflicting information. One classic example of this is for folic acid – an area where there is a vast evidence base in relation to the prevention of neural tube defects but links with cancer development have complicated health messages and the role of fortification. In writing this book I have tried to form balanced, evidence-based conclusions, but inevitably my opinion may sneak in now and again. What is important is that together we move forward, make the most of the evidence that we have available and form prudent, straightforward and consistent recommendations that can be communicated to women in their childbearing years (preferably before they become pregnant!). Folic acid is just one example of a nutrient that is essential to women should they fall pregnant, but there is so much more important information that needs to be communicated.

When writing this book I therefore felt it was important to interpret information in a way that it could be used and applied. As a lecturer, my students are a constant source of inspiration and often tell me (very openly!) what would make a good text. I therefore wanted to write a book that was evidence based but user friendly, not only to students but also to health and medical practitioners. I therefore hope that I have managed to undertake what I set out to achieve. For each chapter, I have included application in practice sections and a summary of key points. Summary tables of dietary and weight gain guidelines and some case study examples are also included in the appendices.

Dedication

I dedicate this book to my grandfather, Arthur Derbyshire.

Acknowledgements

I would not have been able to write this book if I had not met and had support and guidance of, or learnt so much from, the following people: Professor Jill Davies, Professor Michael Hill, Dr Vassiliki Costarelli, Professor John Dickerson, Dr Carrie Ruxton and Professor Gerry Kelleher – thank you; in different ways you have all helped me to complete this mammoth task. Thank you to all of the expectant mothers who have taken part in our research and have also had a valuable input into this book.

I would also like to thank my husband, who is always so patient and supportive, my family and friends. Also, thanks go to Bluey for sitting by my side and keeping me company for the many hours it has taken me to write this book.

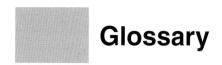

Glossary

Adipocyte Another name for a fat cell.

Adipokines Cytokines (see definition) secreted by fat cells.

Adiponectin A protein produced by fat cells that can regulate the metabolism of glucose and lipids.

Advanced maternal age When women have children later in their childbearing years.

Aflatoxin A toxic substance produced by moulds. Typically grows on crops such as wheat, corn and rice in warm, underdeveloped regions.

Air displacement plethysmography (ADP) When subjects enter a sealed chamber and body fat is calculated using air displacement calculations.

Anencephaly Birth defect when the brain and spinal cord are not well formed.

Anovulation When women of childbearing age do not release eggs from the ovaries.

Antioxidants Substances and/or nutrients that reduce damage caused by free radicals.

Apgar score A practical method used to score the health of the baby after delivery.

Appropriate-for-gestational age (AGA) When an infant's birth weight lies above the 10th percentile for that gestational age and below the 90th percentile.

Basal metabolic rate (BMR) The rate at which energy is used by the body when in a rested state.

Bias Influences on a study that can alter the results and lead to invalid conclusions. Bias may take place when data is collected, analysed, interpreted or reviewed.

Biomarker Markers used to assess nutrition status, usually nutrient levels present in blood and/or urine samples.

Birth length When legs are fully extended, the length of the baby from head to heals. Sometimes referred to as crown–heel length.

Birth weight The weight of the infant at birth. Often used as a marker of foetal nutrient supply/exposure.

Blinding When scientists conducting the study or participants taking part are unaware of the treatment that they are giving or receiving, i.e. whether it is an active or placebo (dummy) treatment. This helps to protect against bias (also see 'Double-blind study').

Body mass index (BMI) Body weight in kilograms divided by height in metres squared. Used to categorise bodyweight.

Caffeine A natural stimulant in coffee beans, tea leaves, cocoa beans (chocolate) and kola nuts (cola). Levels of intake should be monitored in pregnancy.

Calorimetry Equipment that measures levels of heat generated by the body and used to derive energy expenditure.

Cerebral palsy Reduced muscular function and weakness of the limbs.

Choline Classed in the vitamin B complex and an important constituent of biological compounds, i.e. neurotransmitters.

Cleft lip/palate When the infants' lip/roof of the mouth do not fuse together when in utero.

Cohort study When a group of people taking part in a study are followed for a period of time (can be quite lengthy).

Colostrum The milk first produced after birth by the mammary glands. Colostrum is a rich such of nutrients and components that can help to support the infants' immune system.

Confounding factor Factors/data in epidemiological studies that can affect/alter the results leading to ambiguous conclusions, i.e. a study looking at dietary factors and birth weight when smoking is not accounted for (i.e. acting as a confounder).

Constipation Fewer (usually less than three bowel movements per week), hardened stools and straining to go to the toilet are all indicators of constipation.

Cytokines Chemical messengers produced by cells that trigger immune and inflammatory responses.

Dioxins Fat soluble toxic organic compounds (usually from industrial waste) that can accumulate in the food chain and have been associated with increased birth defect risk.

Docosahexaenoic acid (DHA) An essential omega-3 long-chain fatty acid that is needed for brain development in the later stages of pregnancy and after birth.

Double-blind study A study when both the scientist and participant are unaware of whether the active or dummy treatment is given.

Doubly labelled water (DLW) method A method that involves using labelled isotopes to determine energy expenditure.

Dual-energy X-ray absorptiometry (DEXA) When the body is exposed to very low levels of ionising radiation. This method can be used to determine the mineral content of bones as well as body fat and fat free mass measurements.

Early stillbirth Delivery of a stillborn infant before 28 weeks' gestation.

Embryo The term used for the developing child for the first 8 weeks' pregnancy. After this period the term foetus is typically used.

Embryogenesis When cells divide through mitosis, forming an embryo (mass of cells that eventually form tissue and organ systems).

Epigenetics Changes that may indirectly affect the expression of genes without acting on the DNA directly.

Essential fatty acids (EFAs) When fatty acids cannot be manufactured in the body in adequate levels needed for good health and need to be consumed from dietary sources. Linoleic acid (omega-6) and linolenic acid (omega-3) are both EFAs.

Extreme obesity Typically defined as a BMI of 50 or higher and is now a common occurrence amongst women living in more industrial regions.

Extremely low birth weight (ELBW) An infant born that weighs less than 1 kg (1000 g).

Foetal alcohol syndrome (FAS) A syndrome related to alcohol use during pregnancy and characterised by prenatal or postnatal growth retardation, facial anomalies and mental deficiency.

Foetal growth restriction (FGR) Failure of the baby to attain its growth potential.

Foetal–placental unit (FPU) Interaction between the foetus and the placenta to establish a state of hormone balance.

Folate Also known as vitamin B9, naturally occurring in some foods (leafy green vegetables and beans) and essential for DNA synthesis and cell division.

Folic acid The synthetic form of folate added to cereal and typically used in supplements.

Follicle stimulating hormone (FSH) A hormone produced by the anterior pituitary that regulates the production of sex hormones, in both men and women.

Free radical When there is more than one pair of unpaired electrons in an atom making it unstable. These atoms/compounds then have the ability to remove electrons from other compounds leading to chain reactions that can damage the body and lead to disease development.

Functional foods Foods with ingredients that have additional properties which are beneficial to health.

Gestational diabetes mellitus (GDM) Glucose intolerance in pregnancy leading to the development of diabetes in pregnancy.

Gestational weight gain (GWG) Weight gained between conception and delivery, including the weight of the baby and placenta.

Ghrelin A hormone that stimulates appetite – produced by cells in the stomach and pancreas.

Glycaemic index/load The ability of a food to release its sugars and increase blood glucose levels. Glycaemic load also takes into account the amount of food that is ingested.

Goitre Swelling of the thyroid gland, usually caused by iodine deficiency in the diet.

Gold standard A method that is highly regarded.

Head circumference The largest diameter around the infant's head.

Heterocyclic amines Carcinogenic chemicals formed when meat, poultry or fish are cooked at high temperatures.

High-density lipoprotein (HDL) A complex comprised of lipids and proteins that transports cholesterol from tissues back to the liver. Higher levels of this form of blood cholesterol help to improve cardiovascular health.

Homocysteine A naturally occurring amino acid found in the blood which is associated with cardiovascular disease.

Human chorionic gonadotropin (hCG) A protein-based hormone produced by the embryo and placenta early in pregnancy. Pregnancy tests work on the basis of detecting this hormone to confirm pregnancy.

Hyperemesis gravidarum Extreme nausea and excessive vomiting in pregnancy.

Hyperglycaemia Elevated blood glucose levels.

Hypermethylation The addition of methyl groups to DNA bases (adenosine and cytosine) which reduces gene expression.

Hypomethylation When there are fewer methyl groups attached to DNA bases which increase gene expression.

Hypospadia A birth defect with the opening of the urethra is located on the underside of the penis instead of at the tip.

Hypothalamic–pituitary–adrenal (HPA) axis Tightly linked hormone-produced units that work together and interact with each other – the hypothalamus, pituitary and adrenal glands.

Infant A child less than 1 year of age.

Inhibin B A peptide hormone that inhibits the actions of the FSH.

Insulin resistance Decreased ability of the body to respond to the effects of insulin, especially muscle and fat tissue.

Insulin sensitivity How quickly the body responds to the hormone insulin.

Iron-deficiency anaemia (IDA) A decrease in the number of red blood cells in the body caused by too little iron in the diet. It is more accurate to use several markers of iron status when diagnosing IDA rather than just haemoglobin.

Isoflavones A phytoestrogen found in foods, e.g. beans and soy lentils, with potential health benefits.

Lactogenesis Production of milk from the mammary glands after birth.

Large-for-gestational age (LGA) An infant whose birth weight falls above recommended reference standards (usually > 90th percentile).

Late stillbirth Delivery of a stillborn infant after 28 weeks' gestation.

Leptin A protein-based hormone secreted from fat cells that plays a role in regulating long-term appetite and energy expenditure.

Lipomatosis Tumour-like deposits of fat in the tissues.

Lipophilic Substances that are capable of dissolving in lipids and/or are stored in body fat.

Longitudinal study When the same subjects are followed up several times and repeated measurements may be taken during a study.

Low birth weight infant (LBW) An infant born that is less than 2.5 kg (2500 g). Infants may be LBW because they are premature or small-for-gestational age.

Low-density lipoprotein (LDL) A complex comprised of lipids and proteins that transports cholesterol from the liver to tissues and arteries. Higher levels of this form of blood cholesterol contribute to the development of arterial plaques.

Luteinising hormone (LH) A hormone produced by the anterior pituitary which stimulates ovulation in women and testosterone synthesis in men.

Lycopene A red pigment found predominantly in tomatoes with antioxidant properties.

Macronutrient Nutrients consumed in relatively large proportions that provide energy, and include fat, protein and carbohydrate.

Macrosomia A large birth weight baby, typically >4000 g.

Meta-analysis When results from similar studies are pooled and statistical tests undertaken to form firmer conclusions.

Metabolic syndrome A set of risk factors that mean an individual is at risk of heart disease and other medical complications.

Methylmercury A chemical that is toxic to the nervous system, particularly to the developing child in pregnancy.

Micronutrients Essential nutrients required by the body in relatively small proportions, and include vitamins and minerals.

Multiparous When women have already had more than one pregnancy.

Neural tube defect (NTD) A birth defect caused by abnormal development and closure of the neural tube (see 'Spina bifida').

N-nitroso compounds (NOCs) Organic compounds found in foods with potentially carcinogenic properties.

Nulliparous Women that have never given birth.

Nutrient deficiency When an inadequate supply of certain nutrients may impair health.

Ovarian reserve The number and quality off oocytes available for fertilisation in women of childbearing age.

Ovulatory infertility Reproductive problems which mean that the ovaries do not release an egg.

Oxytocin A hormone secreted by the posterior pituitary gland that stimulates both contractions of the uterus in the lead up to giving birth and ejection of milk after delivery.

Parity The number of children previously born to a woman.

Phenylketonuria (PKU) A genetic condition that means the body is unable to metabolise the amino acid phenylalanine. The phenylalanine content of the diet has to be controlled carefully.

Phthalates Man-made chemicals found in plastics and food wrappings that may have health ramifications when ingested.

Pica An eating disorder when non-nutritional objects are eaten.

Placenta previa When the placenta grows lower down in the womb and may bleed or become dislodged.

Polycyclic aromatic hydrocarbons (PAHs) Organic molecules produced by fossil fuel combustion that when ingested can be potentially carcinogenic.

Polycystic ovary syndrome Cysts on the ovaries that may lead to anovulation making conception difficult.

Postnatal depression (PND) A mood disorder that commences after birth which can be caused by hormonal and social changes.

Pre-eclampsia Hypertension in pregnancy and the excretion of protein into urine.

Preterm/premature Delivery before 37 weeks of pregnancy.

Primiparous Women having their first child.

Probiotics Live microorganisms that may confer health benefits.

Prolactin A key hormone that secreted from the anterior pituitary gland that stimulates and maintains the secretion of milk.

Prophylaxis A measure taken to prevent the development of a disease or condition, i.e. supplements of some medications.

Prospective study A study when participants are recruited and followed forward in time when data is collected.

Puerperium The period after birth when the body returns to its pre-pregnancy state.

P-value Whether findings from a study are statistically significant or not. P values less than 0.05 are seen as being statistically significant while those less than 0.001 are highly significant, i.e. findings are less likely to occur by chance.

Randomised controlled trial When people taking part in a study are randomly allocated to groups, i.e. one receives the active treatment and the other a placebo. Findings between the different groups are then compared at a later date.

Reactive oxygen species (ROS) Free radicals and other oxidising species formed through metabolic processes.

Relative risk (RR) A ratio of the probability of an event or a disease occurring in the exposed compared to a non-exposed group.

Relaxin A hormone secreted by the corpus luteum that softens the cervix to help accommodate the developing child.

Reset hypothesis A theory proposing that breastfeeding can help women's metabolic profile return back to what it was before pregnancy, reducing chronic disease risk later in life.

Retrospective study A study that assesses the relationship between a current condition but also uses data/information from the past.

Small-for-gestational age (SGA) An infant whose birth weight falls below recommended reference standards (usually <10th percentile).

Spina bifida When the spinal cord does not close during embryonic development.

Successful pregnancy One that maintains maternal health and well-being and ends in the delivery of a healthy newborn.

Systematic review A review that uses specific methods and set criteria to identify and evaluate research within a particular field.

Total fertility rate The average number of children that would be born to a woman over her lifetime.

Toxoplasmosis An infection caused by a parasite that can invade the tissues of the developing foetus and may lead to permanent damage to the infant.

Transitional milk Milk produced after colostrum and before mature milk is secreted.

Trimester The 9 months of pregnancy that can be divided into 3 separate trimester.

Very low birth weight (VLBW) An infant born less than 1.5 kg (1500 g).

Waist circumference An indicator of the amount of fat stored within the abdomen and useful indicator of long-term health.

Waist-to-hip ratio An indicator of abdominal obesity – waist circumference divided by hip circumference (both in metres).

Zygote After the female egg is fertilised it becomes a zygote.

1 Nutrition and Fertility

Summary

Although genetic and medical conditions may both be common causes of infertility (and subfertility), research shows that certain dietary factors may also affect the chances of conceiving. Over the last few decades, a growing body of literature has been published in this area. There is some evidence to suggest that high alcohol and caffeine intakes and low intakes of antioxidants may be associated with reduced fertility. Equally, both ends of the energy spectrum (under- and overnutrition) appear to have an unfavourable impact on fertility status. For individuals who are overweight or obese, achieving a healthy body weight may help to improve both fertility and the success of reproductive treatments. Overall, simple lifestyle changes such as monitoring alcohol and caffeine intakes and obtaining a healthy body weight are a good start to any pregnancy, as well as helping to improve fertility levels. Imparting these messages to men and women in their childbearing years may help to reduce time to conception and is always worth trying before seeking fertility treatments, which can sometimes be expensive. For those undergoing assisted reproductive technologies, dietary advice may also be effective alongside these treatments when couples are having difficulties conceiving.

Learning Outcomes

- To understand how dietary factors may affect the fertility of both men and women in their childbearing years.
- To be aware of the importance of a healthy body weight when planning a pregnancy, or undergoing assisted reproductive technologies (ARTs).
- To appreciate that simple dietary and lifestyle changes may help to support couples when planning a pregnancy or undergoing reproductive treatments.

1.1 Introduction

Data show that infertility rates are rising, as demonstrated by the rise in fertility treatments such as in vitro fertilisation (IVF) in recent years (HFEA, 2010). There is no doubt that the causes of infertility are multifaceted with older childbearing age, medical and health complications being some underpinning causes. Even though ARTs may go some way towards helping couples conceive, emerging evidence

---

Nutrition in the Childbearing Years, First Edition. Emma Derbyshire.
© 2011 Emma Derbyshire. Published 2011 by Blackwell Publishing Ltd.

suggests that dietary advice may also have an important role to play. For both men and women, there is a strong link between energy balance and reproductive function. In both developed and developing regions, rising body weights are being linked to reduced fertility levels. Although slowly, scientists are starting to uncover how individual dietary components may influence fertility levels. However, this research needs to continue and certainly more carefully designed randomised controlled trials are needed.

Carrying out research during this phase of the life cycle can be difficult for several reasons. Couples planning to have a baby are a difficult population to access, researching time to conception can be stressful for couples and testing the efficacy of dietary interventions can be difficult if patients are already getting reproductive treatments. This chapter has been divided into two sections: the first focusing on nutrition and female fertility and the second part male fertility. The chapter begins by defining the term 'infertility' and related definitions. The role of energy balance, obtaining a healthy body weight and specific nutrients and how these can affect both male and female fertility is then described. Finally, recommendations and guidelines for application in practice will be provided at the end of each section for females and males.

1.2   Nutrition and female fertility

1.2.1   Defining fertility

Fertility, sometimes referred to as fecundity, is the ability to reproduce and conceive naturally. Some couples can get pregnant very easily, but for others, this can take significantly longer than anticipated. The term 'subfertility' is often used to describe any form of reduced fertility and prolonged time to conception (Gnoth et al., 2005). It is estimated that around 10–15% of couples in industrially developed countries have difficulty with conceiving.

When conception fails to precede after 12 months or more of regular, unprotected intercourse, the term 'infertility' is used. For women aged 35 years and over, earlier treatment may be justified when pregnancy has not been achieved after 6 months (American Society for Reproductive Medicine, 2008). There are many different causes underlying fertility problems. These may be genetic, age-related, caused by hormone imbalances or medical problems such as polycystic ovary syndrome (PCOS), as well as dietary and lifestyle factors.

1.2.2   Other definitions

The term 'fertility' is broad and within this there are various subcategories of fertility. We have already defined infertility and subfertility; however, couples may also be defined within primary or secondary infertility, depending on whether a pregnancy has been achieved previously (Table 1.1). Ovulatory infertility accounts for around 30% infertility means that the female partner is having trouble conceiving. Irregular patterns of menstruation (oligomenorrhoea) or the absence of menstrual cycles can be contributing factors, as well as medical conditions such as PCOS (Hamilton-Fairley and Taylor, 2003). When the male partner has reproductive problems, i.e. reduced

Table 1.1   Subcategories of fertility.

Definition	Explanation
Infertility	When pregnancy does not occur, usually after 12 months of unprotected intercourse
Subfertility	When it takes much longer than anticipated to achieve a pregnancy
Primary infertility	When neither partner has achieved a pregnancy previously after having unprotected intercourse
Secondary infertility	When pregnancy has been achieved previously but a second pregnancy is not achieved after 12 months of unprotected intercourse
Ovulatory infertility	When couples are unable to conceive because the female has reproductive problem (usually with ovulation)
Male factor infertility	When couples are unable to conceive because of a problem with the male reproductive system

sperm motility or numbers that can reduce the chances of conception, scientists and doctors usually refer to this as male factor fertility.

Getting Started   Defining the childbearing years

Before discussing the issues around infertility, it is important to attempt to define what may be described as the 'childbearing years', indeed no easy task. Although very distinct age ranges (usually around 16–40 years) have been used in studies, there are always exceptional circumstances!

Falling pregnant too early, or too late, in life can mean that both the diet needs to be tailored and women carefully monitored throughout their pregnancies. Early adolescent childbearing has been defined as 15 years or younger, as the risk of infant mortality, very preterm (born before 32 weeks) and very low birth weight infant deliveries (<1500 g) is higher amongst girls in this age category, stabilising at around age 16 (Phipps and Sowers, 2002).

Equally, more women are also leaving pregnancy until later on in their childbearing years. This is particularly the case in Britain, which has some of the highest birth rates for older women in the world. With advances in fertility treatment and oocyte donation becoming increasingly available, it is not uncommon for women in their 50s, or even the sixth decade of life to fall pregnant (sometimes referred to as advanced reproductive age). These women may also have a higher risk of developing pregnancy complications such as pre-eclampsia, gestational diabetes mellitus and delivering by c-section (Chibber, 2005).

1.2.3   Maternal age

It is well known that the ability to conceive and carry a baby until term declines with age. Pregnancy rates become lower once women reach their mid-thirties and are reduced even further once a woman reaches her forties. Scientists have found that

Table 1.2 How ovarian age can be measured.

Indicator	Explanation
Antral follicle count (AFC)	The AFC is the number of follicles remaining on the ovaries and a good indicator of the number of eggs than can be produced. Doctors can normally count the number of follicles remaining using ultrasound technology.
Levels of follicle stimulating hormone (FSH)	This is the main hormone involved in producing mature eggs in the ovaries. Both high and low levels can reduce fertility. FSH can be measured easily from blood tests.
Inhibin B	A protein hormone produced by the ovarian follicles. The amount produced is an indicator of the number of eggs in the ovaries, i.e. when secreted at lower levels, this indicates that a woman's egg reserves are low. Once again, inhibin B levels can be derived from blood tests.

the number of ova (eggs) and quality of eggs are both reduced as women get older. Women's eggs need to have the right chromosomes and be able to form a viable embryo. With age, the shape of eggs may change and the thickness of their walls becomes thinner. This means that older women not only have reduced fertility levels, but the risk of birth defects and miscarriage is also higher in this group (American Society for Reproductive Medicine, 2002).

On a more positive note, studies have shown that a woman's chronological age does not necessarily determine her ovarian age, sometime referred to as 'ovarian reserve' (the number of eggs remaining in the ovaries). Sometimes, older women may have better quality eggs than younger women, which is where dietary and lifestyle practices may come into play. Scientists have shown that levels of inhibin B (a marker of ovarian ageing; Table 1.2) are lower in women who smoke i.e. ovarian age is more advanced (Waylen *et al.*, 2010). Subjectively, it is also important that such studies control for coital frequency when concluding their findings, as this too decreases with age (Klein and Sauer, 2001) and may affect the results of studies. More research is now needed to study the role of dietary and lifestyle factors and the effect these may have on women's ovarian age. Other markers of ovarian ageing, often used by scientists and researchers, are shown in Table 1.2.

1.2.4 Undernutrition

Reproduction is a costly process requiring significant amounts of energy. When energy intake and expenditure are not in balance, ovulation may be suppressed. There are several theories linking undernutrition to reduced reproductive potential. More than 30 years ago, Rose Frisch, now a Professor at Harvard School of Public Health, was one of the first scientists to link low body weight and fat stores to amenorrhea and reduced fertility. The theory behind this was that a certain level of body fat was needed to convert androgen hormones to oestrogens, hormones needed for female reproductive function. In turn, the potency of these hormones was also thought to be related directly to body weight and fat (Frisch, 1987). Although the science behind this theory still stands, the role of oestrogens in reproductive function is not as vast as once thought.

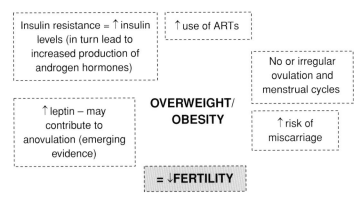

Figure 1.1 Implications of overweight/obesity on a woman's fertility and reproductive health. (Information extracted from Pasquali and Gambineri (2006).)

More recently, it has come to light that body fat, once thought to be a fairly redundant mass, may be involved in the production of another type of hormone, known as adipokines. So far, four key adipokines have been identified: adiponectin, visfatin, omentin and vaspin. Although there remains a lot to be learnt about the role of these hormones, it is thought that they may help to regulate women's menstrual cycles (Bohler *et al.*, 2010) and improve insulin sensitivity (Campos *et al.*, 2008).

Finally, another theory known as the 'metabolic fuel hypothesis' proposes that limited supplies of body fat can lead to altered secretion of key fertility hormones such as gonadotropin-releasing hormone (GnRH) and luteinising hormones (LH). In turn, this can then lead to women having irregular or no menstrual cycle, alter her feelings towards sexual activities and ultimately reduce the ability to conceive (Figure 1.1). Examples of these conditions may include women with eating disorders such as anorexia nervosa or very active females, which can lead to exercise-induced amenorrhea (Mircea *et al.*, 2007).

1.2.5 Overnutrition

Obesity is becoming an increasing health concern in both developed and newly industrialised countries. Overweight/obese women are more likely to have experienced fertility problems than women with a healthy body weight. A considerable proportion of women who are obese have PCOS, which reduces their fertility. Other conditions such as insulin resistance, excess androgen production and irregular ovulation can also make conception more difficult in heavier women (Wilkes and Murdoch, 2009).

Some research has also found that body shape and the distribution of body fat can be used to assess women's likelihood of menstrual irregularities. Research carried out at the University of Bari, Italy, found that about 20% of women with obesity had irregular menstrual cycles. These women also had higher waist circumferences and more fat in the abdominal region (De Pergola *et al.*, 2009).

For overweight/obese women seeking fertility treatment, the British Fertility Society (BFS) advise that women strive to attain a healthy body mass index (BMI) before undergoing these treatments. There are many different reasons for this advice. Firstly,

Table 1.3   Some practical approaches to achieving and maintaining a healthy weight.

NICE (2010) guidelines
1. Base meals on starchy foods (such as potatoes, bread, rice and pasta), choosing wholegrain where possible
2. Eat foods rich in dietary fibre (i.e. fresh fruits and vegetables and wholegrains)
3. Eat at least five portions of fruit and vegetables per day in place of foods higher in fat or calories
4. Eat as little as possible of fried foods, and drinks and confectionary high in sugars and fats
5. Eat breakfast
6. Watch portion size of meals and how often they are eaten

British Fertility Society (2007) guidelines
7. Aim to lose 5–10% body weight before undergoing fertility treatments, or the equivalent to a BMI $<35\,kg/m^2$, or $30\,kg/m^2$ for younger mothers (Balen *et al.*, 2007)

Also incorporate exercise into your daily regime and seek support from relative health practitioners where possible

---

ARTs are not as successful in heavier mothers, which can lead to unnecessary expenses and disappointment. Secondly, if obese/overweight women were to conceive, this may lead to a host of complications in pregnancy and during delivery (see Chapter 9 for further information). Specifically, the BFS advise that women defer their medical treatment until they obtain a BMI of $35\,kg/m^2$ or less, although treatment is preferable in women with a BMI of $30\,kg/m^2$ or less, particularly in the case of younger mothers (Balen *et al.*, 2007). Dieticians, nurses and midwives can play a key role in helping women to achieve these weight loss guidelines and the BFS state that even moderate weight losses of 5–10% may help women to restore their fertility naturally. Most recently, the National Institute for Health and Clinical Excellence have published some useful guidelines to help women of childbearing age maintain a healthy weight (NICE, 2010). These guidelines alongside the BFS recommendations are summarised in Table 1.3.

1.2.6   Dietary components

Scientists from the Harvard School of Public Health have studied whether the consumption of specific dietary constituents has any effect on women's ovulation. Dietary and reproductive assessments were carried out on over 16,000 nurses taking part in the American Nurses Health Study. Nutrition scientists found that carbohydrate-rich foods, especially those with a high glycaemic load, diets rich in animal protein, trans fats and iron, or low in vegetable protein and folic acid were most commonly linked to ovulation problems and subsequent infertility (also see Table 1.4). Authors suggested that swapping just 5% of total energy intake with vegetable rather than animal protein could reduce ovulatory infertility by 50%, possible because it helps to improve insulin sensitivity (Chavarro *et al.*, 2008a). Some other findings from studies carried out by Dr Jorge Chavarro are shown in Table 1.4. Until recently, very few studies have focused on research in this area. It seems that dietary constituents could alter the ovulatory function by modulating either insulin sensitivity or the fat content of the diet. Although the findings from these studies are

Table 1.4   Dietary constituents and ovulatory infertility*.

Dietary constituent under investigation	Findings	Reference
Alcohol	Alcohol intakes were unrelated to ovulatory infertility	Chavarro *et al.* (2009b)
B vitamins	Folic acid (mainly supplied from multivitamins) was associated with a reduced risk of ovulatory infertility	Chavarro *et al.* (2008b)
Caffeine	Intakes of soft caffeinated drinks were associated with ovulatory infertility (but may be unrelated to caffeine)	Chavarro *et al.* (2009b)
Carbohydrate	Risk of ovulatory infertility was higher in women eating carbohydrates with a high glycaemic load	Chavarro *et al.* (2009a)
Dairy produce	Risk of ovulatory infertility was higher in women eating low-fat compared with high-fat dairy foods	Chavarro *et al.* (2007b)
Fat	Risk of ovulatory infertility increased with intakes of trans fats.	Chavarro *et al.* (2007a)
Iron	Women who consumed iron supplements had a reduced risk of ovulatory infertility	Chavarro *et al.* (2006)
Protein	Risk of ovulatory infertility was higher in women consuming animal protein compared with vegetable protein	Chavarro *et al.* (2008a)

Folic acid or iron supplements were associated with a reduced risk of ovulatory infertility. Drinking soft beverages and consuming high-fat dairy foods, foods rich in trans fats or those with a high glycaemic load were linked to ovulatory infertility. Swapping animal for vegetable protein may also help to improve ovulatory function.
*No or irregular ovulation leading to infertility.

very interesting, more research is needed to confirm how these dietary constituents may exert their actions.

Research Highlight   Can dietary fibre influence women's fertility hormone levels?

Dietary fibre, the indigestible part of carbohydrates, may be beneficial to health when consumed at the right levels. Now, a new study suggests that high-fibre diets could influence levels of fertility hormones in childbearing age women.

The American BioCycle Study recruited 250 women aged 18–44 years and monitored their dietary habits and levels of fertility hormones across two menstrual cycles. Scientists found that women eating diets containing more fibre had lower levels of certain hormones. Levels of oestradiol, an active oestrogen hormone, progesterone, LH and FSH were all lower when more fibre was consumed. Ovulation was not likely to occur and menstrual cycles defined as 'anovulatory' if peak progesterone levels were 5 ng/mL or less. Women eating higher levels of dietary fibre, especially soluble fibre were also significantly more likely to experience anovulation (Gaskins *et al.*, 2009).

Whilst there are very interesting results, they are the findings from just one study. Future trials should study women for more than two menstrual cycles and control very carefully for other dietary components, as it can be difficult to separate out the effects of other nutrients. It would also be interesting to study the different fibre forms in further detail, i.e. soluble versus insoluble. An intervention study in the form of a randomised controlled trial would be particularly useful in this sense.

One of the issues that do emerge from these findings is that dietary fibre guidelines for women may need to be tailored when there is more evidence. Whilst dietary fibre may be associated with a spectrum of health benefits related to women's health, i.e. improved cardiovascular well-being and reduced risk or certain cancers, it is possible that upper levels of intake may be warranted. Consuming a diet adequate in fibre should by no means be discouraged; most adults fall short of recommended guidelines. However, women eating diets particularly high in fibre (defined as more than 22 g/day in the present study) who are experiencing difficulties conceiving may consider revising these slightly.

1.2.7   Oxidative stress and antioxidants

Reactive oxygen species (ROS) are highly reactive molecules generated both by metabolic pathways and environmental stresses. An accumulation of ROS can cause cell damage, especially to ova (egg cells). Subsequently, ROS can affect the development of ova and likelihood of fertilisation. Scientists also suggest that increased levels of ROS may contribute to oxidative stress, which can accelerate the age-related decline in fertility levels (Agarwal *et al.*, 2005). There is also some evidence to indicate that the production of ROS may increase the risk of medical complications, such as pre-eclampsia (Ruder *et al.*, 2009).

Several studies have investigated whether antioxidant supplements can reduce the production of ROS and reduce levels of oxidative stress in women of reproductive age. However, these are generally limited in number and use small sample sizes.

An example of such research was carried out by Westphal *et al.* (2006). Ninety-three women aged 24–42 years who were having problems conceiving were asked to take either fertility supplements containing catechins (a source of antioxidants) or placebo over the course of 3 months. After the intervention ended, 26% of women taking the supplement conceived compared with just 10% in the control group. Although levels of oxidative stress were not measured directly in this study, the results do indicate that supplements may go some ways towards improving the chances of conception. Another study carried out by Crha *et al.* (2003) measured levels of ascorbic acid in the follicular fluid of 76 women with fertility problems after half were given 500 mg supplements. Ascorbic acid levels were found to be significantly higher in the follicles of women that had taken vitamin c supplements when compared to the control group. Equally, pregnancy rates were also higher (58% versus 32%) in those taking the vitamin C supplement compared with the control group.

To date, these were the two most relevant studies that could be found within the literature. There seems to be more research investigating how antioxidants can affect male fertility, possible because this is easier to study. The role of antioxidants in female fertility is largely understudied, and this area of research would benefit from further clinical trials.

1.2.8   Alcohol

Increasingly, more young women are drinking higher proportions of alcohol, a trend that is a strong predictor of later consumption (Clemens *et al.*, 2009). For women, the absence of menstruation, failure to ovulate and disruption of the LH spike are just some of the medical problems linked to heavy drinking. When consumed in excess, alcohol can act on the hypothalamic–pituitary–adrenal (HPA) axis, altering the secretion of hormones. Studies have shown that alcohol increases plasma oestradiol and prolactin levels, which may subsequently increase the risk of spontaneous abortion (Teoh and colleagues, 1990). Grodstein *et al.* (1994) interviewed 1050 women from infertility clinics and found that endometriosis was 50% higher in women drinking any level or form of alcohol. Overall, a wealth of research has looked into how alcohol can influence women's fertility, but in this section, we will just focus on the key publications.

In one study, Swedish scientists measured patterns of alcohol consumption, rates and causes of hospital admission in a large sample of over 7000 women over a period of 18 years. Women with higher alcohol intakes were more likely to seek advice from fertility experts, suggesting link between the two (Eggert *et al.*, 2004). In another key study, data extracted from the Danish National Birth Cohort gave a insight into beverage habits and time to conception. The retrospective study of 30,000 pregnant mothers found that wine drinkers had a shorter time to pregnancy when compared with other alcoholic beverages such as beer or spirits. At the other end of the spectrum, drinking no or high levels (>14 alcoholic beverage per week) were linked to longer times to pregnancy (Juhl *et al.*, 2001). These are important research findings, but there is a definite need for well-designed studies controlling for other lifestyle factors that can also affect time to pregnancy, i.e. smoking.

Finally, and as will be discussed in later chapters, it is relatively well known that if alcohol intakes are high and pregnancy occurs, there is a chance that the offspring may develop a foetal alcohol-related disorder (Monsen, 2009). There is even some evidence that alcohol intakes 'before' conception occurs may alter the HPA axis and alter foetal programming when conception occurs (Zhang *et al.*, 2005). More remains to be known about this field of research, but it is possible that this may affect the behaviour, cognitive and immune function of the offspring in the long term. Public health campaigns need to be devised to deliver the message that high levels of alcohol consumption can decrease fertility and if conception does occur, it can impinge upon the health status of the developing child.

1.2.9   Caffeine

Caffeine consumption and its relationship with fertility have been investigated in some detail, with mixed evidence. Animal studies show that the administration of caffeine before fertilisation reduces the eggs ability to implant in the uterus (Pollard *et al.*, 1999). Evidence from human studies is not as consistent, reporting mixed findings. In these epidemiology studies, it is often difficult to separate out the effects of caffeine and smoking and their individual effects on fertility.

To date, the European Study Group on Infertility and Subfecundity is one of the largest investigations studying the effects of caffeine intake on female fertility. In this study, the consumption of caffeinated beverages was monitored in a randomly selected sample of 3187 women recruited from Denmark, Germany, Italy, Poland and Spain (aged 25–44 years). Findings were consistent in all countries: women consuming higher levels of caffeine took longer to conceive (those with intakes over 500 mg/day had an 11% longer time to pregnancy) (Bolumar *et al.*, 1997). More recently, the Oxford Conception Study has started to collect data from 1453 women planning to have a baby. Urinary hormones levels and health and lifestyle information, including measures of caffeine intake have been taken. This research will provide future information about factors influencing time to conception (and fertility) (Pyper *et al.*, 2006).

1.2.10   Physical activity

The female reproductive system is highly sensitive to changes in energy balance. At the extreme end of the energy spectrum, when energy expenditure is high and not matched with an equal energy intake, reproductive disorders may arise. Reduced levels of body fat and altered levels of endocrine hormones (also see Table 1.5), often linked to highly active lifestyles, are common causes of reduced pregnancy rates. In turn and as touched on previously, these physiological changes may lead to irregular menstruation, anovulation and infertility. Scientists generally say that reproductive function should return to normal when energy balance is restored, but more research is needed to confirm this (Redman, 2006).

A number of studies have explored the link between levels of female physical activity and their fertility. One Norwegian study, the North-Trondelag Health Study, recruited 3887 women (45 years or younger) and studied patterns of physical activity and fertility over a ten-year period. After accounting for other factors that could affect fertility, results showed that women active on most days of the week were 3.2 times more likely to experience fertility problems than inactive women. Authors concluded

Table 1.5   Hormonal changes linked with reduced female fertility.

Hormone	Action	Consequence
GnRH	Stimulates the release of LH and FSH	↓ GnRH can suppress the LH surge which normally takes place mid-cycle when conception is most likely to take place
Leptin	Regulates energy balance and reproductive function	↓ leptin occurs when there is a reduction in body fat
Oestrogens	Maintain reproductive cyclicity	↓ oestradiol when body fat levels decline. May result in anovulation (failure to ovulate)
Progesterone	Stimulates the formation of the endometrium lining	↓ progesterone means that implantation of a fertilised ovum is unlikely or may increase the risk of miscarriage

that women taking part in intensive levels of physical activity had the highest risk of infertility. This is an interesting study, but it is important not to discourage women from taking part in regular physical activity.

Overall, evidence seems to suggest that women are mostly at risk of fertility problems when energy expenditure is at the extreme end of the energy spectrum, i.e. women are taking part in high levels of physical activity but not matching this with adequate energy intakes. It is very important that the right health messages are communicated, i.e. when undertaken in moderation, physical activity may be beneficial to reproductive health but women with very active lifestyles should be advised to monitor their energy expenditure and energy intakes if they are planning a pregnancy.

1.2.11   Application in practice

Overall, studies show that dietary factors may influence time to conception and subsequently female fertility. There appears to be relatively consistent evidence from studies investigating the link between alcohol intakes and fertility levels that high alcohol intakes can reduce the likelihood of a successful conception. Scientific studies researching the effects of antioxidants, micronutrients and links with female fertility are generally limited and, there is a clear need for the application of rigorous randomised control trials within this area.

With the development of future research, it is hoped that health messages identifying the importance of dietary, lifestyle factors could go some way towards improving the fertility of women in their childbearing years. This would help to reduce the costs of expensive fertility treatments as well as improving the health and wellbeing of couples. In particular, the importance of being a healthy body weight before conception has many benefits – improved natural fertility, increased success when fertility treatments are sought and improved pregnancy outcomes. However, these benefits do not appear to be well communicated within public sectors. Further work in this area in the form of both research and public health strategies would be a good way forward. Ultimately, achieving a healthy BMI before pregnancy would help to cut the costs of fertility treatments and give women a healthy start to their pregnancies. A summary of key points from the first part of this chapter (nutrition and female fertility) is included in Table 1.6.

LEEDS METROPOLITAN UNIVERSITY LIBRARY

Table 1.6   Nutrition, lifestyle and female fertility – key points.

- Women should be advised to meet NICE (2010) dietary and lifestyle guidelines (Table 1.3).
- This includes achieving a healthy body weight before becoming pregnant, i.e. when planning a pregnancy or undergoing fertility treatments. Ideally, a woman's BMI should be $<35\,kg/m^2$, or $<30\,kg/m^2$ in younger women (Bates *et al.*, 2007).
- Women should get the nutrients they need from a healthy balanced diet, but in certain circumstances, women may benefit from taking an additional antioxidant supplement, i.e. female smokers.
- Older mothers having problems conceiving should be referred to a dietician/nutritionist to ensure that they have the best chances of reproductive success.
- Women should be encouraged to reduce their alcohol intake when planning a pregnancy.
- Women need to be aware that very active lifestyles may encumber fertility.

1.3   Nutrition and male fertility

1.3.1   Trends in male fertility

Data relating to basic sperm parameters can be obtained from as far back as the 1920s, although methods of determining male fertility have changed considerably since then. A controversial paper published in 1992 identified that there had been an overall decline in semen quality over the past 50 years (Swan and Elkin, 1999). Authors proposed that increased rates of testicular cancer, hypospadias (a birth defect of the urethra in males), cyrptorchidism (when one or both testes fail to descend) and increased exposure to oestrogens may all be leading to a reduction in male fertility (Carlsen *et al.*, 1992). This paper was criticised because the methods used to assess fertility were not highly regarded and the same sample of men were not followed through over time, making firm conclusions difficult.

Since then some better designed studies have been carried out. One of these was conducted in New Zealand and it analysed sperm samples of men who were regular sperm donors. Sperm parameters from these samples were analysed over a period of 20 years. Scientists found that the concentration of sperm decreased by an average of 2.5% annually and the volume of semen declined from 3.7 mL to 3.3 mL, but motility remained unchanged (Shine *et al.*, 2008). Even though this was a fairly well-designed study using a large sample of the same men over time and a range of sperm parameters, this still needs to be supported with more research using similar methodological approaches.

1.3.2   Semen – what is normal?

In 1992, the World Health Organisation (WHO) established a set of reference values for a range of semen variables (Table 1.7). Although new papers have been published, identifying ideal reference ranges for certain populations and age ranges, these values still remain to act as a useful guide and are often cited by doctors and researchers as a reference point. The same WHO report also identified and defined a set of nomenclature for different semen variables, which are shown in Table 1.8. More

Table 1.7 Normal values of semen samples.

Test	'Normal' values
Volume	2.0 mL or more
pH	7.2–8.0
Sperm concentration	20×10^6 spermatozoa per mL or more
Total sperm count	40×10^6 spermatozoa per ejaculate or more
Motility	50% or more with forward progression or 25% or more with rapid progression! (within 60 minutes of ejaculation)
Morphology	30% or more with normal forms
Vitality	75% or more live spermatozoa
White blood cells	Fewer than 1×10^6/mL

Source: Adapted from WHO (1992).

Table 1.8 Classifying semen samples (WHO nomenclature).

Terminology used	Explanation
Normozoospermia	Normal, healthy ejaculate
Oligozoospermia	When the sperm concentration is less than 20×10^6 per mL
Asthenozoospermia	When less than 50% spermatozoa move forward, or less than 25% move rapidly!
Teratozoospermia	When less than 30% spermatozoa have a normal morphology
Oligoasthenoteratozoospermia	When all three variables as shown above are affected
Azoospermia	When there are no sperms in the ejaculate
Aspermia	When ejaculate is not produced

Source: Adapted from WHO (1992).

recently, new tests have been developed to assess whether sperms have been exposed to oxidative stress and to determine the stability of nuclear and mitochondrial DNA in sperm cells (Aitken, 2006).

1.3.3 Paternal age

The effects of age-related infertility are not just confined to females. For males, having children later in life may impact upon sperm quality, hormone levels, libido and erectile function. Although age-related changes in semen parameters vary between individuals, it has been suggested that a paternal age of >40 years may contribute to reduced fertility, particular when the female is also older (Kühnert and Nieschlag, 2004).

A recent study analysing the sperm quality of over 400 males found that sperm motility decreased with age, but there were no changes in other parameters (Winkle *et al.*, 2009). It has also been identified that semen ROS levels are often higher in men 40 years and older compared with younger men (Cocuzza *et al.*, 2008). This may in turn increase the risk of DNA damage, which may reduce fertility but could also increase the risk of pregnancy complications and genetic abnormalities in the offspring born to older males (Sartorius and Nieschlag, 2010). Table 1.9 summarises how age may influence male fertility and reproductive health.

1.3.4 Overnutrition

Although more follow-through studies with larger sample sizes are needed, several studies have investigated the effects of male obesity on fertility. It has been reported that men with a BMI over $25 \, kg/m^2$ are less likely to have healthy, mobile sperm cells in their ejaculate (Kort *et al.*, 2006). Equally, medical conditions that are linked to obesity, such as diabetes development may influence men's fertility levels indirectly. Because diabetes can increase blood pressure, reduce the supply of blood to the penis and damage nerve endings, men with diabetes are at particularly high risk

Table 1.9   How can men's age affect their fertility and reproductive health?

↓ libido
↓ erectile function
↓ semen volume
↓ percentage of healthy sperm
↓ sperm motility
↑ DNA damage and ↓ sperm quality
↑ risk of miscarriage after women conceive
↑ risk of genetic medical conditions in the offspring

Men who have waited longer to have children should be advised how simple dietary and lifestyle changes may improve the chances of having a healthy baby.

of erectile dysfunction (Tamler, 2009). Physiologically, there are many reasons as to why obesity may affect reproductive function in males but some of the main explanations are listed below:

- In overweight/obese males, the hormone testosterone may be converted to oestrogen in surplus adipose tissue, leading to reduced testicular function and hormone production.
- Obesity may increase levels of oxidative stress in the testicles. This can lead to reduced sperm production and increased sperm damage.
- An accumulation of fat (particularly in the inner thigh) may cause scrotal temperatures to rise in extreme cases of obesity.
- Levels of inhibin B (a peptide hormone involved in sperm production) may be lower in obese compared to healthy weight males.

Overall, it is certainly not clear, but it seems likely male overweight/obesity could have some affect on fertility. A recent meta-analysis paper by MacDonald et al. (2010) reviewed the finding from 31 studies researching the effects of male obesity on sperm parameters. From the 31 studies that were found, only the results of five were suitable for statistical analysis. Authors concluded that men with a higher BMI had significantly lower testosterone levels. Obesity was not, however, found to affect any semen parameters. Despite these conclusions, small sample sizes and short study timescales mean that continued research is needed in this area.

1.3.5   Metabolic syndrome

Interest in metabolic syndrome, a series of metabolic and cardiovascular risk factors that may precede the development of type 2 diabetes, stroke and heart disease (Ramos and Olden, 2008) has advanced over the last few years. Using the International Diabetes Federation (IDF) classification scale, prevalence of metabolic syndrome is thought to be around 33% amongst men and 35% in women, although this method is thought to slightly overestimate prevalence (Ford, 2005).

Although some research has looked at how the individual components of metabolic syndrome (Table 1.10) may affect male fertility, more work is needed. Canadian scientists Kasturi et al. (2008) have concluded that obesity/overweight, insulin resistance and dylipidemia may increase the chances of infertility in men. The interactions

Table 1.10 Worldwide definition of metabolic syndrome.

Central obesity (waist circumference ≥94 cm for European men and ≥80 cm for women)*
Combined with additional two of the following:
- Raised triglyceride level: >150 mg/dL (1.7 mmol/L)
- Reduced HDL cholesterol: <40 mg/dL (0.9 mmol/L) on males and <50 mg/dL (1.1 mmol/L) in females
- Raised blood pressure: systolic blood pressure ≥130 or diastolic ≥85 mmHg.
- Raised fasting plasma glucose: ≥100 mg/dL (5.6 mmol/L)

Source: International Diabetes Federation (2007).
*Additional cutoffs should be used for other ethnic groups.

between components of metabolic syndrome and male fertility are shown in Figure 1.2. In the Middle East, where this prevalence of male diabetes is high, one study found that over half of the men with diabetes who were infertile were also obese. It was concluded that these combined medical problems along with high rates of smoking may be contributing to the high rates of infertility experienced in this particular population of men (Bener *et al.*, 2009).

1.3.6 Oxidative stress

Over the last 10 years, it has become increasingly known that oxidative DNA damage may be a contributing factor to poor semen quality and infertility. Oxidative stress

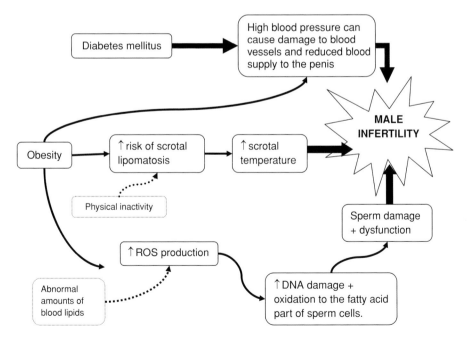

Figure 1.2 How components of metabolic syndrome may affect male fertility. ROS, reactive oxygen species; lipomatosis, an accumulation of fatty deposits which may form a lump of non-malignant fatty tissue. (Adapted and reproduced with permission from Kasturi *et al.* (2008) and the *American Society of Andrology*.)

occurs when there is an imbalance between the generation of ROS and antioxidant levels in the body. ROS may include hydroxyl ions, superoxide, hydrogen peroxide, peroxyl radical and hypochlorite ion, all of which are a natural by-product of ongoing metabolic and physiologic processes (Makker *et al.*, 2009).

Sperm cells are particularly susceptible to ROS because their plasma membrane comprises polyunsaturated fatty acids (PUFA), which oxidise easily. They also lack cytoplasm, the protective layer that surrounds the nucleus, which would normally act as a barrier and help repair damage caused by ROS (Agarwal and Prabakaran, 2005). Although ROS are generated endogenously, additional lifestyle and environmental factors can increase the production of ROS (smoking, alcohol use and environmental pollution) or, equally, protect against the effects of the ROS (antioxidant nutrients). When this balance is not maintained, accumulation of ROS can lead to altered sperm function and DNA damage.

1.3.7   Smoking

Tobacco smoke contains thousands of compounds, including alkaloids, nitrosamines and inorganic substances, many of which act as ROS. Although the trend between smoking and male infertility is well identified, the exact mechanisms of action are not well confirmed. Studies suggest that smoking is associated with modest reductions in semen quality, including sperm concentration, motility and morphology, but large, well-designed studies are lacking. Chemicals and carcinogens found in cigarette smoke may pass directly through the blood–testis barrier, directly affecting sperm function (Vine *et al.*, 1996). Studies have clearly shown that the number of DNA strand breaks is higher in the sperm cells of smokers when compared with non-smokers (Belcheva *et al.*, 2004). Scientists think that fathers who smoke in the run-up to pregnancy could be putting the health of their offspring at risk. Eggs fertilised by male smokers are generally not as viable and the risk of childhood cancers is thought to be higher in offspring born to parents who smoke (Sepaniak *et al.*, 2006). It is clear that smoking can affect male fertility, but larger studies now need to confirm whether a relationship between DNA integrity and childhood health exists. It would also be interesting to study whether stopping smoking helps to improve parameters of sperm function.

1.3.8   Alcohol

Alcohol is known to influence male fertility through several different mechanisms of action. Before describing how alcohol can affect fertility, it is important to describe the function of semeniferous tubules. As the name indicates, these are long tubes where sperm cells and ultimately semen are produced. Alcohol can affect sperm production and quality by acting directly on both Leydig cells inside these tubules, which produce testosterone, and Sertoli cells that line these tubules and play an active role in sperm production. Alcohol can also act on the hypothalamus part of the brain and alter the secretion of hormones that play a key role in male reproduction, namely, LH and FSH (Emanuele and Emanuele, 1998).

Unfortunately, although the physiological mechanisms in which alcohol acts appear to be well established, there is a lack of human trials. A recently published paper has, however, studied the effects of chronic alcoholism on male fertility. Sixty-six male alcoholics were recruited from treatment clinics and 30 non-smoking, non-alcoholic controls were selected. Venous and semen samples were collected from both groups. It was identified that alcoholic patients had elevated LH, FSH and estradiol levels, whilst testosterone and progesterone levels were reduced. Semen volume, sperm count, motility, and the number of healthy sperms were also lower in the sperm samples of alcoholics. In summary, findings from this study demonstrated that heavy drinking can have a detrimental effect on both the secretion of male reproductive hormones and semen quality (Muthusami and Chinnaswamy, 2005).

1.3.9   Polyunsaturated fatty acids

Lipids play an important role in the structure and function of sperm cells. Sperm cells have a high PUFA, which helps them to be fluid, mobile and fertilise the ovuum. Unfortunately, this also makes them susceptible to attack by ROS, which may ultimately affect their viability (Wathes et al., 2007). In some studies, the fatty acid content of sperm samples from healthy and infertile males has been analysed. Interestingly, it has been found that a higher proportion of saturated fatty acids are more likely to be present when either sperm concentration or motility is reduced. Equally, higher proportions of PUFA in sperm samples are found to be associated with improved sperm concentration, motility and morphology (Aksoy et al., 2006; Tavilani et al., 2006).

Overall, these studies show that the type and ratio of fatty acids present in sperm cells may influence their function. More work is now needed to confirm why this may occur and whether there is an 'ideal ratio' of PUFA: SFA (saturated fatty acids) to improve sperm function.

1.3.10   Antioxidants

Seminal plasma contains some natural antioxidant mechanisms that may protect against ROS and damage to spermatozoa to some extent. However, when levels of ROS exceed scavenging activities, sperm defects may occur. Antioxidant nutrients can play a key role in protecting spermatozoa from oxidative stress (Sheweita et al., 2005).

In a large observational study, the Age and Genetic Effects in Sperm (AGES) study set out to establish whether antioxidant intakes (from food and supplement sources) helped to protect against the age-related decline in male fertility. Ninety-seven males aged 20–80 years were recruited and asked to complete food frequency questionnaires. Researchers found that higher antioxidant intakes (particularly vitamins C and E) were significantly associated with increased sperm numbers and motility. Higher intakes of β-carotene improved the concentration of sperm. Overall, it was concluded that a diet containing sufficient amounts of antioxidants may help to offset the age-related decline in sperm quality (Eskenazi et al., 2005). Although several small clinical trails have demonstrated that antioxidants may protect against oxidative damage, evidence that antioxidant supplements may improve measures of semen quality is limited. Well-designed, randomised controlled trials are needed in the future to develop these areas of research.

1.3.11   Selenium

Selenium is an essential nutrient needed for normal testicular development, spermatogenesis, sperm motility and function. Like the antioxidants mentioned previously, selenium can protect against oxidative stress and prevent damage to sperm cells. In addition, the selenium-containing enzyme glutathione peroxidase also has antioxidant properties that help to protect against oxidative damage and improve the viability of sperm cells.

One of the largest randomised controlled trials undertaken to date tested whether supplementation with 200 µg/day selenium or a placebo improved sperm function in 468 infertile men. Supplements were taken daily over a 6-month study period followed by a 30-week treatment-free phase. Blood sample analysis showed that males taking selenium supplements had higher levels of testosterone and inhibin B. Semen parameters (concentration, motility and morphology) also were significantly improved in the group supplementing with selenium (Safarinejad and Safarinejad, 2009).

Overall, given the expense of medical treatment to improve parameters of seminal function, selenium supplementation may be a simple, inexpensive and safe alternative that could be used prior to reproductive technology, or alongside this. Similar well-designed studies are now needed to reinforce findings from this current research.

Research Highlight   Higher levels of ascorbic acid and zinc in semen samples linked to improved sperm quality

Recent research has measured the levels of antioxidant nutrients ascorbic acid and zinc present in the semen samples of both fertile and infertile men. Although larger studies are needed to reconfirm the findings from this research, scientists found that men without fertility problems had significant higher ascorbic acid levels in their sperm samples. In turn, higher levels of ascorbic acid were positively associated with the number of sperm cells present in samples and normal form and structure. Fertile men also had higher levels of zinc in their sperm samples, with smokers having some of the lowest zinc concentrations. The zinc content of sperm samples also correlated with sperm count and normal morphology. Scientists concluded that diets lacking in vitamin C and zinc may be risk factors contributing to reduced sperm quality and male infertility (Colagar and Marzony, 2009; Colagar et al., 2009).

1.3.12   Lycopene

Lycopene (a carotenoid) is a powerful natural antioxidant, mainly obtained from tomatoes and tomato products in the human diet. There is some evidence to suggest that lycopene is important for the body's natural defences and protect against oxidative stress. Studies investigating the role of lycopene supplementation on parameters of sperm function are generally limited, or poorly designed.

In one most recent study, six males were provided with 22.8 mg lycopene per day over a 2-week study period. Blood and seminal lycopene levels were measured at the start and end of the study and analysed using high-performance liquid chromatography. Interestingly, the lycopene in this study was provided from tomato soup and investigators closely monitored the compliance of obliging participants. Scientists found that both blood and seminal levels of lycopene increased after the 2-week study period, but levels of oxidative stress remained unchanged (Goyer *et al.*, 2007).

Although this study gives us some insight into the bioavailability of lycopene and concentration in seminal plasma, considerably more work is needed. Further work is needed to confirm whether improvements in sperm motility and concentration are a direct result of the lycopene or due to the free radical scavenging ability of lycopene.

1.3.13   Isoflavones

Isoflavones are plant-derived polyphenolic compounds that act in a similar manner to oestrogen hormones (they have oestrogenic activity). Animal studies have shown that high levels of isoflavone consumption may be linked to decreased fertility, but few human studies have established whether there is a link between the two.

In one of the largest studies to date, the isoflavone intake of 99 males from couples having problems conceiving were asked to record their isoflavone intake of foods eaten in the previous three months. After accounting for factors that could influence the results, it was found that higher intakes of soy foods (Table 1.11) were associated with reduced sperm concentrations (but not related to motility, morphology or ejaculation volume) (Chavarro *et al.*, 2008c). Although it needs to be confirmed exactly how isoflavones may exert their actions, there does appear to be a relatively strong link between the consumption of soy foods and sperm concentrations.

1.3.14   Phthalates

Phthalates are a group of man-made chemicals that are added to plastics to improve their durability, transparency and flexibility. Such plastics may be used in both household and consumer products, which mainly take the form of food packaging. Animal studies in the past using male rats have shown that exposure to these chemicals can affect the function of the male sex organs directly, reducing fertility.

Table 1.11   Examples of soy foods.

Cereal/energy bars containing soy or soy protein
Cooked green vegetable soybeans
Lecithin, an emulsifier extracted from soybean oil
Meat alternatives – hydrolysed vegetable protein (made from soybeans)
Miso soup
Natto, used as a topping on rice or in miso soup, made from fermented cooked soybeans
Roasted soy nuts and soynut butter
Soy cheese, yoghurt and ice cream
Soy milk and shakes
Soy fibre, from the hulls and pulp of soybeans
Soy flour, made from roasted soybeans ground into a fine flour
Soy sauce
Soy sprouts
Tempeh (a high-protein Indonesian food made from cooked and slightly fermented soybeans)
Tofu and tofu products

Table 1.12 Nutrition, lifestyle and male fertility – key points.

- Men should be guided to achieve a healthy body weight when planning a pregnancy (ideally a BMI less than 25 kg/m^2)
- Men should also be encouraged to consume a healthy, balanced diet that includes at least five daily portions of fruit and vegetables
- Males smokers should ensure that their diet contains antioxidant-rich foods or consider taking a selenium supplement (200 μg/day has been found to have clinical benefits; Safarinejad and Safarinejad, 2009)
- Men should be encouraged to reduce their alcohol intake when planning a pregnancy
- Men should ensure that they are including polyunsaturated fatty acids within their diets (i.e. eating at least two portions of oily fish per week)
- Men with subfertility or infertility (particularly Asian males) may consider monitoring their intakes of isoflavones

One human study comprising 379 men recruited from American infertility clinics found that urinary excretion of phthalate metabolites were directly related to levels of DNA sperm damage, even after controlling for levels of oxidative stress (Hauser *et al.*, 2007). More recently, however, new evidence shows that exposure may also affect the reproductive development of male offspring, leading to medical conditions such as crytorchidism (when the testes fail to descend into the scrotum), hypospadias, a medical complication where the urethra is located on the wrong side of the penis and low-sperm counts (Martino-Andrade and Chahoud, 2010).

1.3.15   Application in practice

Overall, scientific evidence suggests that dietary factors (particularly antioxidants) can play an important role in improving sperm quality and parameters of sperm function. In addition, although better designed studies are needed, rising rates of obesity and diabetes may also be contributing to fertility problems in men, as well as the fact that many couples are waiting longer to have children, particularly in Western regions. It is well known that alcohol can cause oxidative stress, but better designed clinical trials are needed to assess how high intakes directly affect sperm parameters. For other dietary and lifestyle components, such as the role of isofavones and effect of metabolic syndrome, evidence is only just starting to emerge. Although it can be recognised that there are many gaps within the field of nutrition and male fertility, some simple recommendations have been compiled based on the best evidence that is available to date. These are summarised in Table 1.12.

1.4   Conclusion

Infertility and subfertility seem to be becoming an increasingly frequent occurrence, particularly in Western regions. Although this may be attributed to couples waiting longer before they have children, changing dietary and lifestyle habits may have a role to play. For couples who are having problems conceiving, ARTs can be expensive and are not always available to everyone. A thorough evaluation of literature presently available has shown that simple measures such as achieving a healthy body weight and making some simple dietary and lifestyle changes could help couples to achieve a healthy pregnancy. It is hoped that larger, well-designed clinical studies will continue in this important area so that government policies and evidence-base practical guidelines can be imparted to public sectors in the future.

Key Messages

- In Western regions, there is a tendency for couples to wait longer before planning a pregnancy; simple dietary and lifestyle changes may help to improve reproductive health and reduce time to pregnancy.
- For couples seeking the use of ARTs, the success of these fertility treatments may be reduced (particularly for women) if they are overweight or obese.
- Both the BFS and NICE advises that women achieve a healthy body weight before becoming pregnant or when undergoing fertility treatments. Ideally, a woman's BMI should be <35 kg/m² or <30 kg/m² in younger women (Bates *et al.*, 2007).
- Both women and men should avoid consuming large amounts of alcohol when planning a pregnancy.
- For male smokers, although quitting is the best course of action, consuming a diet rich in antioxidants (i.e. vitamin C, selenium and zinc) or taking an antioxidant-containing supplement may be of benefit.
- Nurses and healthcare practitioners can play a key role in supporting couples having trouble conceiving and offering appropriate guidance.
- It is important that healthcare messages are conveyed to women and men of child-bearing age about the benefits a healthy lifestyle can have on fertility and the health of the next generation.
- Overall, a multi-faceted approach should be taken to improve female and male fertility, which involves evaluating diet quality, harmful environmental and occupational risk factors.

Recommended reading

ASRM (American Society for Reproductive Medicine) (2008) Optimizing natural fertility. *Fertility & Sterility* 90(S5), S1–6.

Langley-Evans S (2009) Before life begins. In: *Nutrition. A Lifespan Approach*. Wiley-Blackwell: Oxford.

Wilkes S and Murdoch A (2009) Obesity and female fertility: a primary care perspective. *Journal of Family Planning & Reproduction Health Care* 35(3),181–5.

References

Agarwal A, Gupta S and Sharma RK (2005) Role of oxidative stress in female reproduction. *Reproductive Biology and Endocrinolology* 13, 28.

Agarwal A and Prabakaran SA (2005) Mechanism, measurement, and prevention of oxidative stress in male reproductive physiology. *Indian Journal of Experimental Biology* 43(11), 963–74.

Aitken RJ (2006) Sperm function tests and fertility. *International Journal of Andrology* 29(1), 69–75.

Aksoy Y, Aksoy H, Altinkaynak K, Aydin HR and Ozkan A (2006) Sperm fatty acid composition in subfertile men. *Prostaglandins, Leukotrienes and Essential Fatty Acids* 75, 75–9.

ASRM (American Society for Reproductive Medicine) (2002) Aging and infertility in women: a committee opinion. *Fertility and Sterility* 78, 215–9.

ASRM (American Society for Reproductive Medicine) (2008) Definitions of infertility and recurrent pregnancy loss. *Fertility & Sterility* 89(6), 1603.

Balen AH, Anderson RA; Policy and Practice Committee of the BFS (2007) Impact of obesity on female reproductive health: British Fertility Society, Policy and Practice Guidelines. *Human Fertility (Cambridge)* **10**(4), 195–206.

Bates B, Lennox A and Swan G (2010) *National Diet and Nutrition Survey Headline results from year 1 of the rolling programme (2008–09)*. FSA and the DH: London.

Belcheva A, Ivanova-Kicheva M, Tzvetkova P and Marinov M (2004) Effects of cigarette smoking on sperm plasma membrane integrity and DNA fragmentation. *International Journal of Andrology* **27**(5), 296–300.

Bener A, Al-Ansari AA, Zirie M and Al-Hamaq AA (2009) Is male fertility associated with type 2 diabetes mellitus? *International Urology & Nephrology* **41**(4), 777–84.

Bohler H Jr, Mokshagundam S and Winters SJ (2010) Adipose tissue and reproduction in women. *Fertility & Sterility* **94**(3), 795–825.

Bolumar F, Olsen J, Rebagliato M and Bisanti L (1997) Caffeine intake and delayed conception: a European multicenter study on infertility and subfecundity. European Study Group on Infertility Subfecundity. *American Journal of Epidemiology* **145**(4), 324–34.

Campos DB, Palin MF, Bordignon V and Murphy BD (2008) The 'beneficial' adipokines in reproduction and fertility. *International Journal of Obesity (London)* **32**(2), 223–31.

Carlsen E, Giwercman A, Keiding N and Skakkebaek NE (1992) Evidence for decreasing quality of semen during past 50 years. *British Medical Journal* **305**, 609–13.

Chavarro JE, Rich-Edwards JW and Willett WC (2006) Iron intake and risk of ovulatory infertility. *Obstetrics and Gynaecology* **108**(5), 145–52.

Chavarro JE, Rich-Edwards JW, Rosner BA and Willett WC (2007a) Dietary fatty acid intakes and the risk of ovulatory infertility. *American Journal of Clinical Nutrition* **85**, 231–7.

Chavarro JE, Rich-Edwards JW, Rosner BA and Willett WC (2007b) A prospective study of dairy foods intake and anovulatory infertility. *Human Reproduction* **5**, 1340–7.

Chavarro JE, Rich-Edwards JW, Rosner BA and Willett WC (2008a) Protein intake and ovulatory infertility. *American Journal of Obstetrics & Gynaecology* **198**, 210.e1–7.

Chavarro JE, Rich-Edwards JW, Rosner BA and Willett WC (2008b) Use of multivitamins, intake of B vitamins and risk of ovulatory infertility. *Fertility & Sterility* **89**(3), 668–76.

Chavarro JE, Toth TL, Sadio SM and Hauser R (2008c) Soy food and isoflavone intake in relation to semen quality parameters among men from an infertility clinic. *Human Reproduction* **23**(11), 2584–90.

Chavarro JE, Rich-Edwards JW, Rosner BA and Willett WC (2009a) A prospective study of dietary carbohydrate quantity and quality in relation to risk of ovulatory infertility. *European Journal of Clinical Nutrition* **63**, 78–86.

Chavarro JE, Rich-Edwards JW, Rosner BA and Willett WC (2009b) Caffeinated and alcoholic beverage intake in relation to ovulatory disorder infertility. *Epidemiology* **20**(3), 374–81.

Chibber R (2005) Childbearing beyond age 50: pregnancy outcome in 59 cases "a concern?" *Archives of Gynaecology & Obstetrics* **271**(3), 189–94.

Clemens SL, Grant BM and Matthews SL (2009) A review of the impacts of health and health behaviours on women's alcohol use. *American Journal of Health Behaviour* **33**(4), 400–15.

Cocuzza M, Athayde KS, Agarwal A *et al.* (2008) Age-related increase of reactive oxygen species in neat semen in healthy fertile men. *Urology* **71**(3), 490–4.

Colagar AH and Marzony ET (2009) Ascorbic Acid in human seminal plasma: determination and its relationship to sperm quality. *Journal of Clinical Biochemistry & Nutrition* **45**(2), 144–9.

Colagar AH, Marzony ET and Chaichi MJ (2009) Zinc levels in seminal plasma are associated with sperm quality in fertile and infertile men. *Nutrition Research* **29**(2), 82–8.

Crha I, Hruba D, Ventruba P, Fiala J, Totusek J and Visnova H (2003) Ascorbic acid and infertility treatment. *Central European Journal of Public Health* **11**(2), 63–7.

De Pergola G, Tartagni A, d'Angelo F, Centoducati C, Guida P and Giorgino R (2009) Abdominal fat accumulation, and not insulin resistance is associated to oligomenorrhea in non-hyperandrogenic overweight/obese women. *Journal of Endocrinological Investigation* **32**(2), 98–101.

Eggert J, Theobald H and Engfeldt P (2004) Effects of alcohol consumption on female fertility during an 18-year period. *Fertility & Sterility* **81**(2), 379–83.

Emanuele MA and Emanuele NV (1998) Alcohol's effects on male reproduction. *Alcohol Health & Research World* **22**(2), 195–201.

Eskenazi B, Kidd SA, Marks AR, Sloter E, Block G and Wyrobek AJ (2005) Antioxidant intake is associated with semen quality in healthy men. *Human Reproduction* 20(4), 1006–12.

Frisch RE (1987) Body fat, menarche, fitness and fertility. *Human Reproduction* 2(6), 521–33.

Ford ES (2005) Prevalence of the metabolic syndrome defined by the International Diabetes Federation among adults in the U.S. *Diabetes Care* 28(11), 2745–9.

Gaskins AJ, Mumford SL, Zhang C *et al.* (2009) Effect of daily fiber intake on reproductive function: the BioCycle Study. *American Journal of Clinical Nutrition* 90, 1061–9.

Gnoth C, Godehardt E, Frank-Herrmann P, Friol K, Tigges J and Freundl G (2005) Definition and prevalence of subfertility and infertility. *Human Reproduction* 20, 7.

Goyer A, Chopra M, Lwaleed BA, Birch B and Cooper AJ (2007) The effects of dietary lycopene supplementation on human seminal plasma. *British Journal of Urology International* 99, 1456–60.

Grodstein F, Goldman MB and Cramer DW (1994) Infertility in women and moderate alcohol use. *American Journal of Public Health* 85(7), 1021–2.

Hamilton-Fairley D and Taylor A (2003) Anovulation. *British Medical Journal* 327, 546–9.

Hauser R, Meeker JD, Singh NP *et al.* (2007) DNA damage in human sperm is related to urinary levels of phthalate monoester and oxidative metabolites. *Human Reproduction* 22(3), 688–95.

HFEA (Human Fertilisation Embryology Authority) (2010) Fertility facts and figures. Available at: http://www.hfea.gov.uk/docs/adbcdfh.pdf. (accessed March 2011.)

International Diabetes Federation (IDF) (2007) *The IDF Consensus Worldwide Definition of the Metabolic Syndrome. Part 1: Worldwide Definition for Use in Clinical Practice.* International Diabetes Federation: Belgium.

Juhl M, Nyboe Andersen AM, Grønbaek M and Olsen J (2001) Moderate alcohol consumption and waiting time to pregnancy. *Human Reproduction* 16(12), 2705–9.

Kasturi SS, Tannir J and Brannigan RE (2008) The metabolic syndrome and male fertility. *Journal of Andrology* 29(3), 251–9.

Klein J and Sauer MV (2001) Assessing fertility in women of advanced reproductive age. *American Journal of Obstetrics & Gynaecology* 185, 758–70.

Kort HI, Massey JB, Elsner CW *et al.* (2006) Impact of body mass index values on sperm quantity and quality. *Journal of Andrology* 27(3), 450–2.

Kühnert B and Nieschlag E (2004) Reproductive functions of the ageing male. *Human Reproduction Update* 10(4), 327–39.

MacDonald AA, Herbison GP, Showell M and Farquhar CM (2010) The impact of body mass index on semen parameters and reproductive hormones in human males: a systematic review with meta-analysis. *Human Reproduction Update* 16(3), 293–311.

Makker K, Agarwal A and Sharma R (2009) Oxidative stress and male infertility. *Indian Journal of Medical Research* 129(4), 357–67.

Martino-Andrade AJ and Chahoud I (2010) Reproductive toxicity of phthalate esters. *Molecular Nutrition & Food Research* 54(1), 148–57.

Mircea CN, Lujan ME and Pierson RA (2007) Metabolic fuel and clinical implications for female reproduction. *Journal of Obstetrics & Gynaecology Canada* 29(11), 887–902.

Monsen RB (2009) Prevention is best for fetal alcohol syndrome. *Journal of Paediatric Nursing* 24(1), 60–1.

Muthusami KR and Chinnaswamy P (2005) Effect of chronic alcoholism on male fertility hormones and semen quality. *Fertility & Sterility* 84(4), 919–24.

NICE (National Institute for Health and Clinical Excellence) (2010) *Dietary Interventions and Physical activity Interventions for Weight Management Before, During and After Pregnancy.* NICE: London.

Pasquali R and Gambineri A (2006) Metabolic effects of obesity on reproduction. *Reproductive Biomedicine Online* 12(5), 542–51.

Phipps MG and Sowers M (2002) Defining early adolescent childbearing. *American Journal of Public Health* 92(1), 125–8.

Pollard I, Murray JF, Hiller R, Scaramuzzi RJ and Wilson CA (1999) Effects of preconceptual caffeine exposure on pregnancy and progeny viability. *Journal of Maternal & Fetal Medicine* 8(5), 220–4.

Pyper C, Bromhall L, Dummett S (2006) The Oxford Conception Study design and recruitment experiment. *Paediatric & Perinatal Epidemiology* 20(1), 51–9

Ramos RG and Olden K (2008) The prevalence of metabolic syndrome among US women of child-bearing age. *American Journal of Public Health* 98(6), 1122–7.

Redman LM (2006) Physical activity and its effects on reproduction. *Reproductive Biomedicine Online* **12**(5), 579–86.

Ruder EH, Hartman TJ and Goldman MB (2009) Impact of oxidative stress on female fertility. *Current Opinions in Obstetrics & Gynaecology* **21**(3), 219–22.

Safarinejad MR and Safarinejad S (2009) Efficacy of selenium and/or N-acetyl-cysteine for improving semen parameters in infertile men: a double-blind, placebo-controlled, randomised study. *The Journal of Urology* **181**, 741–51.

Sartorius GA and Nieschlag E (2010) Paternal age and reproduction. *Human Reproduction Update* **16**(1), 65–79.

Sepaniak S, Forges T, Gerard H, Foliguet B, Bene MC and Monnier-Barbarino P (2006) The influence of cigarette smoking on human sperm quality and DNA fragmentation. *Toxicology* **223**(1–2), 54–60.

Sheweita SA, Tilmisany AM and Al-Sawaf H (2005) Mechanisms of male infertility: role of antioxidants. *Current Drug Metabolism* **6**(5), 495–501.

Shine R, Peek J and Birdsall M (2008) Declining sperm quality in New Zealand over 20 years. *New Zealand Medical Journal* **121**(1287), 50–6.

Swan SH and Elkin EP (1999) Declining semen quality: can the past inform the present? *BioEssays* **21**, 614–21.

Tamler R (2009) Diabetes, obesity, and erectile dysfunction. *Gender Medicine* **6**(1), 4–16.

Tavilani H, Doosti M, Abdi K, Vaisiraygani A and Joshaghani HR (2006) Decreased polyunsaturated and increased saturated fatty acid concentration in spermatozoa from asthenozoospermic males as compared with normozoospermic males. *Andrologia* **38**, 173–8.

Teoh SK, Mendelson JH, Mello NK, Skupny A and Ellingboe J (1990) Alcohol effects on hCG-stimulated gonadal hormones in women. *American Society for Pharmacology and Experimental Therapeutics* **254**(2), 407–11.

Vine MF (1996) Smoking and male reproduction: a review. *International Journal of Andrology* **19**(6), 323–37.

Wathes DC, Abayasekara DR and Aitken RJ (2007) Polyunsaturated fatty acids in male and female reproduction. *Biology of Reproduction* **77**(2), 190–201.

Waylen AL, Jones GL and Ledger WL (2010) Effect of cigarette smoking upon reproductive hormones in women of reproductive age: a retrospective analysis. *Reproductive Biomedicine Online* **20**(6), 861–5.

Westphal LM, Polan ML and Trant AS (2006) Double-blind, placebo-controlled study of Fertilityblend: a nutritional supplement for improving fertility in women. *Clinical & Experimental Obstetrics & Gynaecology* **33**(4), 205–8.

WHO (World Health Organisation) (1992) *WHO Laboratory Manual for the Examination of Human Semen and Semen-Cervical Mucus Interaction*, 3rd edition. Cambridge University Press: Cambridge.

Wilkes S and Murdoch A (2009) Obesity and female fertility: a primary care perspective. *Journal of Family Planning & Reproductive Health Care* **35**(3), 181–5.

Winkle T, Rosenbusch B, Gagsteiger F, Paiss T and Zoller N (2009) The correlation between male age, sperm quality and sperm DNA fragmentation in 320 men attending a fertility center. *Journal of Assisted Reproduction & Genetics* **26**(1), 41–6.

Zhang X, Sliwowska JH and Weinberg J (2005) Prenatal alcohol exposure and fetal programming: effects on neuroendocrine and immune function. *Experimental Biology & Medicine* **230**(6), 376–88.

2 Preparing the Body for Pregnancy

Summary

Women may alter their diets throughout the course of their pregnancy, but getting the right nutrients is just as important before pregnancy takes place. Ideally, the body should be prepared before the physiological demands of pregnancy occur. If nutrient reserves are low before pregnancy commences, this may affect the health of the mother and/or child later on. Data from nutrition surveys and studies show that a considerable proportion of women in their childbearing years are not meeting recommended intakes for key nutrients, i.e. iron and folate, and multiple micronutrient deficiencies are common when diets are poor. Poor quality diets and lack of knowledge about what constitutes a 'balanced diet' also mean that women's body weight may not be within recommended ranges when pregnancy begins; a factor that can again have later health consequences for both mother and child. Women need to be guided about the importance of eating a healthy diet and getting body weight into recommended ranges before becoming pregnant. It would also be of benefit if women were aware of certain food safety issues before or in the early stages of their pregnancies. Public health campaigns, nurses, midwives and health practitioners can play a key role in helping to communicate these messages.

Learning Outcomes

- To describe why it is important for women to eat a healthy, balanced diet before pregnancy begins and explain how this may be achieved.
- To provide examples of research investigating women's knowledge of healthy eating guidelines and whether these are being taken on board.
- To recognise the importance of having a healthy body weight before/upon conception and describe the potential role of lifestyle interventions before pregnancy.
- To outline key food safety issues that may arise in pregnancy and discuss the importance of distributing this information in the early stage of pregnancy, if not before.

Nutrition in the Childbearing Years, First Edition. Emma Derbyshire.
© 2011 Emma Derbyshire. Published 2011 by Blackwell Publishing Ltd.

2.1   Introduction

To enhance fertility, support the development of both pregnancy and the growing foetus and promote long-term health, it is important that women consume a diet adequate in the right nutrients before as well as during pregnancy (Cetin *et al.*, 2009). However, even in the twenty-first century, and as we will see from this chapter, it is not uncommon for women to underconsume a variety of nutrients. This is of concern because a considerable proportion of pregnancies are unplanned. European data indicate that the number of planned pregnancies varies across Europe, ranging from just 10–20% up to 85% (EUROCAT Working Group, 2003). Consequently, a considerable proportion of women are starting their pregnancies unprepared from a nutrient perspective. Although, the proportion of unplanned pregnancies is highest amongst girls in their adolescent years, a proportion of women in their middle years also have unplanned pregnancies, as reflected by abortion rates (DH, 2009), possibly because of compliance with contraceptive methods.

This chapter is divided into two sections. The first part covers issues that affect health and nutrition status before pregnancy and focuses on the importance of eating the right balance of nutrients throughout the childbearing years. This is important not only for current health and well-being, but also for future health, both in pregnancy and beyond. The second part of the chapter deals with food safety issues. It can be confusing knowing what foods can be consumed or should be avoided in pregnancy, or what should be advised. This section aims to examine and summate information from recent guidelines and discuss some of the more recent food safety issues.

2.2   Nutrient stores

Being the right body weight and ensuring the mother has optimal nutrient stores before conception can help to give both the mother and the child the best start once pregnancy begins. Like filling up a tank of petrol, it is better to start the journey of pregnancy with adequate reserves. One good example of this relates to low iron stores. Data from UK surveys indicate that around 12% women in their childbearing years are iron-deficient (serum ferritin <15 μg/L), but as many as 58% may have low iron stores (serum ferritin <40 μg/L) (Rushton *et al.*, 2004). As increased blood production, foetal demands and the expansion of maternal tissues all drive up iron requirements during pregnancy (Wahed *et al.*, 2010), it is not surprising that around 1 in 2 women, even amongst educated populations, go on to become anaemic (Kalaivani, 2009).

As can be seen from Figure 2.1, there are a number of factors that can affect women's levels of nutrients in the body before pregnancy. This includes factors such as level of education and socio-economic status, number of children already in the family, body weight before pregnancy, the time intervals between pregnancy (to help recover nutrient stores), levels of physical activity, diet quality and supplement use (Dewey and Cohen, 2007). Every woman is different, but these are important factors to consider when working with or carrying out research with women before/during pregnancy.

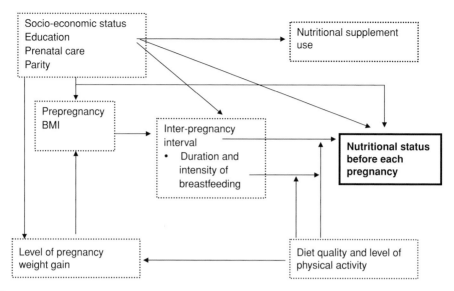

Figure 2.1   Factors influencing maternal nutrient status before pregnancy. (Adapted and printed with permission from Dewey and Cohen (2007) and the *Maternal & Child Nutrition*.)

2.2.1   Pregnancy spacing

Generally, a healthy pregnancy is defined as one that is free from medical complications and leads to the delivery of a healthy baby (ADA, 2002; Figure 2.2). Some studies have researched whether the amount of time between pregnancies can affect the chances of having a healthy baby. Zhu (2005) reported that the relationship between pregnancy spacing and unfavourable pregnancy outcomes generally follows a J-shaped curve, meaning that both very short and long time periods between pregnancies could affect infant health. The same author concluded that a birth interval of 18–23 months appeared to be most favourable in terms of reducing the risk of low birth weight deliveries, preterm birth and small-for-gestational-age (SGA) infants (Zhu, 2005).

If women start pregnancy with inadequate nutrient supplies, a state of biological competition can co-exist between the mother and her foetus. Although the body can adapt to some extent to increased nutrient demands, i.e. slowing transit time to make the absorption of nutrients from foods more efficient, this is not always sufficient. In terms of nutrient supplies, if nutrient deficiencies are severe, the mother is given preference to nutrient supplies, but if marginal deficiencies exist, the foetus is favoured (King, 2003).

> A healthy pregnancy may be defined as one that is "*without physical or psychological pathology in the mother or foetus and results in the delivery of a healthy baby*": ADA (2002).
>
> Ensuring that women eat a balanced diet, containing the correct proportion of nutrients whilst achieving a healthy body weight can go some way to ensuring that women have a pregnancy free from medical complications.

Figure 2.2   Definition of a healthy pregnancy.

Most recently, Dewey and Cohen (2007) have suggested that the term 'recuperative interval', i.e. the period of time during which women are not pregnant or lactating, is perhaps more appropriate than the phrase 'pregnancy spacing'. In scientific terms, as breastfeeding also has extra nutritional demands, this is a much better indicator of whether women have had chance to recover from their pregnancies. In this detailed systematic review paper, Dewey and Cohen (2007) pooled the results from 34 papers studying whether birth spacing could affect nutrition status in mothers and children. Overall, analysis was difficult as so many other confounding factors can influence nutrition status. It was, however, found that short pregnancy intervals of less than 6 months could increase the chances of anaemia in pregnancy. On the whole, this was a very important paper, but studies in the past often fail to control for other factors which can also affect nutrition status.

2.3   Body weight before pregnancy

Being a healthy body weight before becoming pregnant can markedly reduce the risk of complications in pregnancy (see Table 2.1 for body weight categories). Being both underweight and overweight before pregnancy can influence maternal and infant health in different ways. Extremes of body weight follow a U-shaped curve in terms of health effects on the mother and baby. Being underweight is associated with poor foetal growth and pregnancy loss, whilst being overweight is more commonly linked to the development of medical complications in pregnancy, miscarriage, stillbirth and high birth weight deliveries (Davies, 2006). In one study, women who put on weight rapidly (between 2.3 and 10 kg/year) before falling pregnant were 2.5 times more likely to develop gestational diabetes in pregnancy (Hedderson *et al.*, 2008).

One of the main adverse consequences of obesity and an area that is being studied increasingly is metabolic syndrome (a range of medical conditions that affect later health). There is good evidence that the incidence of metabolic syndrome is rising amongst women in their childbearing years and concern that this may affect health in pregnancy, metabolic programming of the foetus and the offspring's health in later life (Ramos and Olden, 2008). There is already some evidence to show that elevated glucose levels in pregnancy (one medical condition linked to metabolic syndrome) can affect the growth of the foetus and increase the chances of obesity and glucose intolerance of the offspring in adulthood (McMillen *et al.*, 2009). However, more remains to be known about the effect of metabolic syndrome on the health of the mother and next generation of offspring.

Table 2.1   Categorising body weight before pregnancy.

BMI category	Prepregnancy BMI
Underweight	<18.5
Normal weight	18.5–24.9
Overweight	25.0–29.9
Obese	≥30.0

Source: Rasmussen and Yaktine (2009).
BMI, weight (kg)/height (m²).

Research Highlight   The lifestyle study

In the Netherlands, around 30% of women with fertility problems are overweight or obese. Small trials have shown that weight loss may help not only to improve fertility but also reduce medical complications in pregnancy and improve health in childhood. To test this theory more rigorously, Dutch scientists have carefully designed a randomised controlled trial (RCT) to determine whether a 6-month lifestyle programme can help to promote weight loss. Women taking part in the programme receive normal fertility care after they have taken part in the lifestyle programme (Mutsaerts *et al.*, 2010). It is hoped that such interventions could reduce the need for fertility treatments while helping to reduce the risk of pregnancy complications.

2.4   The importance of a balanced diet

Guidelines in terms of what constitutes a balanced diet vary slightly between international organisations. No single food contains all of the nutrients that the body needs, so eating a balanced diet means eating a wide variety of foods in proportions needed for good health (NHS, 2011). In essence, a well-balanced diet should contain plenty of starchy foods such as wholegrain bread, pasta and rice, fruit and vegetables and some protein foods such as lean meat, fish, eggs and lentils. Intakes of saturated fat, salt and alcohol should be carefully monitored and eaten in smaller proportions. Many nations have developed conceptual ways to represent the ideal diet, often using visual models. These help to support nutrient recommendations which are often poorly understood and need to be put into context by health professionals. Visual models such as the pyramid system, plate model and traffic light system can help to get healthy eating messages across to women in their childbearing years.

The Scientific Advisory Committee on Nutrition (SACN) (2008) compiled a useful summary of dietary guidelines so that nutrients intakes from UK surveys could be compared against these targets (Table 2.2). Analysis of data from UK surveys showed that young women aged 19–24 years were only eating an average of $1^1/_2$ portions of fruit/vegetables each day and 83% consumed more than 6 g salt on a daily basis. Dietary intakes of fibre (analysed as non-starch polysaccharide (NSP)) were just 11 g/day and 25% women had low biochemical status for vitamin D. Iron deficiency was also common with 42% women consuming less than 8 mg iron per day and 27% defining having low iron status, defined using biochemical markers.

2.5   What are women eating?

In a review paper of more than 110 published research studies and reports, Ruxton and Derbyshire (2010) reviewed the diets of UK women. For women in their childbearing years, it was found that around 1 in 5 women did not get enough iron from their diets, 11% had inadequate intakes of vitamin B_2 and 9% failed to consume enough magnesium. Although presently there are no vitamin D recommendations for non-pregnant women, the European Commission recommends a daily intake of 5 μg for labelling purposes (EC, 2008). Mean intakes from UK dietary surveys

Table 2.2 Summary of dietary recommendations.

Recommendation	Level of intake
Fruit and vegetables	At least 5 × 80 g portions/day (400 g)
Oily fish	At least 1 portion/week (140 g)
Fat	35% food energy (maximum)
Saturated fat	11% food energy (maximum)
NSP	An average intake of 18 g/day
Alcohol	No more than 2–3 units/day*. Women planning a pregnancy should drink no more than 1–2 units twice per week (DoH, 2004).
Salt (sodium chloride)	Maximum of 6 g/day (2.4 g sodium/day)

Source: SACN (2008).
*Women aged 18+, 1 unit (8 g alcohol) is equivalent to approximately half a pint of beer, lager or cider, or a single measure (25 mL) spirits, or a small glass (125 mL) of wine, sherry, port or other fortified wine.

were found to be, on average 2.1 μg vitamin D per day, significantly below these cutoffs. This is of concern as there is evidence that vitamin D intakes between 7 and 41 μg/day (depending on the level of sun exposure) may be needed to maintain serum vitamin D levels in the ranges needed for good health (Cashman *et al.*, 2008).

The European Commission also recently instigated the development of the first European Nutrition and Health Report, combining nutrition and health data from 14 different European countries (Elmadfa *et al.*, 2009). Although the age categories extend slightly beyond what is normally constituted as childbearing age, average daily intakes of selected nutrients from this survey are summarised in Table 2.3. As data is presented as ranges, women generally appear to meet dietary guidelines for most nutrients. However, women seem to fall below requirements for iron, even at the upper end of the range, and iodine (aged 14–24 years). Intakes of total fat, alcohol and sodium should be continuously monitored as the range of intake is quite broad and exceed dietary guidelines in some circumstances.

2.6 A note on dietary recommendations

Different countries use different standards to define good health, which can be confusing. In the United Kingdom, the Department of Health (DH) published Dietary Reference Values (DRVs) for Food Energy and Nutrients in 1991 (DH, 1991). DRVs are a guide to whether diets are meeting targets that will help to maintain good health. DRVs can be divided into three main categories: (1) reference nutrient intakes (RNI) – the amount of a nutrient that should meet the requirements of most (about 97.5%) people, (2) estimated average requirement (EAR) – nutrients consumed at this level of intake are generally enough for average person (about 50% people) and (3) lower reference nutrient intake (LRNI) – the nutrient level/cut-off below which deficiencies are most likely to occur. Although these are a useful guide, a wealth of evidence has accumulated since these were compiled.

For this reason, the European Food Safety Authority (EFSA) is in the process of compiling new dietary guidelines. This will be of benefit as countries across Europe

Table 2.3   Daily intakes of selected nutrients in European women.

Nutrient*	Intakes – data presented as ranges (min.–max.)		UK DRVs non-pregnant women 19–50 years (DH, 1991)
	14–24 years	**18–64 years**	
Protein (%EI)	12–17	13–19	–
Carbohydrates (%EI)	42–55	38–53	50
Fat (%EI)	29–40	30–48	35
SFA (%EI)	12–16	9–17	11
PUFA (%EI)	4–7	4–9	–
Dietary fibre (g)	14–22	16–26	18 (average intake)
Alcohol (%EI)	0.3–2	0.3–6	5
Vitamin D (μg)	1.5–3.4	2.0–5.1	–
Calcium (mg)	659–1121	579–1467	700
Sodium (g)	2.2–3.2	2.0–6.4	2.4
Folate (μg)	161–266	194–359	200
Iron (mg)	8.9–12.8	7.1–12.8	14.8
Iodine (μg)	78–106	80–235	140

Source: Data extracted from Elmadfa and Freisling (2009).
DRV, dietary reference value.
*Reference nutrient intake (RNI) shown for micronutrients.

should then be able to compare data against the same cut-offs for which there is currently no consensus. So far, new guidelines have been compiled for carbohydrate (45–60% EI), fat (20–35% EI), dietary fibre (25 g/day) and water (Section 5.9; EFSA, 2010). Revised recommendations for micronutrients are to follow shortly. It is also hoped that new guidelines will be compiled for vitamin D for which there is currently no UK recommendation for women. Also, present DRVs and RNIs hardly include any increments for pregnancy, or target the nutritional needs at the different trimesters, which should to be considered in the future (Wynn and Wynn, 2000).

2.7   Compliance with current recommendations

The Southampton Women's Survey is one of the largest investigations to date that has studied the diet, body composition, lifestyle and social circumstances of over 12,000 women from before pregnancy until after they have had children (Inskip *et al.*, 2006; Figure 2.3). Analysis of data from the study has provided many interesting findings. Crozier *et al.* (2009) found that 54% non-pregnant women aged 20–34 years drank more than 4 units of alcohol per week, 39% had daily caffeine intakes >300 mg/day and only 47% women ate a minimum of 5 portions of fruit and vegetables a day. In terms of combined recommendations, Inskip *et al.* (2009) found that only 0.06% women who were not yet pregnant took 400 μg folic acid daily, or drank less than 4 units of alcohol in a week. Younger women with fewer educational qualifications were the least likely to meet public health recommendations.

Taken together, evidence from this work indicates that nutrition and health recommendations may need to be better promoted amongst women in their childbearing years. At present, a large proportion of women before pregnancy fail to meet even

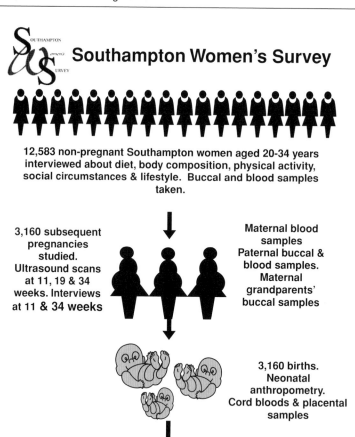

Figure 2.3   Cohort profile: The Southampton Women's Survey. (Provided with permission from Inskip *et al.* (2006).)

basic diet and lifestyle guidelines. This is of particular concern when pregnancies are unplanned and nutrient status is inadequate at the start of pregnancy.

Research Highlight   Mothers' interpretations of dietary recommendations

Setting dietary targets is one way to help women improve the quality of their diets. However, women may have trouble interpreting and applying such guidelines to their daily lifestyles. A recent study carried out at Cardiff University found that women's descriptions of balanced diets were not in line with official definitions.

Family doctors from local health centres interviewed a sample of 46 mothers with children aged 16 years or younger and questioned them about balanced diets and the main reasons for ill health. Television programmes and advertisements were found to be the main sources of dietary advice. Although the basic health promotion slogans were easily recited, understanding did not extend much beyond this. Misunderstandings were apparent and practical constraints such as time, money and family preferences were all barriers to healthy eating. Women also seemed to adapt their understanding of advice to suit their personal preferences and reality of their lives (Wood *et al.*, 2010).

Clearly, a better and deeper understanding of dietary recommendations is needed. Improving women's understanding of a good diet may also have nutritional benefits that could extend to the whole family. It seems that being exposed to health messages alone is not enough to produce lasting, behavioural changes, and perceptions of 'healthy eating' are far from official recommendations. Similar studies in different groups of women, i.e. different age, ethnic and income groups, would be of benefit.

2.8   A focus on alcohol

For women in their childbearing years, not drinking alcohol is a preventable cause of birth defects and developmental disabilities (Floyd *et al.*, 2009). There is inconsistent evidence about the impact alcohol intake can have on fertility, but excessive alcohol consumption is certainly harmful to the foetus (NICE, 2004). Prenatal alcohol exposure can also affect the development and function of the placenta. Alcohol exposure has been linked to reduced placental size, impaired blood flow and nutrient transport, hormonal changes and increased rates of stillbirth and low birth weight deliveries (Burd *et al.*, 2007).

Increasingly, it has been documented that women in their childbearing years may be exceeding alcohol guidelines. In the United Kingdom, over 22% of women fall into the category of 'heavy drinkers' (drinking >6 units on one survey day), with young women aged 19–24 years reporting some of the highest intakes (Henderson *et al.*, 2003).

For women who are trying to become pregnant, they should be advised to drink no more than 1 or 2 units of alcohol twice per week. Episodes of intoxication should be avoided to reduce the risk of harming the developing child (DH, 2004). Women are most at risk when they drink heavily and pregnancy is unplanned. Additional research on placental development from populations with heavy alcohol exposure should be encouraged; one way to do this may be through the use of tissue banks holding placentas and documenting exposures to alcohol, smoking and other relevant data variables (Burd *et al.*, 2007).

2.9   A focus on caffeine

Caffeine is one of the most frequently ingested pharmacologically active substances in the world. It is most commonly found in beverages (tea, coffee and soft drinks), products containing cocoa or chocolates and in some medications (Kuczkowski, 2009). Women may benefit from reducing their caffeine intakes to 200 mg/day during pregnancy (FSA, 2008; discussed further in Chapter 8). This is equivalent to about two mugs of instant coffee, two mugs of tea, five cans of cola, two cans of energy drink or four (50 g) bars of plain chocolate (Table 2.4). Therefore, a pregnant women eating a bar of plain chocolate and drinking two cups of tea will have probably reached the 200 mg guidelines.

For non-pregnant women in their reproductive years, very few large, well-designed studies have been undertaken to study the effects of caffeine consumption on female health before conception. Presently, the National Institute on Clinical

Table 2.4 Caffeine content of common food and beverage sources.

Food/beverage source	Caffeine content (mg)
1 μg instant coffee	100
1 μg filter coffee	140
1 μg of tea	75
1 can of cola	Up to 40
1 can of 'energy drink'	Up to 80
1 × 50 g bar of plain chocolate	Up to 50
1 × 50 g bar of milk chocolate	Up to 25

Source: Adapted from FSA (2008).

Evidence (NICE) (2004) have stated that there is no consistent evidence of an association between the consumption of caffeinated beverages and fertility problems. More work is needed to see if women planning a pregnancy may benefit from the same guidelines as pregnant mothers.

2.10   A focus on calcium

A diet rich in calcium is essential for many physiological processes. These include blood pressure, body weight regulation and the prevention of osteoporosis (Heaney, 2006). In terms of women's health, there is some evidence that a calcium-rich diet may be one way to help maintain and regulate body weight, although this theory has been contested recently (Teegarden and Gunther, 2008). A recent Cochrane review comprising 13 high-quality RCTs found that risk of pre-eclampsia was halved and the risk of premature deliveries and infant death was reduced amongst women taking supplements containing 1 g calcium (Hofmeyr *et al.*, 2010).

Although calcium may be mobilised from the mother's skeleton during pregnancy to support foetal growth, there is mixed evidence about whether calcium intakes can affect the degree of utilisation. Olausson *et al.* (2008) monitored calcium intakes and changes in the bone mineral content (BMC) in 34 pregnant women using dual-energy X-ray absorptiometry (DEXA) measurements. Results were compared with non-pregnant controls and showed that BMC reduced in pregnancy, but calcium intakes had no effect on skeletal changes. This is an interesting study, but it is possible that the range of calcium intakes was not varied enough to observe measurable differences.

On the whole, there remain to be many 'grey areas' when it comes to the benefits of calcium intake on women's health. However, women should at least aim to meet dietary targets for calcium (700 mg/day; DH, 1991) before pregnancy until these guidelines are revisited.

2.11   A focus on folate

In the United States and Canada, food fortification with folic acid has been found to be one way to improve red blood cell folate levels. US figures show that the prevalence of low red blood cell levels (less than 140 ng/mL) reduced from 37.6% in 1988–1994 to 4.5% in 2005–2006 amongst women of childbearing age (McDowell *et al.*, 2008). This study shows that food fortification appears to play a key role in helping to improve women's folate status, but some scientists suggest that supplements may still be needed alongside this. Canadian scientists measured red blood cell folate

Table 2.5 Folic acid requirements for women before and in the first 12 weeks of pregnancy.

Who?	Folic acid requirement
Healthy woman	400 µg/day
Woman with diabetes	5 mg/day
Woman who have had a NTD affected pregnancy previously	5 mg/day

Source: SACN (2006).

levels in 95 fasted women who had consumed fortified foods as part of their daily diets. Whilst no women were deficient in folate, scientists found that only 14% women had blood folate levels in the right range to reduce neural tube defect (NTD) risk. Authors conclude that folate status seems to have improved after fortification strategies have been put into place, but this may still not be sufficient in terms of protecting against NTDs. For this reason, scientists concluded that women of childbearing age should be advised to continue taking a supplement containing folic acid (Shuaibi *et al.*, 2008).

For countries where foods are not yet fortified, women should be advised to take a supplement containing 400 µg folic acid per day both pre-conceptually and in the first trimester of pregnancy to support the closure of the neural tube (SACN, 2006; Table 2.5). Evidence from a recent UK study showed that only 12% women took folic acid supplements before falling pregnant and only 17% before neural tube closure. Women from lower social groups and with lower levels of education were least likely to use folic acid and take it at the appropriate time point (Brough *et al.*, 2009).

Overall, the importance of taking a daily folic acid supplement needs to be communicated to women in their childbearing years. To increase compliance, alternative means of delivery, i.e. fortified foods, may be one way forward for women who cannot afford and are unlikely to comply with taking a daily supplement. More remains to be understood about why women do not take, or comply with, supplement regimes. Also, although a difficult area to study, more work is needed to establish whether women would benefit from taking certain supplements before conception and how long these should be taken for.

Research Highlight   Low folate status early in pregnancy linked to hyperactivity in the offspring

It is well known that folate is needed early in pregnancy to help during periods of rapid cell division and brain development. Now, a new study has found that lower levels of maternal red blood cell folate and intakes of folate (from dietary and supplement sources) measured at 14 weeks into pregnancy were associated with higher levels of hyperactivity and other peer problems when children born to these mothers were followed up 8 years later. These findings were still present even when data was adjusted for smoking and drinking alcohol during pregnancy (Schlotz *et al.*, 2010). Overall, these are interesting findings although it must be considered that the associations were only small and other factors may have influenced the findings.

2.11.1 Diabetes and folate requirements

Women with diabetes before pregnancy are a special group that require individual attention. Correct dietary advice can help women to achieve good glycaemic control and reduce the risk of complications should pregnancy occur. Standard healthy eating advice should be followed and foods consumed at regular intervals. For women who are overweight, or obese and diabetic, weight loss strategies should ideally be employed before pregnancy occurs, to help women achieve a healthy pre-pregnancy body mass index (BMI), as discussed in Section 2.3. After conceiving, women should monitor their rate of weight gain carefully, staying within recommended ranges (Chapter 9).

It is advised that women with diabetes should take extra folic acid both before and in the early stages of pregnancy. Women with diabetes are at higher risk of having a baby with NTDs because hyperglycaemia (elevated blood sugar levels) may have teratogenic effects on the developing foetus (Allen et al., 2007). For this reason, nutrition scientists recommend that these women take 5 mg folic acid before and in the early stages of pregnancy (SACN, 2006; Table 2.5). There is also some evidence that dietary supplements containing antioxidant vitamins E and C can reduce the risk of birth defects in women with gestational diabetes. These antioxidants may help to counteract levels of oxidative stress which is thought to be higher in women with gestational diabetes and a possible cause of birth defects (Dheen et al., 2009).

Overall, health professionals playing an active role in pre-conception programmes can help guide women already diagnosed with diabetes to monitor their blood sugar levels, body weight and intake of folic acid when planning to have a child. Research has shown that pre-conception counselling may help to increase awareness about the importance and use of folic acid supplements in women with diabetes (Tripathi et al., 2009).

2.12   A focus on iron

In the United Kingdom, women in their childbearing years (19–45) have an average iron intake of 9.4 mg/day (Henderson et al., 2003) and women from low-income groups about 8.6 mg/day (Nelson et al., 2007). In less developed regions such as India, mean intakes (around 9.5 mg/day) are not dissimilar to levels consumed in industrialised regions. Rates of iron deficiency, however, in these regions pose significant health problems and as many as 39% women aged 18–35 are anaemic and 62% are iron deficient (Thankachan et al., 2007).

A whole host of factors can affect iron stores and the risk of low iron status or deficiency symptoms (Figure 2.4) and contributing factors vary for each woman. However, the consumption of non-heme food sources such as cereals, pulses and vegetables, which contain iron but in a less bioavailable form (about 2.8% bioavailability), can mean that even if dietary iron intakes are sufficient and meeting recommended targets (Table 2.6), this is not necessarily being utilised and absorbed inside the body. Women should be made aware that simple strategies such as soaking beans, lentils and drinking orange juice with meals, i.e. cereal-based breakfast, may go some way towards improving the amount of iron that is absorbed (Gibson et al., 2006).

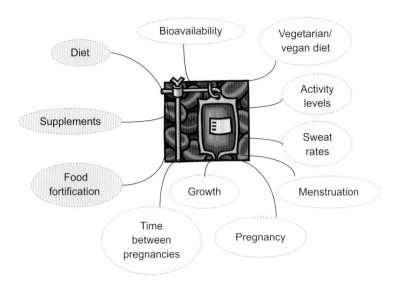

Figure 2.4   Factors affecting iron status.

Table 2.6   Recommended iron intakes for non-pregnant women.

Country	Age range (years)	Recommended intake (mg/day)	Upper intake/limit	Source
United Kingdom	15–50	14.8	–	DH (1991)
United States	19–50	18	–	FDA (2004)
Australia/New Zealand	19–50	18	45	NHMARC (2006)
Japan	15–49	10.5–13.5	40–45	Sasaki (2008)

Research Highlight   Cereal consumption may help to improve nutrient status before pregnancy

Research suggests that eating cereals could be one simple, safe and effective way to improve diet quality before and in the early stages of pregnancy. In an American study, over 500 low-income American women less than 20 weeks into their pregnancy were asked to recall their dietary habits from the previous 3 months using food frequency questionnaires. Women eating cereals regularly (at least three times per week) had higher intakes of folate, iron, zinc, calcium, fibre and vitamins A, C, D and E and were 65–90% less likely to fall short of dietary requirements.

These are very interesting findings and show that women planning a pregnancy may benefit from regular cereal consumption. This appears to be a simple, safe and cost-effective way for women to optimise their nutrient intakes should pregnancy occur (Parrott *et al.*, 2008).

2.13 Emerging interest in choline

Choline is often classed as a B vitamin and is an important part of many biological molecules. There is emerging evidence suggesting that the development of the central nervous system may be particularly sensitive to choline availability and deficiencies may affect neural tube closure and later cognitive function. The need for additional choline during pregnancy and lactation has been demonstrated in research studies showing that newborns have choline blood levels three times higher than their mothers and large amounts are also present in human breast milk. In the United States, an Adequate Intake (AI) level of 425 mg/day has been set for non-pregnant women, increasing by an extra 25 mg/day for pregnancy and 125 mg/day for lactating mothers. From the evidence available, however, women do not appear to be achieving target levels of intake and certain genetic variants may increase choline requirements beyond current recommendations for some individuals (Caudill, 2010).

2.14 Multivitamin and mineral supplements

For women who eat a balanced, nutrient-rich diet, multivitamin and mineral supplements may not be required. However, in some circumstances, supplements are recommended (Table 2.7). It is not yet understood exactly how micronutrient supplementation can affect pregnancy outcomes, but improved immune function and energy metabolism, reduced risk of infections and intrauterine growth restriction are some of the proposed mechanisms (Keen et al., 2003). Bhutta and Haider (2009) suggest that women living in less developed regions may benefit from supplementation with multimicronutrients rather than just iron and folic acid.

One meta-analysis paper written by scientists from the University of Toronto evaluated the findings from 13 research papers to determine whether prenatal supplementation had any effect on pregnancy outcomes. Scientists found that the risk of women delivering LBW (low birth weight) infants was significantly reduced when women took multimicronutrient supplements before birth, compared with women who just took iron–folic acid supplements (Shah et al., 2009). Clearly, it seems that women may benefit from taking multimicronutrient supplements rather than single-dose supplements, particularly in regions where multiple micronutrient deficiencies are common. However, at the other end of the spectrum, for women whose diets are sufficient in nutrients, more work is needed to evaluate the safety of dietary supplements in relation to pregnancy outcomes. At present, dietary recommendations for

Table 2.7 Women that may benefit from multivitamin and mineral supplementation before pregnancy.

Women who smoke, abuse alcohol or drugs

Women with iron-deficiency anaemia

Women with poor quality diets, i.e those not consuming animal sourced foods, such as vegans. A supplement containing vitamin B_{12} is important in these instances, particularly as folic acid supplementation can mask symptoms of B_{12} deficiency.

Women carrying a multiple number of foetuses

Source: ADA (2002).

women in the periconceptual period are lacking and safe upper limits have not been developed specifically for this phase of the female lifecycle.

2.15   Application in practice

The importance of women's diets and nutrient status before pregnancy is an area that has been overlooked in the past. However, emerging scientific evidence shows that getting body weight into the right ranges and eating a balanced diet can not only improve fertility but also help to give both mother and child a head start to the physiological demands of pregnancy that lie ahead. Findings from scientific studies clearly demonstrate that women's knowledge of nutrition and lifestyle guidelines is limited and there is room for improvement. It is now important that health campaigns promote messages about the importance of nutrient adequacy in the periconceptual period before women attend antenatal appointments, when the benefits of dietary and lifestyle modifications may be too late. Supplements do have a role to play but women should first be guided to improve their overall diet quality before pregnancy, focusing on their diet as whole.

2.16   Food safety

During pregnancy, a woman's immune system undergoes considerable changes. The immune system has to adapt to accommodate and prevent rejection of the foetus (Hanson and Silfverdal, 2009). In turn, these immunological changes mean that expectant mothers may become susceptible to infectious diseases such as listeriosis, salmonella and toxoplasmosis (Jamieson et al., 2006). In addition, dietary intakes of some fat-soluble vitamins (namely, vitamin A) and environmental contaminants present in food sources may also need to be monitored during pregnancy. This section aims to describe which foods may contain pathogens that could cause illness, or toxicity symptoms, during pregnancy. At the end of this section, questions relating to common food concerns are answered.

2.16.1   Listeriosis

Listeriosis is an infection caused by eating food containing *Listeria monocytogenes*. These bacteria reside in the digestive tract of animals, which can lead to the contamination of meat and dairy products, especially when unpasteurised, and fruit and vegetables, when animal manure is used to fertilise (Delgado, 2008). Because a pregnant woman's immune system is weaker than that of an average adult, the risk of getting listeriosis is significantly higher. When infected during pregnancy, there is evidence to suggest that it can increase the risk of miscarriage, delivering stillborn babies, prematurely, and newborns are also at risk of infection (Benshushan et al., 2002; CDC, 2009a). However, some simple lifestyle and food preparation amendments can help to minimise the risk of infection.

As prevention is better than cure, pregnant women should avoid eating foods displayed in Table 2.8. As a rule of thumb, all fruit and vegetables should be washed thoroughly. Vegetables, raw meat and fish must be cooked at high temperatures to destroy bacteria. Knives, chopping boards and other kitchen utensils should be washed after use with uncooked meat and fish.

Table 2.8 Foods most likely to be contaminated with *Listeria monocytogenes*.

Cold patés or meat spreads
Dairy products made with raw (unpasteurised) milk
Hot dogs and cold/deli meats (must be steaming hot when served)
Raw smoked seafood (unless it is part of a steaming hot cooked dish)
Soft, blue-veined or Mexican-style cheeses – brie, feta, goats cheese, Roquefort and queso fresco/blanco (unless heated until bubbling)

Source: CDC (2009a).

2.16.2   Salmonella

Salmonella is caused by ingesting contagious bacteria (*Salmonella enterica*) that can cause infection, fever and gastroenteritis-like symptoms (Pejcic-Karapetrovic *et al.*, 2007). Salmonella can infect the ovaries of hens before the shells are formed, or live in the intestinal tracts of animals and birds, causing external faecal contamination of egg shells (CDC, 2009b). Although this condition is not as common now as it once was, several food safety practises should be employed to avoid infection.

In terms of preventing salmonella poisoning, in the United Kingdom, the Lion Quality Code of Practice (marking egg shells and boxes that have been produced using the highest food safety standards) has successfully reduced the number of UK cases. Even though eggs are produced to a better standard, only eggs cooked thoroughly should be eaten in pregnancy. Expectant mothers should avoid all foods made from raw eggs such as mayonnaise, Caesar salad dressing, mousses, homemade ice cream and some sauces such as hollandaise (also see Table 2.9). Raw meat, particularly chicken, should also be well cooked and again utensils used for preparation should be washed properly (CDC, 2009a).

2.16.3   Toxoplasmosis

Toxoplasma gondii is a parasite that can infect pregnant women, often without symptoms and can be transmitted to the foetus, with severe consequences. The infection usually results from the consumption of undercooked meat, contact with soil, or cat litter. Tissue cysts often found in undercooked meat lead to the production of oocysts that house the parasite. These can be eaten directly when meat is undercooked

Table 2.9 Foods most likely to be contaminated with *Salmonella enterica*.

Avoid eating raw eggs
Avoid eating foods containing raw eggs – mayonnaise, Caesar salad dressing, mousses, homemade ice cream, eggnog and hollandaise sauce.
Commercial products are generally safe because they use pasteurised eggs
Avoid restaurant dishes made with raw or undercooked eggs
Make sure that raw meat is cooked all the way through
Do not eat food prepared on a contaminated chopping board (previously used to prepare raw foods)

Source: CDC (2009a).

Table 2.10   Advice for pregnant women to reduce the risk of toxoplasmosis.

Avoid eating undercooked meat

Avoid eating unpasteurised goat's milk

Change the cat litter regularly wearing gloves whilst doing so

Keep cats indoors where possible throughout pregnancy and do not feed them undercooked meat

Wash all raw fruit and vegetables before consumption (particularly if home grown)

Wash hands and utensils thoroughly after handling raw meat

Wear gloves when gardening or working in soil. Wash hands thoroughly afterwards

Source: Based on findings by Kravetz and Federman (2005).

or ingested through the faecal–oral route (i.e. handling cat litter) (Kravetz and Federman, 2005).

Eating infected, undercooked meat, food or water contaminated with *T. gondii* parasite can lead to toxoplasmosis (also see Table 2.10). When transmitted to the foetus, this may result in a range of manifestations, from seizures, visual and hearing loss to mental retardation, haematological abnormalities, enlargement of the liver and spleen to death (Montoya and Remington, 2008). Studies have shown that the risk of toxoplasmosis infection increases from 0–9% in the first trimester to 35–59% in the third trimester (Montoya and Liesenfeld, 2004). Unfortunately, when infection occurs early in pregnancy, this is more likely to be detrimental to the health of the foetus. Early diagnosis during pregnancy can significantly reduce the risk of these unfavourable outcomes.

2.17   Vitamin A

Whilst vitamin A is needed to support the immune system during pregnancy, excess vitamin A may have teratogenic effects on the foetus. Hypervitaminosis vitamin A usually occurs when single-dose supplements are taken (Azais-Braesco and Pascal, 2000). For women living in developing regions, supplementation may be necessary, but for those living in industrialised countries, vitamin A should be obtained from the diet when possible (Miller *et al.*, 1998). The EFSA (2006) recommended that women of childbearing age (including pregnant mothers) consume no more than 3000 µg/day vitamin A from food and supplement sources.

Vitamin A may be provided from animal sources (retinol) or plant derived (beta carotene). Generally, beta-carotene appears to be less teratogenic than animal food sources (Miller *et al.*, 1998). As vitamin A is stored in the liver, pregnant women should avoid consuming liver or liver-derived products such as paté in pregnancy (Table 2.11). Equally, although fish oils may be beneficial during pregnancy, supplements containing cod liver oil should not be taken. Individual cod liver oil supplements contain about 800 µg retinol (FSA, 2006).

2.18   Fish consumption

Oily fish are a good source of long-chain omega-3 polyunsaturated fatty acids that can help to support the development of the infants' central nervous system during pregnancy (SACN/CoT, 2004). However, there are concerns that the oily fish

Table 2.11   Vitamin A-rich foods that should be avoided in pregnancy.

Food source	Retinol (µg per 100 g)
Boiled haggis	1,800
Cod liver oil	18,000
Faggots in gravy	1,100
Fried calf liver	25,200
Fried chicken liver	10,500
Fried lamb liver	19,700
Liver paté	7,300
Liver sausage	2,600

Source: FSA (2006).

Table 2.12   FDA and EPA (2004) guidelines for fish consumption during pregnancy.

Do not eat fish that has a high mercury content. This includes shark, swordfish, king mackerel and tilefish
Eat up to two portions of fish per week (a portion is roughly the size of a fist). Fish that are lower in mercury include canned tuna (excludes albacore), salmon, shrimp, pollock and catfish
Check local advisories about the safety of fish caught from local lakes, rivers or coastal areas. If information is not available, eat no more than 170 g per 6 oz/week

consumption may increase the mothers' exposure to methyl mercury and dioxin-like compounds during pregnancy (environment contaminants that may pass through the placenta) (Sioen *et al.*, 2007). As some contaminants have a long half-life (methyl mercury) or lipophilic properties (polychlorinated dioxins), even fish intake before pregnancy may determine foetal exposure to these compounds (SACN/CoT, 2004).

In one of the largest studies to date, the Avon Longitudinal Study of Parents and Children (ALSPAC) assessed the benefits and ramifications of eating different amounts of seafood during pregnancy. Researchers found that eating at least 340 g seafood each week during pregnancy was most beneficial to childhood development. Authors concluded that the risks of not consuming essential nutrients found in fish outweighed any risk linked to the exposure of contaminants (Hibbeln *et al.*, 2007). The US Food and Drug Administration (FDA) and Environmental Protection Agency (EPA) have developed three key recommendations for pregnant mothers (Table 2.12).

2.19   Peanut allergy

Where there is a family history of food allergies on either the mother's or father's side – whether asthma, hay fever or food allergies – then pregnant and breastfeeding women should avoid eating peanuts, or foods containing peanuts. By avoiding these foods, women can reduce the risk of the baby developing anaphylaxis (fatal allergic reactions). In non-allergic individuals, the foetus may become sensitised in utero to the proteins in peanuts, which can cross the placenta or pass into breast milk (Theobald, 2007).

2.20   Food additives and ingredients

Food additives, substances used to colour, conserve and flavour foods and beverages, are used in a vast array of foods. For the majority of individuals, food additives are ingested in marginal proportions and ingredients sold in supermarkets must be declared safe to use by EU law, although much depend on the level of research that is available. Some studies suggest that foetal exposure to additives in the early stages of pregnancy could lead to changes at the cellular level, affecting the offspring's risk of disease when they move through into adulthood. A few animal (rat/mice) studies have shown that certain food colouring may contribute to growth retardation (Banderali *et al.*, 2007), but overall findings are difficult to extrapolate to adults and better quality evidence is needed before firm guidance can be given to women.

Checking labels, eating a varied diet and more fresh produce, sweetening foods, i.e. with pasteurised honey, or opting for organic foods, which can generally contain lower levels of additives (although 5% non-organic ingredients may be added), are some ways that women can minimise their intakes of foods additives.

2.21   Organic food

The term organic can be applied to a wide range of products, but from a farming perspective, a strict set of standards define what organic farmers need to comply with in order for their produce to be sold as organic. Generally, to be labelled as an organic food, the use of pesticides is restricted, artificial chemical fertilisers cannot be used and the use of drugs, antibiotics and wormers is not permitted. Instead, preventative strategies need to be used, i.e. smaller herd sizes. Genetically modified (GM) crops are also banned from carrying the organic label (Soil Association, 2010).

There has been much debate over whether organic foods are better from a nutrition and health perspective. Now, there is more evidence to suggest that organic fruit and vegetables tend to contain higher levels of vitamin C, iron, magnesium and phosphorous than that of non-organic versions of the same foods. Organic foods may also provide higher levels of antioxidant phytochemicals such as anthocyanins, carotenoids and flavonoids although it is important to consider that the nutrient content of crops can also vary seasonally and regionally (Crinnion, 2010). More work is now needed to see if this can affect individual's biochemical levels of nutrients once consumed and whether this could have any implications for health.

2.22   Other concerns

As food market evolves, this brings new food safety issues to light. Increasingly, probiotics are being taken during pregnancy for their health benefits. This is an area that has been studied increasingly over the last few years and has been linked to significant improvements in health, i.e. reduced incidence of gestational diabetes from 34% in the control group to 13% in those improving their diets and taking probiotic supplement (Luoto *et al.*, 2010). Because of these possible health benefits, the safety of probiotic use in vulnerable populations such as pregnant women has needed to be studied further. In one RCT, various strains of probiotic bacteria were taken by women in the last trimester of pregnancy and their infants for the first 6 months of life. Also, some symptoms were observed in a small proportion of the mothers and infants and these were not thought to be caused by the probiotic supplement and scientists regarded their use as safe (see Allen *et al.* (2010) for full study). In more detail, a review paper weighed the findings from 11 studies testing probiotic use in pregnancy. Research scientists concluded that *lactobacillus* and *bifidobacterium* had no effect on infant birth weight, delivery date or the mode of delivery. As the safety of *Saccharomyces* is not yet well established, caution should be taken until more evidence is available (Dugoua *et al.*, 2009). A list of common food safety concerns and some points for consideration are further included in Appendix I.

2.23   Application in practice

There are many misconceptions surrounding areas of food safety in pregnancy. Taken as a whole, safe food preparation methods, i.e. good hand washing practices, cooking food until piping hot and steering away from certain foods (liver and fish with a high mercury content) can help to minimise the risk of food-borne illnesses in pregnancy, which can both be unpleasant and potentially dangerous to the developing foetus. Sharing these key messages with women in the early stages of pregnancy, or preferably before pregnancy, could help to reduce problems in pregnancy itself when awareness of these issues can be too late.

2.24   Conclusion

The phase before pregnancy is a critical time period that is often overlooked. Improving knowledge of good nutrition, lifestyle and food safety practices at this point in time is not only a good opportunity to improve women's health in general but also beneficial in pregnancy and for the health of the next generation. From a financial perspective, simple dietary and lifestyle improvements before pregnancy could significantly help to reduce costs and pressures currently placed on health services, usually in the form of medical treatment and aftercare. Unfortunately, the fact that a considerable proportion of pregnancies are planned makes the problem of getting nutrient status right before pregnancy somewhat of a challenge. Equally, not all women have access to nutritious food, or have the knowledge to make suitable food choices. For these reasons, fortification strategies such as those used in the United States and Canada (folic acid fortification) could be a good way forward.

Key Messages

- Nutrition status before pregnancy determines whether a woman has sufficient nutrient reserves when she enters pregnancy.
- Compared to the wealth of information that is available for pregnancy, considerably less is known or communicated about the importance of good nutrition practices before pregnancy.
- It is important that women's body weight is brought into a healthy range before conception to minimise health risks in pregnancy (NICE, 2009).
- Food-related infections in pregnancy can easily be prevented provided that enough information and guidance is given early on.
- The education of women in their childbearing years about the importance of an adequate diet and food safety/preparation practices for improved pregnancy outcomes should be a priority.

- More research needs to study the dietary habits and nutrient status of women in the periconceptual period. Collecting data for this life phase is no easy task, and it would be extremely valuable if scientists were to collaborate, fathom suitable methods and undertake large studies with enough statistical power.
- More work is needed to determine if/how long supplements should be taken before pregnancy.

Recommended reading

Berry RJ, Bailey L, Mulinare J, Bower C and the Folic Acid Working Group (2010) Fortification of flour with folic acid. *Food and Nutrition Bulletin* **31**(1S), S22–35.

Caudill MA (2010) Pre- and postnatal health: evidence of increased choline needs. *Journal of the American Dietetic Association* **110**(8), 1198–206.

Langley-Evans S (2009) Before life begins. In: *Nutrition a Lifespan Approach*, pp. 23–46. Wiley-Blackwell: Oxford.

NICE (National Institute for Health and Clinical Excellence) (2009) *Dietary Interventions and Physical Activity Interventions for Weight Management Before, During and After Pregnancy.* NICE: London.

Ruxton CHS and Derbyshire EJ (2010) Women's diet quality in the UK. *Nutrition Bulletin* **35**(2), 126–37.

References

ADA (American Dietetic Association) (2002) Position of the American Dietetic Association: nutrition for a healthy pregnancy outcome. *Journal of the American Dietetic Association* **102**(10), 1479–90.

Allen SJ, Jordan S, Storey M *et al.* (2010) Dietary supplementation with lactobacilli and bifidobacteria is well tolerated and not associated with adverse events during late pregnancy and early infancy. *Journal of Nutrition* **140**(3), 483–8.

Allen VM, Armson BA, Wilson RD *et al.* (2007) Teratogenicity associated with pre-existing and gestational diabetes. *Journal of Obstetrics and Gynaecology Canada* **29**(11), 927–44.

Azais-Braesco V and Pascal G (2000) Vitamin A in pregnancy: requirements and safety limits. *American Journal of Clinical Nutrition* **71**, 1325S–33S.

Banderali G, Carmine V, Rossi S and Giovannini M (2007) Food additives: effects on pregnancy and lactation. *Acta Biomed Ateneo Parmense* **71**(S1), 589–92 [Abstract only].

Benshushan A, Tsafrir A, Arbel R *et al.* (2002) Listeria infection during pregnancy: a 10-year experience. *Israel Medical Association* **4**(10), 776–80.

Bhutta ZA and Haider BA (2009) Prenatal micronutrient supplementation: are we there yet? *Canadian Medical Association Journal* **180**(12), 1188–9.

Brough L, Rees GA, Crawford MA and Dorman EK (2009) Social and ethnic differences in folic acid use during preconception and early pregnancy in the UK: effect on maternal folate status. *Journal of Human Nutrition and Dietetics* **22**, 100–107.

Burd L, Roberts D, Olson M and Odendaal H (2007) Ethanol and the placenta: a review. *Journal of Maternal Fetal and Neonatal Medicine* **20**(5), 361–75.

Cashman KD, Hill TR, Lucey AJ *et al.* (2008) Estimation of the dietary requirement for vitamin D in healthy adults. *American Journal of Clinical Nutrition* **88**(6),1535–42.

Caudill MA (2010) Pre- and postnatal health: evidence of increased choline needs. *Journal of the American Dietetic Association* **110**(8), 1198–206.

CDC (Centres for Disease Control and Prevention) (2009a) Listeriosis available information and FAQs. Available: http://www.cdc.gov/nczved/dfbmd/disease_listing/listeriosis_gi.html (accessed September 2010).

CDC (Centres for Disease Control and Prevention) (2009b) *Salmonella enteritidis* available information and FAQs. Available: http://www.cdc.gov/ncidod/dbmd/diseaseinfo/salment_g.htm (accessed September 2010).

Cetin I, Berti C and Calabrese S (2009) Role of micronutrients in the periconceptional period. *Human Reproduction Update* **16**(1), 80–95.

Crinnion WJ (2010) Organic foods contain higher levels of certain nutrients, lower levels of pesticides, and may provide health benefits for the consumer. *Alternative Medicine Review* **15**(1), 4–12.

Crozier SR, Robinson SM, Borland SE and the SWS Study Group (2009) Do women change their health behaviours in pregnancy? Findings from the Southampton Women's Survey. *Paediatric and Perinatal Epidemiology* **23**, 446–53.

Davies MJ (2006) Evidence for effects of weight on reproduction in women. *Reproductive Biomedicine Online* **12**(5), 552–61.

DCAC (Diabetes Care Advisory Committee) (2003) National subcommittee of the diabetes care advisory committee of diabetes UK. The implementation of nutritional advice for people with diabetes. *Diabetic Medicine* **20**, 786–807.

Delgado AR (2008) Listeriosis in pregnancy. *Journal of Midwifery and Women's Health* **53**(3), 255–9.

Dewey KG and Cohen RJ (2007) Does birth spacing affect maternal or child nutritional status? A systematic literature review. *Maternal and Child Nutrition* **3**, 151–73.

DH (Department of Health) (1991) *Dietary Reference Values for Food Energy and Nutrients for the United Kingdom*, 2nd edition. *Report on Social Subjects no. 41*. The Stationery Office: London.

DH (Department of Health) (2004) Sensible drinking. The report of an inter-departmental working group. Available: www.doh,gov.uk/alcohol/pdf/sensibledrinking.pdf (accessed September 2010).

DH (Department of Health) (2009) *Abortion Statistics, England and Wales: 2008*. Department of Health: London.

Dheen ST, Tay SS, Boran J *et al.* (2009) Recent studies on neural tube defects in embryos of diabetic pregnancy: an overview. *Current Medicinal Chemistry* **16**(18), 2345–54.

Dugoua JJ, Machado M, Zhu X *et al.* (2009) Probiotic safety in pregnancy: a systematic review and meta-analysis of randomized controlled trials of Lactobacillus, Bifidobacterium, and Saccharomyces spp. *Journal of Obstetrics and Gynaecology Canada* **31**(6), 542–52.

EC (European Commission) (2008) Commission Directive 2008/100/EC amending Council Directive 90/496/EEC on nutrition labelling for foodstuffs as regards recommended daily allowances, energy conversion factors and definitions. *Official Journal of the European Union* L285/9. Available: http://eur-lex.europa.eu/LexUriServ/LexUriServ.do?uri= OJ:L:2008:285:0009:0012:EN:PDF. (accessed March 2011).

EFSA (European Food Safety Authority) (2006) Tolerable upper intake levels of vitamins and minerals by the Scientific Panel on Dietetic Products, Nutrition and Allergies (NDA) and Scientific Committee on Food (SCF). Available at: http://www.efsa.europa.eu/fr/scdocs/ oldsc/upper_level_opinions_full-part33.pdf (accessed March 2011).

EFSA (European Food Safety Authority) (2010) EFSA sets European dietary reference values for nutrient intakes. Available at: http://www.efsa.europa.eu/en/press/news/nda100326.htm (accessed September 2010).

Elmadfa I, Meyer A, Nowak V *et al.* (2009) European nutrition and health report 2009. *Annals of Nutrition and Metabolism* **55**(S2), 1–40.

EUROCAT Working Group (2003) *Special Report: Prevention of Neural Tube Defects by Periconceptional Folic Acid Supplementation in Europe*. University of Ulster.

FDA (Food and Drugs Administration) and EPA (Environmental Protection Agency) (2004) EPA and FDA advice for women who might become pregnant, women who are pregnant, nursing mothers and young children. Available at: http://www.fda.gov/food/foodsafety/ product-specificinformation/seafood/foodbornepathogenscontaminants/methylmercury/ucm 115662.htm (accessed March 2011).

Floyd RL, Weber MK, Denny C and O'Connor MJ (2009) Prevention of fetal alcohol spectrum disorders. *Developmental Disabilities* **15**, 193–9.

FSA (Food Standards Agency) (2006) *McCance and Widdowson's, the Composition of Foods*, 6th edition. Royal Society of Chemistry: London.

FSA (Food Standards Agency) (2008) Food Standards Agency publishes new caffeine advice for pregnant women. Available at: http://www.food.gov.uk/news/pressreleases/2008/nov/caffeineadvice (accessed March 2009).

Gibson RS, Perlas L and Hotz C (2006) Improving the bioavailability of nutrients in plant foods at the household level. *Proceedings of the Nutrition Society* **65**(2),160–8.

Hanson LA and Silfverdal SA (2009) The mother's immune system is a balanced threat to the foetus, turning to protection of the neonate. *Acta Paediatrica* **98**, 221–8.

Heaney RP (2006) Calcium intake and disease prevention. *Arquivos Brasileiros de Endocrinologia* **50**(4), 685–93.

Hedderson MM, Williams MA, Holt VL, Weiss NS and Ferrara A (2008) Body mass index and weight gain prior to pregnancy and risk of gestational diabetes mellitus. *American Journal of Obstetrics and Gynaecology* **198**(4), 409.e1–7.

Henderson L, Gregory J, Irving K *et al.* (2003) *National Diet and Nutrition Survey: Adults Aged 19–64 years. Volume 2: Energy, Protein, Carbohydrate, Fat and Alcohol Intake*. The Stationery Office: London.

Hibbeln JR, Davis JM, Steer C *et al.* (2007) Maternal seafood consumption in pregnancy and neurodevelopmental outcomes in childhood (ALSPAC study): an observational cohort. *Lancet* **369**, 578–85.

Hofmeyr GJ, Lawrie TA, Atallah AN and Duley L (2010) Calcium supplementation during pregnancy for preventing hypertensive disorders and related problems. *Cochrane Database Systematic Reviews* **8**, CD001059.

Inskip HM, Crozier SR, Godfrey KM and the SWS Study Group (2009) Women's compliance with nutrition and lifestyle recommendations before pregnancy: general population cohort study. *British Medical Journal* **338**, b481.

Inskip HM, Godfrey KM, Robinson SM and the SWS Study Group (2006) Cohort profile: the Southampton Women's Survey. *International Journal of Epidemiology* **35**, 42–8.

Jamieson DJ, Theiler RN and Rasmussen SA (2006) Emerging infections and pregnancy. *Emerging Infectious Diseases* **12**(11), 1638–43.

Kalaivani K (2009) Prevalence and consequences of anaemia in pregnancy. *Indian Journal of Medical Research* **130**(5), 627–33.

Keen CL, Clegg MS, Hanna LA *et al.* (2003) The plausibility of micronutrient deficiencies being a significant contributing factor to the occurrence of pregnancy complications. *Journal of Nutrition* **133**(S2), 159S–605S.

King JC. (2003) The risk of maternal nutritional depletion and poor pregnancy outcomes increases in early or closely spaced pregnancies. *Journal of Nutrition* **133**(5 S2), 1732S–6S.

Kravetz JD and Federman DG (2005) Prevention of toxoplasmosis in pregnancy: knowledge of risk factors. *Infectious Diseases in Obstetrics and Gynaecology* **13**(3), 161–5.

Kuczkowski KM (2009) Caffeine in pregnancy. *Archives of Gynaecology and Obstetrics* **280**(5), 695–8.

Luoto R, Laitinen K, Nermes M and Isolauri E (2010) Impact of maternal probiotic-supplemented dietary counselling on pregnancy outcome and prenatal and postnatal growth: a double-blind, placebo-controlled study. *British Journal of Nutrition* **103**(12),1792–9.

McDowell MA, Lacher DA, Pfeiffer CM *et al.* (2008) Blood folate levels: the latest NHANES results. *National Centre for Health Statistics Data Brief* **6**, 1–12.

McMillen IC, Rattanatray L, Duffield JA *et al.* (2009) The early origins of later obesity: pathways and mechanisms. *Advances in Experimental Medicine and Biology* **646**, 71–81.

Miller RK, Hendrickx AG, Mills JL, Hummler H and Wiegand UW (1998) Periconceptional vitamin A use: how much is teratogenic? *Reproductive Toxicology* **12**(1), 75–88.

Montoya JG and Liesenfeld O (2004) Toxoplasmosis. *Lancet* **363**, 1965–76.

Montoya JG and Remington JS (2008) Management of *Toxoplasma gondii* during pregnancy. *Clinical Infectious Diseases* **47**(4), 554–66.

Mutsaerts MA, Groen H, ter Bogt NC *et al.* (2010) The LIFESTYLE study: costs and effects of a structured lifestyle program in overweight and obese subfertile women to reduce the need for fertility treatment and improve reproductive outcome. A randomised controlled trial. *BMC Womens Health* **10**, 22.

NHS (2011) NHS Choices: Food and Diet. Available at: http://www.nhs.uk/LiveWell/Goodfood/Pages/Goodfoodhome.aspx (accessed March 2011).

NICE (National Institute of Clinical Excellence) (2004) *Fertility Assessment and Treatment for People with Fertility Problems*. RCOG Press: London.

NICE (National Institute for Health and Clinical Excellence) (2009) *Dietary Interventions and Physical Activity Interventions for Weight Management Before, During and After Pregnancy*. NICE: London.

Nelson M, Erens B, Bates B *et al.* (2007) *Low Income Diet and Nutrition Survey. Three Volume Survey, Executive Summary*. The Stationery Office: London.

NHMRC (National Health and Medical Research Council) (2006) *Nutrient Reference Values for Australia and New Zealand*. NHMRC publications: Australia.

Olausson H, Laskey MA, Goldberg GR and Prentice A (2008) Changes in bone mineral status and bone size during pregnancy and the influences of body weight and calcium intake. *American Journal of Clinical Nutrition* 88(4), 1032–9.

Parrott MS, Bodnar LM, Simhan HN *et al.* (2008) Maternal cereal consumption and adequacy of micronutrient intake in the periconceptional period. *Public Health Nutrition* 12(8), 1276–83.

Pejcic-Karapetrovic B, Gurnani K, Russell MS, Finlay BB, Sad S, Krishnan L (2007) Pregnancy impairs the innate immune resistance to *Salmonella typhimurium* leading to rapid fatal infection. *The Journal of Immunology* 179, 6088–96.

Ramos RG and Olden K (2008) The prevalence of metabolic syndrome among US women of childbearing age. *American Journal of Public Health* 98(6), 1122–7.

Rasmussen KM and Yaktine AL (2009) *Weight gain during pregnancy: re-examining the guidelines*. The National Academies Press: Washington DC.

Ruston D, Hoare J, Henderson L *et al.* (2004) *National Diet and Nutrition Survey: Adults Aged 19–64 Years. Volume 4: Nutritional Status (Anthropometry and Blood Analytes), Blood Pressure and Physical Activity*. The Stationery Office: London.

Ruxton CHS and Derbyshire EJ (2010) Women's diet quality in the UK. *Nutrition Bulletin* 35(2), 126–37.

SACN (Scientific Advisory Committee on Nutrition) (2008) *The Nutritional Wellbeing of the British Population*. The Stationery Office: London.

Sasaki S (2008) Dietary reference intakes (DRIs) in Japan. *Asia Pacific Journal of Clinical Nutrition* 17(S2), 420–44.

SACN (Scientific Advisory Committee on Nutrition) (SACN) (2006) *Folate and Disease Prevention*. The Stationery Office, London.

SACN/CoT (Scientific Advisory Committee on Nutrition/Committee on Nutrition/Committee on Toxicity) (2004), *Advice on Fish Consumption: Benefits and Risks*. The Stationery Office: London.

Schlotz W, Jones A, Phillips DI, Gale CR, Robinson SM and Godfrey KM (2010) Lower maternal folate status in early pregnancy is associated with childhood hyperactivity and peer problems in offspring. *Journal of Childhood Psychology and Psychiatry* 51(5), 594–602.

Shah PS and Ohlsson A (2009) Effects of prenatal multimicronutrient supplementation on pregnancy outcomes: a meta-analysis. *Canadian Medical Association Journal* 180(12), E99–108.

Shuaibi AM, House JD and Sevenhuysen GP (2008) Folate status of young Canadian women after folic acid fortification of grain products. *Journal of the American Dietetic Association* 108(12), 2090–4.

Sioen I, De Henauw S and Van Camp J (2007) Evaluation of benefits and risks related to seafood consumption. *Verh K Acad Geneeskd Belg* 69, 249–89.

Soil Association (2010) *What is organic?* Available: http://www.soilassociation.org (accessed September 2010).

Teegarden D and Gunther CW (2008) Can the controversial relationship between dietary calcium and body weight be mechanistically explained by alterations in appetite and food intake? *Nutrition Reviews* 66(10), 601–5.

Thankachan P, Muthayya S, Walczyk T, Kurpad AV and Hurrell RF (2007) An analysis of the etiology of anemia and iron deficiency in young women of low socioeconomic status in Bangalore, India. *Food and Nutrition Bulletin* 28(3), 328–36.

Theobald HE (2007) Eating for pregnancy and breastfeeding. *Journal of Family Health Care* 17(2), 45–9.

Tripathi A, Rankin J, Aarvold J, Chandler C and Bell R (2009) Preconception counselling in women with diabetes – a population-based study in the North of England. *Diabetes Care* 33(3), 586–8.

Wahed F, Latif SA, Nessa A *et al.* (2010) Gestational anaemia. *Mymensingh Medical Journal* 19(3), 462–8.

Wilson RD, Désilets V, Wyatt P *et al.* (2007) Pre-conception vitamin/folic acid supplementation 2007: the use of folic acid in combination with a multivitamin supplement for the prevention of neural tube defects and other congenital anomalies. *Journal of Obstetrics and Gynaecology Canada* 138, 1003–13.

Wood F, Robling M and Prout H (2010) A question of balance: a qualitative study of mothers' interpretations of dietary recommendations. *Annals of Family Medicine* 8(1), 51–7.

Wynn M and Wynn A (2000) New nutrient intake recommendations are needed for child-bearing. *Nutrition and Health* **13**, 199–211.

Zhu BP (2005) Effect of interpregnancy interval on birth outcomes: findings from three recent US studies. *International Journal of Gynaecology and Obstetrics* **89**, S25–33.

3 Hormonal and Physiological Changes

Summary

The hormonal and physiological changes that take place during pregnancy are vast and generally not experienced at any other healthy life phase. The changes that occur help the mother's body to accommodate the growing child and create a suitable environment to support its development. During this time, most body systems undergo a degree of change that can lead to a range of different symptoms and side effects. Changes in appetite, mood, body weight and bowel habits, amongst others, are not uncommon in pregnancy and are often underpinned by the physiological, hormonal and metabolic changes that are taking place. Sometimes, if the mother has health problems before pregnancy, this can place additional demands on the body and lead to medical conditions in pregnancy or affect the health of the offspring. For example, overweight and obese women have a higher risk of gestational diabetes and pre-eclampsia in pregnancy, which can also have health implications for the offspring. This chapter sets out to explain the main hormonal and physiological changes that take place during pregnancy. The role that diet can play in helping to alleviate some of the symptoms exhibited in pregnancy will also be discussed where appropriate.

Learning Outcomes

- To be familiar with key hormonal and physiological changes that occur in pregnancy.
- To understand why these changes occur and how they can impact upon the health and well-being of the mother.
- To discuss briefly how the physiological changes associated with pregnancy may affect the nutritional needs of the mother.

3.1 Introduction

One of the most renowned obstetricians Professor Frank Hytten explained that 'during pregnancy the body is subject to physiological turmoil on a scale not otherwise experienced in healthy adult life' (Hytten, 1995). From a medical viewpoint, pregnancy is a separate and important life phase during which a women's body is

Nutrition in the Childbearing Years, First Edition. Emma Derbyshire.
© 2011 Emma Derbyshire. Published 2011 by Blackwell Publishing Ltd.

in a dynamic state of change. It is important that nurses, midwives and other health practitioners are aware of how the body changes physiologically as this is often the cause of symptoms and side effects so often experienced in pregnancy. An awareness of the physiological processes of childbearing can also help to prevent maternal morbidity and mortality, improving health outcomes for the mother and child. From a nutrition perspective, ensuring that women consume the right proportion and balance of nutrients can also help to support the physiological changes that are taking placing. This chapter will first begin by briefly explaining the physiological processes of childbearing before and after conception. The chapter will then go on to describe the hormonal changes of pregnancy in more detail and how pregnancy affects the different systems of a woman's body.

3.2   Before conception

Before describing the physiology of pregnancy, it is important to understand the different stages of the menstrual cycle and when conception can take place. Typically, each menstrual cycle occurs every 26–30 days over the childbearing period. The menstrual cycle normally begins with a series of interactions between a number of key hormones produced by three organs of the body: (1) the hypothalamus, (2) pituitary gland and (3) the ovaries (Silberstein and Merriam, 2000). The interaction between these three body parts, often referred to as the hypothalamic–pituitary–ovarian (HPO) axis, in healthy women leads to the monthly release of an egg (ovum). The menstrual cycle is divided into several key stages and typically occurs over a period of 28 days with ovulation (and potentially fertilisation) taking place 14 days before the next menstrual cycle (Table 3.1).

Table 3.1 Phases of the menstrual cycle.

Phase	Days	What takes place?
Menstrual phase	1–2	The lining of the uterus breaks down and menstruation takes place. Menstrual flow usually lasts between 2 and 5 days but varies between individuals.
Follicular phase	6–14	Cells mature inside cavities (follicles) that eventually become eggs. The FSH helps eggs to mature while LH stimulates the release eggs from the follicles.
Ovulation phase	14	There is a surge in LH on day 14 and the most mature eggs are released from the follicles and move down the follicle tubes. If the egg is fertilised, *pregnancy will take place*.
Luteal phase	15–27	If fertilisation has taken place, the corpus luteum secretes oestrogen and progesterone, which help to maintain the pregnancy.
		If fertilisation has not taken place, oestrogen and progesterone levels drop, the uterus lining breaks down and menstrual bleeding occurs.

Women usually ovulate 14 days before their next cycle. For example, women with a 28-day cycle will ovulate on day 14, whereas women with a 32-day cycle would ovulate on day 18. The 'fertile period' is typically two days before and after ovulation.
FSH, follicle-stimulating hormone; LH, luteinising hormone; corpus luteum, the ruptured sac left behind once the egg has been released.

3.2.1   Fertilisation

Fertilisation is when the male and female sex cells fuse to form a zygote, a specialised sex cell that then divides to form a ball of cells known as a blastocyst. This then implants and attaches itself to the wall of the uterus, usually about 6–12 days after ovulation. This is generally referred to as the 'implantation window'. Once this attachment has taken place, the placenta can start to establish itself.

Indeed, there are many factors that can affect the chances of fertilisation. From a nutrition perspective, there is some evidence that diet quality in the 'periconceptional period', the period of time just before and in the early stages of pregnancy, can affect the chances of conception, foetal organogenesis and placental function. For example, certain micronutrient deficiencies, particularly low habitual intakes of B vitamins and antioxidants, may contribute to elevated levels of homocysteine and reactive oxygen species, both of which can subsequently affect the chances of conception and the processes of embryogenesis and organogenesis (Cetin *et al.*, 2010). Research is needed to concentrate on which micronutrients are particularly important in the periconceptional period and to determine whether micronutrient requirements are higher during this time.

3.3   After conception

3.3.1   Embryo or foetus?

Once the ova is fertilised, the cell divides and passes through different stages of division. The dividing cell is usually referred to as a blastocyst at 6 days after fertilisation and attaches to the uterine epithelium where an inner mass of cells form the embryonic pole and the placenta starts to establish. Surrounding tissues then develop further, forming a trophoblast, which helps to protect and nourish the embryo. As a rule of thumb, the term embryo is usually used to refer an organism in its early stages of development (also known as embryogenesis) before it reaches a recognisable form. The term foetus is used at about 8 weeks after fertilisation or 10 weeks after the first day of the last menstrual cycle (SACN, 2010). This is the point in time when the body structures starts to become recognisable and organ systems begin to develop (also known as organogenesis).

From a different viewpoint, there is much debate about when the cutoff for abortion should be and phases of foetal development have been important in determining this in the past. One of the main issues with abortion is when human life begins and moral status is acquired. There are many opposing views with some suggesting that the embryo is a potential person after fertilisation and others suggesting that the development of brain is the most morally significant phase of development (rapid brain growth normally occurs between 20 and 32 weeks into pregnancy). The current abortion time limit is set at 24 weeks, but there is discussion this could be too late, particularly as pregnancies may be viable at this stage (BMA, 2005).

Carnegie Stages

Carnegie stages are a series of 23 different phases used to unify and categorise the development of the embryo. Although other methods can also be (*continued overleaf*)

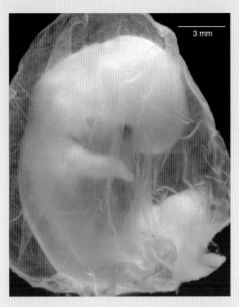

Figure 3.1 Carnegie Stage 19. (Reproduced with permission from Bradley Smith, University of Michigan.)

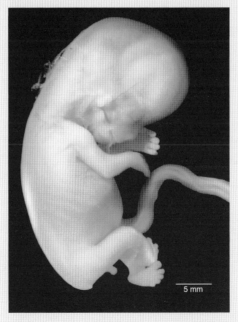

Figure 3.2 Carnegie Stage 23. (Reproduced with permission from Bradley Smith, University of Michigan.)

used, this is probably this is probably the most widely known. Each stage is based on the development of the embryos structures rather than its size, making it a useful system for comparing embryonic development. The 23 Carnegie stages only cover the first 60 days of embryogenesis, starting from the last day of ovulation before pregnancy. As mentioned previously, the term foetus is generally used after this time period once the embryos organ systems are well established. Some of the later phases of embryogenesis are shown in Figures 3.1 and 3.2, Carnegie stages 19 and 23, respectively. This is about 46 and 56 days since the last day of ovulation and conception.

3.3.2   Placental function

After fertilisation has taken place, the placenta begins to establish. The placenta is a highly complex, temporary organ that acts as an important passageway for the exchange of metabolic products between the foetus and mother. The placenta establishes rapidly in the early stages of pregnancy but also acts as an important endocrine gland, synthesising a number of key hormones. Once the foetus and placenta begin to interact, this may be referred to as the foeto–placental unit (FPU). Amongst other functions (Figure 3.3), this is the main site of protein and steroid hormone secretion and some of the physiological changes that take place in pregnancy are often a result of hormonal signals generated from the FPU (Burney *et al.*, 2008).

There is great interest in placental function, the passage of nutrients and how these can affect foetal growth. It is thought that the placenta's ability to adapt and meet

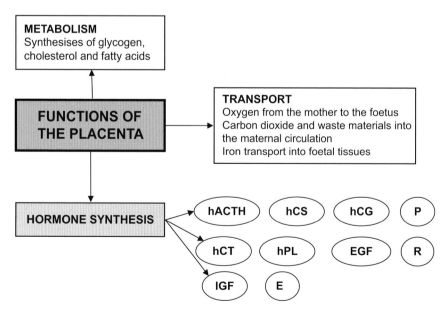

Figure 3.3 Functions of the placenta. E, estrogen; EGF, endothelial growth factor; hACTH, human chrorionic adrenocorticotropin; hCT, human chorionic thyrotropin; hCG, human chorionic gonadotropin; hPL, human placental lactogen; IGF, insulin-like growth factor; p, progesterone; R, relaxin.

foetal demands may affect the growth and composition of the foetus, resulting in lifelong programming at certain set points after conception (Sibley *et al.*, 2010). There is also emerging evidence that foetal uptake of certain nutrients, for example long chain polyunsaturated fatty acids, not only depends on maternal metabolism, but also on placental function (Cetin *et al.*, 2009), i.e. nutrients needs to be consumed, metabolised and then transferred effectively for the foetus to have full benefits. There is now good evidence that altered nutrient and hormone metabolism and placenta growth may all have important effects on foetal programming – permanent changes in foetal tissue structure and function that can affect lifelong health (Godfrey *et al.*, 2002). It seems likely that finding future ways to improve placental function could be of permanent benefit to the developing child.

Scientific Highlight   Can placental function affect later risk of cardiovascular disease?

In Western nations, cardiovascular disease remains to be one of the leading causes of death. Although its causes are multfactorial and can be attributed to a host of genetic and lifestyle factors, there is evidence to suggest that the size and function of the placenta when *in utero* may also contribute to its development.

A number of studies have identified that there is a U-shaped relationship between placental-to-foetal weight. This means that if the placenta is smaller or larger than average, this may lead to altered foetal growth. Findings from animal studies go some way towards helping to explain these findings. For example, research mainly using rats has shown that mycocardial walls surrounding the heart are undergrown when the placenta has been small or malformed. Equally, muscular heart cells known as cardiomyocytes have been found to be fewer in number and not as well formed when the placenta has developed insufficiently (Thornburg *et al.*, 2010). Taken together, the findings from these important human and animal studies suggest that cardiovascular health may start as early as *in utero*, which appears to be influenced, if not closely regulated by the placenta.

3.4   Formation of the neural tube

The term neurulation is often used to describe the processes leading to the development of the neural tube (Figure 3.4). Neurulation encompasses the formation of the neural plate, neural fold and the neural tube, which will then go on to form the brain and spinal cord. As this is a period of rapid cell division, folic acid requirements are significantly higher in the early stages of pregnancy. For these reasons, it is important that women consume sufficient levels of folate from the diet or folic acid from supplement sources, at least during the first 12 weeks of pregnancy when the neural tube should have formed. Inadequate intakes may mean that the neural tube does not form or close correctly leading to neural tube defects. More work is needed to confirm how long women should take folic acid before pregnancy or if there are benefits for continued supplementation throughout the later stages of pregnancy.

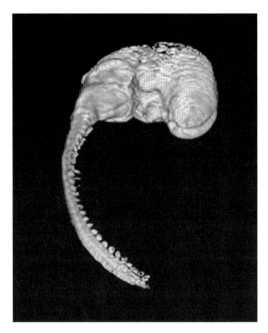

Figure 3.4 Neural tube, Carnegie Stage 23. (Reproduced with permission from Bradley Smith, University of Michigan.)

3.5 Foetal growth

A ready supply of nutrients is needed from the mother to meet foetal demands and achieve healthy growth and development of the foetus. When the balance between the foetal supply and demand for nutrients is altered, this can have potential consequences for long-term health (Constancia *et al.*, 2005). Physiologically and metabolically, the mother does have some ability to ensure there is a steady supply of nutrients reaching the foetus, but equally mothers also needs nutrients for their own needs. For a successful pregnancy to occur, women need to be able to draw on their own reserves and sustain the nutrient demands of the foetus throughout pregnancy. When this does not occur, i.e. during times of reduced accessibility to food, this may have implications for foetal growth.

It is well established that energy and protein restriction during critical periods of development can lead to reduced foetal growth, but the role of individual micronutrients is not as well established (Christian and Stewart, 2010). There is now over two decades worth of literature linking reduced foetal growth to a range of health complications later in life (Figure 3.5), but most recently reduced maternal–foetal nutrition during early- to mid-pregnancy has been linked to an increased risk of overweight and altered metabolic profile in the offspring. It is thought that when women are not adequately nourished in pregnancy, this may programme foetal adipose tissue to upregulate its number of fat (adipose) tissue cells. In turn, later in life, this may increase the risk of metabolic syndrome and predispose towards obesity when the progeny are exposed to the extrauterine environment (Symonds *et al.*, 2009).

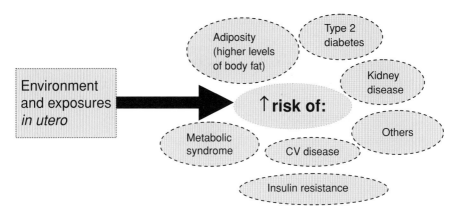

Figure 3.5 How reduced foetal growth, placental function and nutritional exposures *in utero* may affect health in later life.

3.6   Key hormones

A vast array of hormones are secreted during pregnancy. Normal maternal secretion of extra hormones is produced by the corpus luteum and then by the FPU once pregnancy is established. A woman's body will experience a range of physical and physiological changes that are brought about by changes in these hormone levels. Every hormone has a different function and the levels change considerably through-out the course of pregnancy. The main aim of the next section is to explain the patterns of secretion and roles of key hormones in pregnancy as well as how these may affect women from a physiological viewpoint.

3.6.1   Oestrogens and progesterone

Oestrogen is not one single hormone, but there are actually three different forms (oestradiol, oestriol and oestrone). These hormones along with progesterone are produced by the corpus luteum from early pregnancy. Levels of oestrogen rise steadily throughout the course of pregnancy (Figure 3.6), whilst progesterone levels plateau

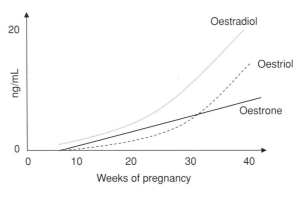

Figure 3.6 Levels of oestrogen hormones increase as pregnancy proceeds, reaching their highest levels in the third trimester.

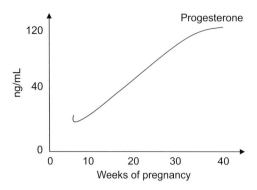

Figure 3.7 Levels of progesterone rise as pregnancy progresses, reaching their highest levels in the third trimester.

towards the end of pregnancy (Figure 3.7). Eventually, levels of these hormones secreted during pregnancy overtake and are higher than levels produced in non-pregnant menstruating women (Wald *et al.*, 1982).

Past animal studies using gastrointestinal (GI) tissue samples have shown that progesterone slows down the muscular contractions that normally take place, propelling food through the intestine. Oestrogen hormones also seem to play a role in the relaxation of intestinal tissue (Ryan and Bhojwani, 1986). When taken together, it seems that both oestrogen and progesterone hormones play a key role in slowing transit time. This means that food in the gut has a longer time period over which nutrients can be absorbed. It is thought that this may be the body's way of adapting physiologically to ensure that nutrients are absorbed during a time when requirements are higher.

3.6.2   Follicle-stimulating and luteinising hormone

Follicle-stimulating hormone (FSH) and luteinising hormone (LH) both belong to a family known as gonadotrophins, hormones that stimulate the reproductive glands. Both hormones are secreted by cells called gonadotrophs located in the brain's pituitary glands and are glycoprotein molecules containing a carbohydrate and protein portion.

FSH is more important in the run-up to pregnancy, helping the follicles holding the eggs to grow and mature (Howles, 2000). Once pregnancy has taken place, FSH levels decline and remain low throughout the duration of pregnancy. Levels of LH hormones surge mid-cycle, and once fertilisation has taken place, LH is needed to maintain and sustain the corpus luteum, the sac left behind once the egg has been released. With the help of the LH, the corpus luteum continues to produce oestrogen hormones and progesterone throughout pregnancy.

3.6.3   Human chorionic gonadotrophin

Human chorionic gonadotrophin, generally abbreviated to hCG, is a protein produced by the placenta in early pregnancy. This protein may be present in urine just a few days after conception has taken place and forms the basis of many pregnancy tests. Serum concentrations rise rapidly in early pregnancy and peak at around

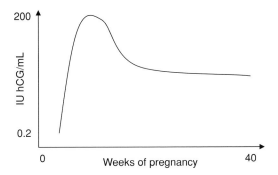

Figure 3.8 Levels of hCG rise in early pregnancy and form the basis of most pregnancy tests.

60 days after fertilisation (Figure 3.8). After this point in time, serum levels decline and low serum levels are maintained until delivery (King, 2000). It is thought that the rapid rise in hCG in early pregnancy may represent the growth of the trophoblast, the outer layer of the blastocyst that attaches the fertilised ovum to the uterine wall and serves as a nutritive pathway for the embryo.

3.6.4 Prolactin and oxytocin

A few days after conception has taken place, levels of prolactin start to rise. As its name indicates, this hormone starts to prepare the body for lactation after birth. The hormone is produced and secreted from the anterior lobe of the pituitary gland and works closely with another hormone secreted by the placenta, placental lactogen. Although prolactin levels remain low during early- to mid-pregnancy, this neurohormone (a hormone that acts on neurons) plays a key role in preparing the breasts for milk production after birth. Levels of this hormone are closely regulated by a short-loop negative-feedback mechanism (Figure 3.9). Placental lactogen helps to maintain low levels of prolactin in early pregnancy by stimulating this negative feedback loop. Prolactin, when secreted, stimulates brain neurones known as tuberoinfundibular dopamine (TIDA) neurones to produce dopamine, which then enters the pituitary portal bloodstream, detected by receptors and then prolactin secretion is inhibited (Grattan *et al.*, 2008).

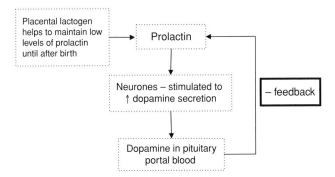

Figure 3.9 Placental lactogen works with prolactin to help the body prepare for milk production after birth. Levels of prolactin, however, are closely regulated by the neurotransmitter dopamine.

Oxytocin is secreted by the posterior lobe of the pituitary gland and is another example of a neurohormone. The hormone is released in spurts at the end of gestation and targets the uterus, stimulating contractions (Petraglia *et al.*, 2010). As discussed later in Chapter 11, oxytocin is also released when the breast is suckled by breastfed infants after birth and is an important part of the let-down reflex.

3.6.5 Relaxin

Relaxin is a protein-based hormone and as its name indicates plays a key role in helping to relax certain body tissues. For example, relaxin helps to promote the growth and softening of the cervix, easing the passage of the child during delivery (Sherwood, 2004). Relaxin levels rise in early pregnancy, peak at around 10–14 weeks after conception and decline after then (Wathen *et al.*, 1995). Some authors believe that the hormones relaxin and progesterone work together to help relax the tissues and uterus during pregnancy (Tincello *et al.*, 2003). This helps the body to accommodate the child but can also contribute to constipation symptoms often experienced in pregnancy by relaxing the GI tract (Bonapace and Fisher, 1998).

A number of studies have observed whether high (hyperrelaxinemia) or low (hyporelaxinemia) relaxin levels could affect the length or pregnancy or maternal health. Elevated relaxin levels have been associated with premature deliveries, whilst lower relaxin levels have been linked to insulin resistance, which could be a risk factor for diabetes development in pregnancy (Goldsmith and Weiss, 2009).

3.6.6 Leptin

Leptin is derived from the Greek word 'leptos' meaning thin. It is a satiety hormone secreted by fat cells (adipocytes) and acts on the hypothalamus of the brain, normally helping to regulate body fat levels around a set point. Normally, higher leptin levels suppress appetite, whilst lower levels increase feelings of hunger. Pregnancy studies mainly carried out on animals show that the feedback loop between leptin and appetite suppression is disrupted and a state of leptin resistance takes place, i.e. the body does not respond as readily to the hormone (Ladyman, 2008).

As leptin is also produced by the FPU, scientists believe that it may help to regulate foetal growth and body composition (namely, body fat levels). Over the last decade, scientists have started to uncover the actions of leptin and it seems likely that much is still undiscovered (Hauguel-de Mouzon *et al.*, 2006).

3.6.7 Ghrelin

Ghrelin is a hormone produced by the stomach and pancreas that is thought to stimulate hunger. Only a limited amount of research has studied the role of ghrelin in pregnancy. Ghrelin levels rise in the first part of pregnancy, peak mid-pregnancy and decline in the second half of pregnancy. As with leptin, ghrelin is another example of a hormone that plays a role in appetite regulation. In pregnancy, the secretion of ghrelin appears to be closely related to foetal growth, but further studies are needed to understand exactly how it may exert its actions (Fuglsang, 2008).

3.6.8   Thyroid hormone

The thyroid gland produces two key hormones: thyroxine (T$_4$) and triiodothyronine (T$_3$), which help to regulate the body's metabolism during pregnancy. Iodine is an important component of these hormones. Therefore, adequate intakes of iodine are needed to meet the levels required to produce these hormones.

There is good evidence to suggest that inadequate supplies of iodine during pregnancy may cause permanent damage to the foetal brain, contributing to the development of learning difficulties in childhood (de Escobar *et al.*, 2007). Also, inadequate iodine status in pregnancy may affect the function of the foetus's thyroid glands that are still developing (Glinoer, 2007). Therefore, inadequate iodine intakes in pregnancy can lead to the development of goitre (swelling of the thyroid glands) both in pregnancy and also in the newborn. Generally, goiters formed during pregnancy only partially regress after birth (Glinoer, 1999).

3.7   Key physiological changes

The physiological changes that take place in pregnancy are vast and books alone may be and have been dedicated to the alterations that take place. This next section therefore only aims to summarise the main changes that occur and explain how these change affect women's well-being in pregnancy.

3.7.1   Amniotic fluid

Amniotic fluid is a straw-coloured liquid comprised mainly of water (about 98%). This was once considered to be stagnant pool of very little importance. Scientific views, however, are now changing and it is thought that amniotic fluid may help to maintain the fluid balance of the foetus – swallowing of amniotic fluid and excretion of foetal urine are two of the main processes involved in the clearance and formation of amniotic fluid. For this reason, levels of amniotic fluid are now being used increasingly as an indicator of foetal kidney function (Modena and Fieni, 2004).

There are times in pregnancy when women may have too little (oligohydramnios) or too much (polyhydramnios) amniotic fluid. If amniotic membranes rupture prematurely, this has been linked to oligohydramnios and increased risk of preterm deliveries and foetal growth restriction. There are many different causes of polyhydramnios, but women with diabetes in pregnancy or having twins may be more likely to have excess amniotic fluid (Volante *et al.*, 2004).

3.7.2   Blood volume

Blood volume includes the plasma (yellow, fluid component of blood) and red blood cells. It is important that changes in blood volume that occur during pregnancy prepare for the blood losses that take place during delivery (about 500–1200 mL). Blood volume changes are also needed to ensure that the uterus, baby, placenta and mother's tissues all have a continuous supply of oxygen. On average, for women having a single baby, blood volume increases by about 35–40%, when expressed as a percentage of the non-pregnant volume (Picciano, 2003).

Maternal side	Foetal side
↑ Macrophages	↑ Maternal T-cells (down regulate)
↑ Natural killer cells	↑ Anti-inflammatory effects
↑ Oestrogen and Progesterone	↑ Cytokines
↑ Anti-inflammatory effects	
↑ Cytokines	

Figure 3.10   A summary of immunological changes that take place in pregnancy.

Generally, about 6 weeks into pregnancy, the mother's blood volume starts to rise slowly. After this, blood volume increases proportionately with the growth of the baby, reaching a peak in the third trimester (about 32 weeks into pregnancy). To help sustain the changes in pregnancy blood volume, the cardiovascular system also has to adapt – maternal heart rate and cardiac both increase in pregnancy to help pump the extra blood volume around the body (Torgersen and Curran, 2006).

3.7.3   The immune system

As the foetus is not genetically identical to the mother, several immunological changes must occur to prevent rejection by the immune system (Miller, 2009). Immunity is regulated on both sides of the placenta (Figure 3.10), namely through the actions of the placenta. On the mother's side, there is a rise in the number of macrophages and natural killer cells, cells that help to destroy foreign materials. The hormones oestrogen and progesterone also promote anti-inflammatory responses. In combination, these are thought to play a significant role in preventing rejection of the placenta and foetus. On the foetal side, maternal T-cells are largely inactive, helping to sustain the pregnancy and cytokines also help to maintain the uterine environment (Poole and Claman, 2004).

From an immunological perspective, pregnancy is a unique challenge. The foetus develops in its own confined specialised organ (the uterus), where it is protected by its own mucosal barrier (the deciduas) and secretes its own products that can regulate the immune system of the mother (a range of hormones, lipids and cytokines) and infuse into her bloodstream. Taken together, even though these immunological mechanisms are in place, the foetus can be at risk of infections, which may increase the risk of miscarriage, premature labour, growth defects and sometimes intrauterine death (Sacks *et al.*, 1999).

Innate versus adaptive immunity

Immunity may be non-specific or specific. Non-specific immunity (innate) immediately protects the body from a range of substances, whilst specific immunity (adaptive) acts specifically against particular invaders. Whilst innate immunity is immediate, i.e. surface barriers such as the skin and mucus membranes filter out antigens, or the inflammatory response blocks their entry, adaptive immunity can take time to develop (Stables and Rankin, 2006).

Research studying the immunity of pregnant women has shown that innate immunity is increased during pregnancy, whilst the ability to respond to infections (adaptive immunity) is reduced (Miller, 2009). The reasons behind this are largely unknown, although it is thought that regulating adaptive immunity may help to prevent an immune overreaction to the foetus or could act as an energy saving mechanism (Lochmiller and Deerenberg, 2000). The activated innate system may also be linked to help problems that may arise in pregnancy. Although the causes of pre-eclampsia are multifaceted, it is possible that there may also be an immunological basis, i.e. women at risk may have an increasingly active immune system (Saito et al., 2007).

Autoimmune disorders

Autoimmune disorders occur when the immune system reacts and attacks healthy body tissue (a form of a hypersensitivity reaction). In pregnancy, connective tissue diseases (CTDs) such as rheumatoid arthritis, sclerosis, Sjogren syndrome and systemic lupus erythematosus (SLE) are most common in young women between the ages of 20 and 40. Explanations of these conditions are found in Table 3.2. Women with these conditions that fall pregnant or are planning to conceive are considered 'at risk populations' because their autoimmune condition may flare during pregnancy or their medications may have teratogenic effects (Mecacci et al., 2007).

3.7.4   The GI tract

Changes in GI function are a common cause of complaint in expectant mothers and symptoms can be particularly uncomfortable and often embarrassing. In pregnancy, the combined effects of hormonal and physiological changes mean that expectant mothers become increasingly susceptible to a range of GI symptoms. These can vary between individuals but range from mild symptoms of nausea to hyperemisis gravidarium (severe sickness and vomiting), heartburn, constipation and haemorrhoids (Keller et al., 2008). Although prevalence rates vary between countries and study populations, around 25% pregnant women may experience constipation at some phase in their pregnancy (Bradley et al., 2007). Equally, heartburn may occur in 30–50% pregnancy and in some populations incidence may be as high as 80% (Richter, 2003).

Table 3.2   Autoimmune disorders that may occur in pregnancy.

Autoimmune disorder	Definition
Rheumatoid arthritis	A chronic inflammatory disorder that affects tissues and organs, damaging cartilage and joints
Sclerosis	When organ-specific tissue is replaced with connective tissue causing it to stiffen
Sjogren syndrome	When immune cells attack and destroy the glands that produce tears and saliva
Systemic lupus erythematosus	The immune system attacks the body's cells and tissue causing inflammation and tissue damage. Periods of occurrence are referred to as 'flares'.

Nausea and vomiting

Around 75–80% of women experience nausea and vomiting in pregnancy (NVP), typically in the first trimester and early stages of the second trimester. The aetiology of NVP is generally not well understood but certain hormones, *Helicobacter plyori* infection and psychological factors are all thought to be involved (Badell *et al.*, 2006). One theory with the most standing is that the secretion of hCG may be related to NVP, as both peak at around 12–14 weeks into pregnancy (Furneaux *et al.*, 2001). It is also thought that morning sickness may be a natural mechanism, to help protect the developing embryo from foods and chemicals that may be potentially teratogenic, or induce early miscarriage. This theory is now well supported and literature strongly demonstrates the following:

- NVP peaks when the embryo is most vulnerable to chemical disruption (weeks 6–18).
- NVP reduces the risk of miscarriage.
- Women experiencing vomiting are less likely to miscarry when compared to those with nausea alone.
- Women develop aversions to foods that may be teratogenic (Flaxman and Sherman, 2000).

Overall, it can be seen that NVP is a natural mechanism, possibly brought about by the rise in hCG. Symptoms of NVP in the early stages of pregnancy may help prevent ingestion of foods that could be potentially harmful to the developing child, optimising the chances of a successful pregnancy outcome.

Research Highlight   NVP may modify dietary intakes

A recent study carried out by scientists from the University of Turku, Finland, studied the dietary habits and nutrient intakes of women with and without NVP. Women with NVP ($n = 134$) had higher intakes of grain and milk products, margarine, vegetable oils, sugar and sweets and consumed less meat than the 53 controls. Although it is difficult to establish whether different nutrient intakes were a result of poorer quality diets or a consequence of nausea and vomiting, dietary intakes of vitamin B_{12}, magnesium and zinc were lower amongst women experiencing higher rates of nausea and vomiting. Women experiencing severe NVP had shorter pregnancies, but levels of pregnancy weight gain, infant weight and length were unaffected (Latva-Pukkila *et al.*, 2010). Similar findings have also been reported by Lee *et al.* (2004) who also found that morning sickness in pregnancy led to poor dietary diversity and lower intakes of energy, protein and micronutrients, with reduced intakes been directly related to the severity of morning sickness.

Together, the findings from the studies show that although NVP may be an inbuilt mechanism to help protect the developing foetus from potentially harmful substances, NVP can also lead to reduced intakes of certain nutrients that may have its own implications for foetal growth, programming and later health. Considerably, more remains to be known about the clinical and dietary impacts of NVP.

Nausea and Vomiting – What Helps?

Nausea, retching and vomiting can be unpleasant to experience in pregnancy and can make everyday regimes more challenging. From a nutrition perspective, both ginger and vitamin B_6 have been thought to help alleviate these symptoms, but until recently evidence has not been thoroughly reviewed. In one study, 67 pregnant women, all experiencing nausea and vomiting took either ginger (250 mg) or control capsules over a period of 4 days. This helped to reduce symptoms of nausea and frequency of vomiting (Ozgoli et al., 2009), but the length of the intervention period was short and the sample size comparatively small.

Most recently, a systematic review of 27 randomised controlled trials comprising 4041 women evaluated the evidence from studies investigating the efficacy of interventions used to alleviate symptoms of nausea and vomiting. Authors concluded that the use of ginger products may be helpful to women, but evidence from studies to date is inconsistent. Evidence to support the use of vitamin B_6 was more limited with a clear need for larger, well-designed clinical trials (Matthews et al., 2010).

Hyperemesis gravidarium

Around 0.3–2% of pregnant women may develop hyperemesis gravidarium (severe sickness and vomiting) in pregnancy (Philip, 2003). The causes of this condition are largely unknown but it has been suggested that the condition may have a genetic aetiology. In an American study, data relating to family history was collected from 1224 females diagnosed with hyperemesis gravidarium. Of these cases, 28% reported that their mothers and 19% said their sisters had similar experiences (Fejzo et al., 2008).

Whilst NVP may be beneficial to pregnancy outcome, hyperemesis gravidarium may pose health risks to both mother and baby. Infants born to mothers with the condition may be low birth weight (LBW) and smaller at term (Bailit, 2005). It is, however, yet to be confirmed whether this is caused by hyperemesis gravidarium per se or physiological changes related to the condition. Dodds et al. (2006) found that poor level of weight gain in mothers with hyperemesis gravidarium was the likely cause of adverse pregnancy outcomes (LBW and preterm deliveries). Equally, Tan et al. (2007) found that metabolic and biochemical indices including hypokalemia and elevated creatine levels were linked to adverse pregnancy outcomes (emergency operative delivery and induction of labour), rather than the condition itself. More work is needed within this field to reinforce the findings from these studies. Until this is undertaken, the causes and consequences of this condition will remain to be under question.

Research Highlight   Extreme weight loss, hyperemesis gravidarium and pregnancy outcome

In a recent study, 819 women who had given birth were questioned about their own health in pregnancy and their infant's health status. All women taking part in the study had experienced extreme weight loss since giving birth, defined as more than 15% of their pre-pregnancy weight i.e. if a woman was 70 kg before birth, she would weigh less than 59.5 kg.

Scientists observed that extreme weight loss was strongly related to symptoms of hyperemesis gravidarium in pregnancy, with 22% women reporting that symptoms lasted throughout pregnancy. Just over 9% of women who had experienced extreme weight loss had children with behavioural disorder, premature and LBW deliveries (Fejzo *et al.*, 2009). Overall, it seems that hyperemesis gravidarium may be a risk factor for extreme weight loss during and after pregnancy. This may have long-term effects not only for the infant but also for the mother's health.

Gums and teeth

Changes in hormonal concentrations may increase women's susceptibility to periodontal disease in pregnancy. Rising levels of oestrogen and progesterone in particular increase blood flow to the gums and can lead to gingivitis development (Soory, 2000). Gingivitis in pregnancy is characterised by dark red, swollen and smooth gums that bleed easily. Generally, symptoms recede after delivery but some women may develop gingival enlargements, which may require medical attention. When oral flora is transferred to the infant, this may increase the risk of dental caries in the offspring and unfavourable pregnancy outcomes, i.e. preterm and small-for-gestational-age deliveries (Boggess and Edelstein, 2006)

It is also commonly thought that teeth soften in pregnancy because of calcium and mineral mobilisation, but this theory now lacks standing. Scientists now believe that changes in the pH and composition of saliva may be more likely causes of predisposition to dental caries and erosion in pregnancy (Laine, 2002). More work is needed to understand the physiological changes related to oral health in pregnancy. However, scientists and dental practitioners do appear to have reached a consensus: that the importance of good oral health should be promoted in pregnancy (Boggess and Edelstein, 2006).

A Note on Appetite in Pregnancy

During pregnancy, women become increasingly hungry (hyperphagia), which helps to meet the energy needs of the growing foetus and prepare for the metabolically demanding process of lactation after birth. Contradictory to common belief, metabolism does not always slow during pregnancy; instead, energy needs can be met by increasing energy intakes to the levels needed, through changes in appetite levels. The mechanisms underlying the changes in appetite levels during pregnancy are not well understood but several theories have been put forward.

It is thought that the hormones oxytocin and progesterone may be involved (Douglas *et al.*, 2007), but further confirmation is needed. Animal studies also indicate that the hormone leptin may help to increase appetite and food intake in pregnancy (Johnstone and Higuchi, 2001). Normally, leptin levels upregulate as a mechanism to promote satiety and reduce food intake, but leptin levels are reduced in pregnancy. Most recently, it has been proposed that the secretion of the hormone placental lactogen may block the body's response to leptin in pregnancy (Lady man *et al.*, 2010). This means that feelings of hunger are not switched off as effectively and feelings of hunger may still persist in pregnancy. Women will therefore still feel hungry, allowing for additional energy intake to fuel both pregnancy and lactation.

Oesophagus and heartburn

Heartburn typically occurs in around 30–50% of expectant mothers (Richter, 2003) with symptoms generally increasing as pregnancy proceeds (from 22% in the first trimester to 73% in the third; Marrero *et al.*, 1992). Although increased intra-abdominal pressure because of the expanding uterus is the traditional explanation for the initiation of heartburn, this theory has been disparaged (Feeney, 1982) and it is thought that hormones, namely progesterone, are more likely to be linked to its onset. One of the earliest studies to investigate the effects of progesterone of symptoms of heartburn was carried out by van Thiel *et al.* (1977). Lower oesophageal pressure (LES) was measured in four previously asymptomatic pregnant patients at weeks 12, 24 and 36 of pregnancy and 1–4 weeks after birth. LES pressure was reduced in pregnancy and returned to normal after birth. It was thought that surges in progesterone were responsible for these reduced sphincter pressures, hence the increase in heartburn in the third trimester when sphincter pressures were at their lowest and decrease postpartum when sphincter pressures return to non-pregnant levels.

Intestinal function

The GI tract undergoes dramatic physiological alterations to support the nutritional needs of the mother and her developing child. Several factors may influence GI function in pregnancy as displayed in Figure 3.11. As discussed previously, rising levels of female sex hormones can influence GI function in pregnancy. Although these hormones (progesterone in particular) promote tissue laxity to help accommodate the developing child, they can have an unfavourable effect on the GI tract by mainly causing motility disturbances caused by increased levels of female sex hormones (Keller *et al.*, 2008). Consequently, constipation is a common occurrence in pregnancy with around 35–39% women experiencing symptoms in the first two and 21% in the third trimester (Derbyshire *et al.*, 2007). Reported rates of constipation vary between studies and depend largely on the country of origin and methods used to define the condition. The Rome II diagnostic criterion (Table 3.3) uses a range

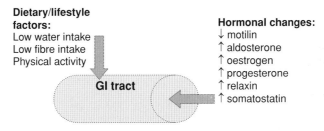

Figure 3.11   Factors influencing GI function in pregnancy.

Table 3.3   Rome II criteria.

Women may be defined as functionally constipated if two or more of the following are present
Defecation frequency <3/week Incomplete evacuation in ≥25% of defecations Lumpy, hard stools Straining to finish in ≥25% of defecations Straining to start in ≥25% of defecations

Source: (Thompson *et al.*, 1999).
If two of more of the following are present, individuals are likely to be constipated. Ideally, bowel habit data should be collected over a 12-week period. This method is thought to be more accurate than previous subjective definitions such as 'altered bowel habits'.

of bowel habit parameters to diagnose constipation and is most highly regarded (Thompson *et al.*, 1999). Although hormonal changes are the most likely cause of constipation, movement of the intestinal tract and uterus in pregnancy may also be contributing causes (Wald, 2003).

Fibre, Fluid and GI Function

Physiological and hormonal changes associated with pregnancy can lead to increased nutritional requirements. For example, a diet adequate in dietary fibre that is supplemented with sufficient fluid may help to ease some of the GI problems often experienced in pregnancy. Higher intakes of fibre can increase stool water absorption, promote the expansion of bacterial populations and help form bulky stools that stimulate the defecation reflex (James *et al.*, 2003). Eating a diet sufficient in dietary fibre, i.e. at least the recommended 18 g/day (DH, 1991), may help to reduce symptoms of constipation and other uncomfortable bowel habit problems, including bloating, haemorrhoids and anal fissures (enlarged veins in the anal canal that may tear).

In terms of fluid consumption, low water intakes can lead to hardened stools and constipation (Arnaud, 2003). Reducing intakes of caffeinated beverages that act as diuretics and consuming enough water from food and fluids (about 2.3 L; EFSA, 2010) may help to soften stools and promote healthy bowel habits during pregnancy. On the whole, simple dietary amendments may help to make bowel habits more comfortable in pregnancy. Pregnant mothers, however, with persistent GI problems should seek referral to a dietician and/or GP.

3.7.5   Application in practice

Nurses, midwives and general practitioners can play an important role in helping women to understand the changes that are going to be taking place to her body. Women should be encouraged to drink enough water throughout pregnancy to replace fluids lost through nausea and vomiting, support the expansion of extracellular fluids and help to make bowel habit movements more comfortable. Consuming sufficient levels of dietary fibre, i.e. from wholegrain foods, may also help to promote healthy bowel function. Presently, there is a lack of evidence supporting the use of

Table 3.4 Summary of pregnancy symptoms linked to hormonal and physiological changes.

Trimester	Weeks	Symptoms
First	0–14	Breast tenderness, morning sickness, increased micturition, fatigue
Second	15–28	Fainting/dizziness
Second and third	15+	Constipation, heartburn, dyspnoea, varicose veins, oedema, weight gain, leg cramps, restless leg syndrome, carpal tunnel syndrome
Third	29+	Slight nausea, heartburn, constipation, haemorrhoids, increased micturition
Throughout pregnancy	Emotional changes	Mood swings, changing body image, depression, fearful
Throughout pregnancy	Physical changes	Skin changes, backache, headache, stuffy nose, bleeding gums

Source: From Stable and Rankin (2006), with permission.

vitamin B_6 and ginger supplements, but ginger food-based products may be helpful in some instances.

3.8 Conclusion

The body makes tremendous adaptations to accommodate the developing child and provide the best environment for the foetus during pregnancy. The physiological and hormonal changes that take place, combined with the growth of the foetus, means that a range of symptoms are often experienced by women during pregnancy (Table 3.4). Although there is a lack of evidence, some simple dietary amendments, i.e. consuming recommended levels of fibre and fluid, may help to improve bowel habits in pregnancy. For nausea and vomiting, evidence from studies is currently inconsistent, but ginger products may be helpful in alleviating some symptoms. On the whole, simple changes to dietary and lifestyle habits that are needed anyway for good health may be beneficial in pregnancy, helping to make pregnancy more comfortable during a time that should be enjoyed to the utmost

Key Messages

- A spectrum of hormonal and physiological changes take place in pregnancy, affecting most body systems.
- The conceptus is referred to as an embryo in the early stages of pregnancy and as a foetus once the organ systems are established (about 8 weeks after fertilisation).
- The placenta is a temporary but important organ regulating not only the passage of nutrients, but also producing and secreting a range of hormones.
- Reduced foetal growth, a result of limited nutrition supplies, has been associated with a range of health complications later in life.
- Hormones play an important role in pregnancy, regulating appetite, softening tissues and helping the body to accommodate the child.
- Hormonal changes can, however, lead to mood swings, constipation, emotional and other physical changes in pregnancy.

- NVP may help to protect the embryo from agents that could cause damage but can also lead to reduced nutrient intakes, which may, in turn, have implications for foetal growth.
- Hyperemesis gravidarium may take place in some pregnancies and has been linked to weight loss and unfavourable pregnancy outcomes, i.e. lower birth weight infants.
- Simple dietary amendments, i.e. eating recommended amounts of fibre (18 g/day; DH, 1991) and consuming enough water (2.3 L/day; EFSA, 2010), may help to alleviate some of the painful bowel problems that often come hand-in-hand with the physiological and hormonal changes of pregnancy.

Recommended reading

Blackburn ST (2003) *Maternal, Fetal and Neonatal Physiology: A Clinical Perspective*, 2nd edition. WB Saunders: Philadelphia.
SACN (Scientific Advisory Committee on Nutrition) (2010) *The SACN Subgroup on Maternal and Child Nutrition (SMCN): The Influence of Maternal, Fetal and Child Nutrition on the Development of Chronic Disease in Later Life*. The Stationery Office: London.
Stables D and Rankin J (2006) *Physiology in Childbearing*. Elsevier: London.

References

Arnaud MJ (2003) Mild dehydration: a risk factor of constipation. *European Journal of Clinical Nutrition* **57**, S88–95.
Badell ML, Ramin SM and Smith JA (2006) Treatment options for nausea and vomiting during pregnancy. *Pharmacotherapy* **26**(9), 1273–87.
Bailit JL (2005) Hyperemesis gravidarium: epidemiologic findings from a large cohort. *American Journal of Obstetrics & Gynaecology* **193**(3 Pt 1), 811–14.
BMA (British Medical Association) (2005) *Abortion Time Limits: A Briefing Paper from the BMA*. BMA: London.
Boggess KA and Edelstein BL (2006) Oral health in women during preconception and pregnancy: implications for birth outcomes and infant oral health. *Maternal & Child Health Journal* **10**(5), S169–4.
Bonapace ES and Fisher RS (1998) Constipation and diarrhoea in pregnancy. *Gastroenterology Clinics of North America* **27**, 197–211.
Bradley CS, Kennedy CM, Turcea AM, Rao SS and Nygaard IE (2007) Constipation in pregnancy: prevalence, symptoms, and risk factors. *Obstetrics & Gynaecology* **110**(6), 1351–7.
Burney RO, Mooney SB and Giudice LC (2008) *Endocrinology of Pregnancy*. Available at: http://www.endotext.org/female/female13/femaleframe13.htm. (accessed March 2011.)
Cetin I, Alvino G and Cardellicchio M (2009) Long chain fatty acids and dietary fats in fetal nutrition. *Journal of Physiology* **587**(Pt 14), 3441–51.
Cetin I, Berti C and Calabrese S (2010) Role of micronutrients in the periconceptional period. *Human Reproduction Update* **16**(1), 80–95.
Christian P and Stewart CP (2010) Maternal micronutrient deficiency, fetal development, and the risk of chronic disease. *Journal of Nutrition* **140**(3), 437–45.
Constancia M, Angiolini E, Sandovici I *et al.* (2005) Adaptation of nutrient supply to fetal demand in the mouse involves interaction between the Igf2 gene and placental transporter systems. *Proceedings of the National Academy of Sciences* **102**, 19219–24.
de Escobar GM, Obregón MJ and del Rey FE (2007) Iodine deficiency and brain development in the first half of pregnancy. *Public Health Nutrition* **10**(12A), 1554–70.
Derbyshire EJ, Davies GJ, Costarelli V and Dettmar PW (2007) Changes in bowel function: pregnancy and the puerperium. *Digestive Diseases and Sciences* **52**(2), 324–8.
DH (Department of Health) (1991) *Dietary Reference Values for Food Energy and Nutrients for the United Kingdom*, 2nd edition. *Report on Social Subjects* no. 41. The Stationery Office: London.

Dodds L, Fell DB, Joseph KS, Allen VM and Butler B (2006) Outcomes of pregnancies complicated by hyperemesis gravidarium. *Obstetrics and Gynaecology* **107**(2 Pt 1), 285–92.

Doughty DB (2002) When fibre is not enough: current thinking on constipation management. *Ostomy/Wound Management* **48**, 30–41.

Douglas AJ, Johnstone LE and Leng G (2007) Neuroendocrine mechanisms of change in food intake during pregnancy: a potential role for brain oxytocin. *Physiology & Behaviour* **91**(4), 352–65.

EFSA (European Food Standards Agency) (2010) Scientific opinion on dietary reference values for water. *EFSA Journal* **8**(3), 1459.

Feeney JG (1982) Heartburn in pregnancy. *British Medical Journal* **284**, 1138–9.

Fejzo MS, Ingles SA, Wilson M *et al.* (2008) High prevalence of severe nausea and vomiting of pregnancy and hyperemesis gravidarium among relatives of affected individuals. *European Journal of Obstetrics and Gynaecology and Reproductive Biology* **141**(1), 13–7.

Fejzo MS, Poursharif B, Korst LM *et al.* (2009) Symptoms and pregnancy outcomes associated with extreme weight loss among women with hyperemesis gravidarum. *Journal of Women's Health (Larchmt)* **18**(12), 1981–7.

Flaxman SM and Sherman PW (2000) Morning sickness: a mechanism for protecting mother and embryo. *Quarterly Review of Biology* **75**(2), 113–48.

Fuglsang J (2008) Ghrelin in pregnancy and lactation. *Vitamins & Hormones* **77**, 259–84.

Furneaux EC, Langley-Evans AJ and Langley-Evans SC (2001) Nausea and vomiting of pregnancy: endocrine basis and contribution to pregnancy outcome. *Obstetrical & Gynaecological Survey* **56**(12), 775–82.

Glinoer D (1999) What happens to the normal thyroid during pregnancy? *Thyroid* **9**(7), 631–5.

Glinoer D (2007) The importance of iodine nutrition during pregnancy. *Public Health Nutrition* **10**(12A), 1542–6.

Godfrey KM (2002) The role of the placenta in fetal programming – a review. *Placenta* **22**(16), S20–7.

Goldsmith LT and Weiss G (2009) Relaxin in human pregnancy. *Annals of the New York Academy of Sciences* **1160**, 130–5.

Grattan DR, Steyn FJ, Kokay IC, Anderson GM and Bunn SJ (2008) Pregnancy-induced adaptation in the neuroendocrine control of prolactin secretion. *Journal of Neuroendocrinology* **20**(4), 497–507.

Hauguel-de Mouzon S, Lepercq J and Catalano P (2006) The known and unknown of leptin in pregnancy. *American Journal of Obstetrics & Gynaecology* **194**(6), 1537–45.

Herrera E (2000) Metabolic adaptations in pregnancy and their implications for the availability of substrates to the fetus. *European Journal of Clinical Nutrition* **54**(S1), S47–51.

Howles CM (2000) Role of LH and FSH in ovarian function. *Molecular & Cellular Endocrinology* **161**, 25–30.

Hytten F (1995) *The Clinical Physiology of the Puerperium*. Farrand Press: London.

Hytten FE and Chamberlain G (1991) *Clinical Physiology in Obstetrics*. Blackwell Scientific Publications: Oxford.

James SL, Muir JG, Curtis SL and Gibson PR (2003) Dietary fibre: a roughage guide. *Internal Medicine Journal* **33**, 291–6.

Johnstone LE and Higuchi T (2001) Food intake and leptin during pregnancy and lactation. *Progress in Brain Research* **133**, 215–27.

Keller J, Frederking D and Layer P (2008) The spectrum and treatment of gastrointestinal disorders during pregnancy. *Nature Clinical Practice Gastroenterology & Hepatology* **5**(8), 430–3.

King JC (2000) Physiology of pregnancy and nutrient metabolism. *American Journal of Clinical nutrition* **71**, 1218S–25S.

Ladyman SR (2008) Leptin resistance during pregnancy in the rat. *Journal of Neuroendocrinology* **20**(2), 269–77.

Ladyman SR, Augustine RA and Grattan DR (2010) Hormone interactions regulating energy balance during pregnancy. *Journal of Neuroendocrinology* **22**(7), 805–17.

Laine MA (2002) Effect of pregnancy on peridontal and dental health. *Acta Odontologica Scandinavica* **60**(5), 257–64.

Latva-Pukkila U, Isolauri E and Laitinen K (2010) Dietary and clinical impacts of nausea and vomiting during pregnancy. *Journal of Human Nutrition & Dietetics* **23**(1), 69–77.

Lee JI, Lee JA and Lim HS (2004) Morning sickness reduces dietary diversity, nutrient intakes, and infant outcome of pregnant women. *Nutrition Research* **24**, 531–40.

Lochmiller RL and Deerenberg C (2000) Trade-offs in evolutionary immunology: just what is the cost of immunity? *Okios* **88**, 87–98.

Marrero JM, Goggin PM, de Caestecker JS, Pearce JM and Maxwell JD (1992) Determinants of pregnancy heartburn. *British Journal of Obstetrics and Gynaecology* **99**, 731–4.

Matthews A, Dowswell T, Haas DM, Doyle M and O'Mathúna DP (2010) Interventions for nausea and vomiting in early pregnancy. *Cochrane Database of Systematic Reviews* **9**, CD007575.

Mecacci F, Pieralli A, Bianchi B and Paidas MJ (2007) The impact of autoimmune disorders and adverse pregnancy outcome. *Seminars in Perinatology* **31**, 223–6.

Miller EM (2009) Changes in serum immunity during pregnancy. *American Journal of Human Biology* **21**, 401–3.

Modena AB and Fieni S (2004) Amniotic fluid dynamics. *Acta Bio Medica Ateneo Parmense* **75**(1), 11–13.

Ozgoli G, Goli M and Simbar M (2009) Effects of ginger capsules on pregnancy, nausea, and vomiting. *Journal of Alternative & Complementary Medicine* **15**(3), 243–6.

Petraglia F, Imperatore A and Challis JR (2010) Neuroendocrine mechanisms in pregnancy and parturition. *Endocrine Reviews* **31**(6), 783–816.

Philip B (2003) Hyperemesis gravidarium: literature review. *Wisconsin Medical Journal* **102**(3), 46–51.

Picciano MF (2003) Pregnancy and lactation: physiological adjustments, nutritional requirements and the role of dietary supplements. *Journal of Nutrition* **133**(6), 1997S–2002S.

Poole JA and Claman HN (2004) Immunology of pregnancy. Implications for the mother. *Clinical Reviews in Allergy & Immunology* **26**, 161–70.

Richter JE (2003) Gastroesophageal reflux disease during pregnancy. *Gastroenterology Clinics of North America* **32**(1), 235–61.

Ryan JP and Bhojwani A (1986) Colonic transit in rats: effect of ovariectomy, sex steroid hormones, and pregnancy. *American Journal of Physiology* **251**, G46–50.

Sacks G, Sargent I and Redman C (1999) An innate view of human pregnancy. *Viewpoint Immunology Today* **20**(3), 114–18.

SACN (Scientific Advisory Committee on Nutrition) (2010) *The SACN Subgroup on Maternal and Child Nutrition (SMCN): The Influence of Maternal, Fetal and Child Nutrition on the Development of Chronic Disease in Later Life*. The Stationery Office: London.

Saito S, Shiozaki A, Nakashima A, Sakai M and Sasaki Y (2007) The role of the immune system in pre-eclampsia. *Molecular Aspects of Medicine* **28**(2), 192–209.

Sherwood OD (2004) Relaxin's physiological roles and other diverse actions. *Endocrine Reviews* **25**(2), 205–34.

Sibley CP, Brownbill P, Dilworth M and Glazier JD (2010) Review: Adaptation in placental nutrient supply to meet fetal growth demand: implications for programming. *Placenta* **31**, S70–4.

Silberstein SD and Merriam GR (2000) Physiology of the menstrual cycle. *Cephalalgia* **20**(3), 148–54

Soory M (2000) Hormonal factors in periodontal disease. *Dental Update* **27**(8), 380–3.

Stables D and Rankin J (2006) *Physiology in Childbearing*. Elsevier: London.

Symonds ME, Sebert SP, Hyatt MA and Budge H (2009) Nutritional programming of the metabolic syndrome. *Nature Reviews Endocrinology* **5**(11), 604–10.

Tan PC, Jacob R, Quek KF and Omar SZ (2007) Pregnancy outcome in hyperemesis gravidarium and the effect of laboratory clinical indicators of hyperemesis severity. *Journal of Obstetrics & Gynaecological Research* **33**(4), 457–64.

Thompson WG, Longstreth GF, Drossman DA, Heaton KW, Irvine EJ and Müller Lissner SA (1999) Functional bowel disorders and functional abdominal pain. *Gut* **45**(SII), 1143–7.

Thornburg KL, Tierney PFO and Louey S (2010) Review: The placenta is a programming agent for cardiovascular disease. *Placenta* **31**(24), S54–9.

Tincello DG, Teare J and Fraser WD (2003) Second trimester concentration of relaxin and pregnancy related incontinence. *European Journal of Obstetrics and Gynaecology and Reproductive Biology* **106**, 237–8.

Torgersen CKL and Curran CA (2006) A systematic approach to the physiologic adaptations of pregnancy. *Critical Care Nursing Quarterly* **29**(1), 2–19.

Van Thiel DH, Gavaler JS, Joshi SN, Sara RK and Stremple J (1977) Heartburn of Pregnancy *Gastroenterology* **72**, 666–8.

Volante E, Gramellini D, Moretti S, Kaihura C and Bevilacqua G (2004) Alteration of the amniotic fluid and neonatal outcome. *Acta Bio Medica Ateneo Parmense* **75**(1), 71–5.

Wald A (2003) Constipation, diarrhoea, and symptomatic hemorrhoids during pregnancy. *Gastroenterology Clinics of North America* **32**, 309–22.

Wald A, Van Thiel D, Hoechstetter L *et al.* (1982) Effect of pregnancy on gastrointestinal transit. *Digestive Diseases and Sciences* **27**, 1015–18.

Wathen NC, Perry LA, Gunn L, Campbell DJ and Chard T (1995) Relaxin levels in amniotic fluid, extraembryonic coelomic fluid and maternal serum in early human pregnancy. *Early Human Development* **43**, 71–4.

4 Nutrient Metabolism in Pregnancy

Summary

Metabolic changes throughout pregnancy are extensive and not the same for every expectant mother. Nutritional status before pregnancy, genetic factors and maternal lifestyle can all influence the metabolic changes that occur during pregnancy. From a nutritional perspective, metabolic adjustments take place to help regulate energy balance and the exchange of nutrients between the mother and her foetus. In the early phases of pregnancy, the body is in an 'anabolic state', accruing tissue reserves, but this shifts towards a 'catabolic state' in the later stages of pregnancy with nutrients becoming increasingly available for foetal growth. Although these processes are tightly regulated to promote maternal and foetal well-being when metabolic pathways are not regulated, this can impact upon maternal health and result in poor pregnancy outcomes. The main aim of this chapter is to discuss how energy balance and nutrient pathways are regulated throughout pregnancy.

Learning Outcomes

- To identify and discuss some of the main metabolic changes that take place to nutrient pathways in pregnancy.
- To discuss findings from key scientists and some current research papers within this field of work.
- To recognise how these metabolic pathways may contribute to maternal/foetal well-being.

4.1 Introduction

During pregnancy, a spectrum of metabolic changes takes place to meet the changing demands of the mother, as well as the foetus and placenta. Energy metabolism, mainly in the form of reduced energy expenditure, is needed to meet the energy needs of the growing foetus. Carbohydrate metabolism adapts to meet the demands of the

Nutrition in the Childbearing Years, First Edition. Emma Derbyshire.
© 2011 Emma Derbyshire. Published 2011 by Blackwell Publishing Ltd.

growing foetus – glucose is the main energy source for the foetus in early pregnancy and protein metabolism is enhanced, to provide substrates to help support maternal tissue expansion and foetal growth. Changes in fat metabolism in pregnancy also mean that levels of most blood lipids are elevated in pregnancy.

There are also changes to important micronutrient pathways – calcium, vitamin D, iron and folate status all modify in pregnancy to help meet foetal demands. If maternal reserves are low before pregnancy and nutrient intakes inadequate in pregnancy, metabolic pathways generally do not operate as efficiently as they should. As mentioned earlier, this chapter sets out to give a broad overview of how energy balance and nutrient pathways are regulated during pregnancy. The chapter will also touch on some of the implications to maternal/foetal well-being that may occur if these pathways are not in balance or functioning as they should.

4.2 Energy metabolism

Energy metabolism changes significantly throughout gestation. Only a few key studies have measured energy metabolism in pregnancy, when compared to research undertaken with non-pregnant women. This is mainly because pregnant women are an intricate population to study. Obtaining data for the first trimester can be difficult, with many pregnancies not being confirmed until later on in this trimester. Acquiring data for each trimester can also be difficult, as women may withdraw from research studies before the end of their pregnancies. When combined with the fact that pregnancy is a 'dynamic state' where physiological and metabolic changes take place continuously and inter-relate, it can be seen that this is a complex area to study. Therefore, the aim of this section is to give a broad overview of energy metabolism in pregnancy, although it should be considered that this varies between women.

4.2.1 Some basic principles

To maintain energy balance and regulate body weight, the basic principles of energy balance need to exist, i.e. energy intake = energy expenditure. However, in pregnancy, this is not always the case. Most women are generally in a state of positive energy balance with either energy intakes increasing or levels of energy expenditure/physical activity reducing. In some cases, however, states of negative energy balance may exist. In some less developed regions, seasonal food shortages combined with the physically demanding agricultural work can mean that energy intakes are lower than the levels of energy used.

The amount of energy expended on a daily basis is therefore a combination of several different factors. This includes not only the energy expenditure through physical activities (also known as active energy expenditure) but also the energy needed to fuel the body's basic metabolic processes (basal metabolic rate (BMR)) and to heat the body and digest food (diet-induced thermogenesis). For pregnant women, there is a fourth component to consider – the energy costs needed to synthesise expanding maternal and foetal tissues (Figure 4.1). As a result, in pregnancy, total energy expenditure (TEE; the sum of these) comprise four rather than three energy components (Forsum and Lof, 2007).

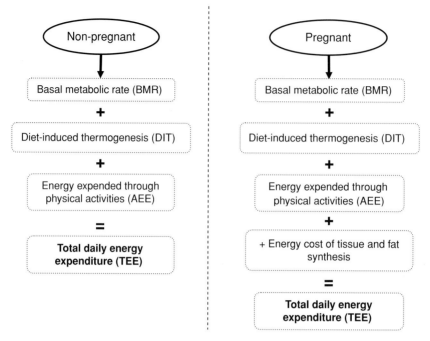

Figure 4.1   Components of total energy expenditure.

4.2.2   Basal metabolic rate

BMR constitutes a large proportion of energy expenditure in pregnancy. On average, compared to before pregnancy, BMR is 4.5, 10.8 and 24.9% higher in the first, second and third trimesters of pregnancy, respectively (Butte and King, 2005). However, rates of BMR appear to vary geographically and the energy cost of pregnancy may be related to body composition before pregnancy.

In one study, Lof *et al.* (2005) studied which factors (body weight, body fat, fat-free mass, insulin-like growth factor and thyroid hormones) were most likely to influence BMR in 22 healthy pregnant women. It was found that both weight and body fat levels before pregnancy were most likely to result in a higher BMR in pregnancy (by up to 40%). Although more work is needed to explain these findings, it appears that pregnancy is a unique condition where BMR is regulated by maternal adipose reserves (rather than fat-free mass, as is usually the case in non-pregnant women).

4.2.3   Thermogenesis and active energy expenditure

The energy cost of digestion, absorption, transport and storage of food is around 10% of the daily energy intake. For pregnant mothers, it is thought that changes in metabolic substrate routing may reduce energy expended from these processes in pregnancy (Bronstein *et al.*, 1995).

In terms of energy expended through daily activities, the energy costs of non-weight activities are similar to non-pregnant women. Energy expended through weight-bearing activities is higher, however, in pregnancy, mainly because of the rise in body weight. Overall, scientists and physiologists believe that the increased energy costs of physical activity are offset by a decrease in the amount of time spent in weight-bearing activities and change in the type of activities that are undertaken in pregnancy (King, 2000), i.e. women may take part in physical activities for less time but be expending higher levels of energy because body weight is higher.

4.2.4 Total energy expenditure

Scientists have used a combination of calorimetry and the doubly labelled water (DLW) method to measure the amount of energy expended on a daily basis in pregnancy. Using this method, Lof and Forsum (2006) measured the TEE of 23 Swedish women, before and at weeks 14 and 32 of pregnancy. Scientists found that both BMR and TEE increased with pregnancy. TEE increased slightly in the first trimester, but the largest change was found in the third trimester (11,760 KJ/24 hours compared to 10,510 KJ/24 hours before pregnancy). It was concluded by authors that BMR can contribute significantly to the rise in TEE as pregnancy proceeds and when patterns of physical activity are maintained.

4.2.5 Energy costs

It has been estimated the total energy cost for women gaining around 12.0 kg weight in pregnancy is around 77,000 calories (Butte and King, 2005). When calculated for the three trimesters of pregnancy, it can be seen that the energy costs of pregnancy and calorie requirements increase as pregnancy proceeds (Table 4.1). However, in reality, it is considered unlikely that women need extra energy in the first trimester of pregnancy and lower energy expenditures later in pregnancy means that energy intakes do not necessarily need to change. For these reasons, the Scientific Advisory Committee on Nutrition (SACN) (2009) recommend the EAR (Estimated Average Requirement) for pregnancy originally established by COMA (Committee on Medical Aspects of Food and Nutrition Policy), an additional intake of 0.8 MJ/day (191 kcal/day) in the last trimester remain appropriate. Women who are overweight when they enter pregnancy may not need to increase their energy intakes, but there is currently not enough data to make a firm recommendation.

Table 4.1 Estimated pregnancy energy costs in each trimester.

	Energy cost (KJ/d)	Kcals/trimester	Kcals extra /d*
First trimester	375	7885	89
Second trimester	1200	25,340	285
Third trimester	1950	41,110	462

Source: Data calculated using figures from Butte &and King (2005).
SACN (2009) recommend that energy intakes only need to change in the third trimester, i.e. an additional intake of 0.8 MJ/day (191 kcal/day) is advised.
*Length of gestation taken to be 266 days (and each trimester 89 days).

4.2.6   Measuring energy expenditure

As mentioned previously, measuring energy expenditure accurately can be difficult in pregnancy. For such reasons, scientists in the past have used a combination of methods to obtain the data that they need. Controlled environments are better from a scientific perspective, but these are generally not representative of daily life. The main methods used to derived levels of energy expenditure (calories used on a daily basis) are given below:

- Indirect calorimetry – when oxygen consumption and carbon dioxide production are measured and energy expenditure is calculated using standard calculations. These usually involve participants lying down whilst wearing a mask or hood to collect expired air.
- Direct calorimetry – when the rate of heat lost from the human body to the calorimeter is measured and used to calculate energy expenditure. These are usually chamber-based systems, which may be more accurate but do not reflect real life.
- DLW method – when water labelled with isotopes is administered and rates of clearance measured. Saliva, urine and blood samples are taken regularly to determine this. This enables energy expenditure to be measured in free-living subjects, which is more realistic.

Although at present DLW method is regarded as being the 'gold standard' for measuring TEE, there are also limitations with this method. This method is expensive and invasive – particularly for pregnant women and does not always account for all components of energy expenditure (i.e. digestion). Consequently, even this method may under-report energy expenditure to some extent (Levine, 2005).

4.3   Carbohydrate metabolism

In healthy mothers, the secretion of insulin may be 50–70% lower later in pregnancy compared to levels in non-pregnant mothers (Butte, 2000). Although reduced levels of insulin, also known as 'insulin resistance', appear to serve a biological purpose – to shunt ingested nutrients (particularly glucose) to the foetus – hyperglycaemia may also contribute to the development of gestational diabetes mellitus (GDM) in late pregnancy (Figure 4.2). When combined with the rising rates of obesity, GDM is becoming an increasingly frequent occurrence in pregnancy (Sathyapalan *et al.*, 2010).

4.3.1   Insulin sensitivity

Levels of insulin insensitivity are a tale of two stories in pregnancy (Table 4.2). In the early stages of pregnancy, muscle, fat and liver cells are more responsive to the hormone insulin. As a result, plasma glucose, amino acid and free fatty acid levels reduce and glycogen is synthesised. However, as pregnancy progresses, insulin sensitivity decreases and carbohydrate metabolism switches over into a state of 'insulin resistance'. When this takes place, fat stores in adipose tissue become

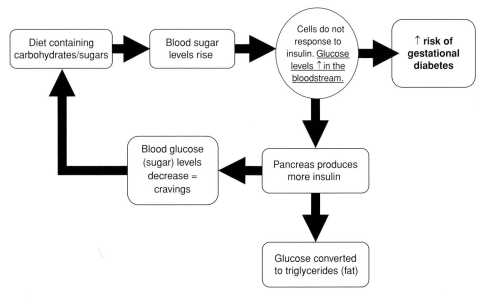

Figure 4.2 Insulin resistance in pregnancy.

mobilised, glycogen synthesis is impaired and blood glucose and amino acid levels become elevated (Lain and Catalano, 2007).

It is thought that rises in levels of several hormones may contribute to insulin resistance in pregnancy. Most recently, it has been proposed that the hormone oestradiol may act directly on beta cells in the pancreas, stimulating insulin synthesis and production in early pregnancy (Nadal *et al.*, 2009), whilst a change in the way that insulin binds to red blood cells may contribute to insulin resistance in late pregnancy (Lázaro *et al.*, 2002). These are interesting theories, but more work is needed to determine the mechanisms involved in the change in insulin metabolism that take place in pregnancy.

4.3.2 Hyperglycaemia

It is becoming increasingly known that hyperglycaemia and gestational diabetes may be detrimental to the health of the offspring. After birth, infants need to adapt rapidly to regulate their own blood sugar levels. There is evidence to suggest that exposure to

Table 4.2 Changes in insulin sensitivity in pregnancy.

Early pregnancy	Late pregnancy
Increased insulin sensitivity	Increased insulin resistance
The body is in an anabolic state	The body is in a catabolic state
Lipid, protein and glycogen stores accumulate	Lipid, protein and glycogen stores are utilised
	Elevated blood glucose and amino levels. In severe cases may cause gestational diabetes.

high blood sugar levels during pregnancy may mean that the offspring are susceptible to glucose intolerance and diabetes later in life. This has recently been demonstrated in a study that followed up 514 children born to Indian mothers who had diabetes in pregnancy. The offspring of diabetic mothers had higher adipose tissue reserves and elevated glucose and insulin levels. Authors concluded that exposure to maternal diabetes *in utero* increased diabetes and cardiovascular risk, independently to genetic factors (Krishnaveni *et al.*, 2010).

4.3.3 Carbohydrate transfer to the foetus

Glucose is the main source of fuel for the foetus, providing around 50–80% of its energy. Glucose is supplied to the foetus continuously by the mother who can increase her glucose production by 15–30% in late pregnancy. Glucose is transferred from the mother's bloodstream, across the placenta and to the foetus with the aid of glucose transporters, known as GLUT 1 and 4. These transporters play an important role in ensuring that the foetus receives a constant supply of energy.

During times when the mother has low blood sugar levels (hypoglycaemic), these transporters are upregulated and when the mother has high blood sugar levels (hyperglycaemic), this can be down-regulated (Hay, 2006a). These homoeostatic mechanisms help to ensure that the foetus is provided with a steady supply of glucose. Once the glucose passes across the placenta, this is then converted to liver/muscle glycogen or storage lipids, which will help to maintain glucose homeostasis in the infant after delivery. Although the foetus has the ability to adapt to changes in glucose supply to some extent, such changes may underlie certain metabolic disorders such as insulin resistance, obesity and diabetes mellitus later in life (Hay, 2006b).

4.4   Lipid metabolism

Pregnancy has a profound effect on lipid metabolism. Most recently, the use of stable, non-radioactive isotopes together with glucose and insulin clamps has enabled the field of lipid metabolism to be studied in detail (Butte, 2000). Overall, studies have shown that fat accrues during the first two-thirds of pregnancy but then switches in the last trimester when fat reserves are mobilised to provide a supply of free fatty acids to the foetus. Therefore, blood lipid levels are usually elevated in the later stages of pregnancy (Herrera, 2002a).

4.4.1 Body fat stores

During pregnancy, most of the subcutaneous fat is deposited centrally (between the mid-thorax and mid-thigh). This was demonstrated in a large follow-through study undertaken by Sidebottom *et al.* (2001). In this study, skin-fold thickness was measured in each trimester of pregnancy and after birth. Body fat stores did not change in the first 6 weeks of pregnancy, but subcutaneous tricep stores increased by 1.5 mm, subscapular fat (above the shoulder blade) by 4.2 mm and thigh stores by 7.3 mm by 35 weeks into pregnancy. Women having their first child, or carrying males gained significantly more weight at the thigh and subscapular sites than other women. Overall, the findings from this study demonstrate that body fat is generally deposited later in pregnancy, although this may vary between individuals.

4.4.2   Fatty acid profile

Lipid metabolism has been studied exhaustively during pregnancy. Most aspects of lipid metabolism adjust in pregnancy and changes are complex. Therefore, this section aims to discuss findings from the most recent and relevant studies.

In a recent Italian study, Lippi *et al.* (2007) undertook a comprehensive lipid and lipoprotein analysis from 57 women, each at the different phases of pregnancy. Lipid profile varied considerably when women from different trimesters of pregnancy were compared. Total cholesterol, low- and high-density lipoprotein cholesterol levels were all significantly higher later in pregnancy when compared to samples taken in early pregnancy or from non-pregnant controls.

Similar findings have been reported amongst women from developing regions. In Bangladesh, total cholesterol, high- and low-density lipoprotein levels were also elevated in the second and third trimesters of pregnancy when compared to serum levels analysed from non-pregnant women (Husain *et al.*, 2008, 2009). New studies now need to follow women up after birth to see if these metabolism changes still persist and for how long.

Research Highlight   Can dietary fibre in early pregnancy reduce pre-eclampsia risk?

A wealth of evidence from epidemiological and experimental studies have shown that fibre-rich diets play an important role in preventing chronic diseases such as diabetes, coronary heart disease, obesity and disorders of the bowel, although conflicting definitions can make interpretations from such studies difficult (Mann and Cummings, 2009).

Now, there is also some evidence to suggest that eating fibre-rich foods in early pregnancy may help to reduce the risk of pre-eclampsia later on. Scientists from the Swedish Medical Centre in Seattle studied the dietary habits of 1538 pregnant women before and in early pregnancy using a food frequency questionnaire to derive their fibre intakes. A cross-section of mothers also had their plasma lipid and lipoprotein levels measured.

Results showed that mothers reporting higher dietary fibre intakes in early pregnancy were less likely to develop pre-eclampsia later on. Both higher intakes of water-soluble and insoluble fibre were associated with reduced pre-eclampsia risk (relative risk of 0.30 and 0.35, respectively) and had a favourable effect on lipoprotein profile; women eating 21.2 g fibre/day or more had significantly lower mean triglyceride levels ($\downarrow$ by 11.9 mg/dL) and significantly higher levels of high-density lipoprotein cholesterol ($\uparrow$ by 2.6 mg/dL), helping to promote cardiovascular health. The findings from this study demonstrate that a diet adequate in dietary fibre may help to regulate levels of blood lipids, protecting against the development of pre-eclampsia later in pregnancy. It is, however, important to consider that further trials are needed to reinforce the findings from this research. Further randomised controlled trials (RCTs) using dietary fibre interventions would be useful.

A Note on Relative Risk

Relative risks are a form of statistical test used to determine the risk of developing a disease or certain side effects. Relative risks are presented as a number falling below or above 1 and compares the risk of developing a disease or side effect in people receiving an intervention, i.e. a supplement, functional food or medication to those not receiving treatment (the control/placebo group). As a rule of thumb

- A relative risk of 1 means the risk of developing a disease or side effects is no different between groups.
- A relative risk less than (<) 1 means the risk is less likely to occur in the intervention than the control group.
- A relative risk greater than (>) 1 means the risk is more likely to occur in the intervention than in the control group.

4.4.3   The role of fat cells

Most recently, scientists are beginning to study the role that adipocytes may play in lipid metabolism. Adipocytes (fat cells) were once thought to be relatively biologically redundant with roles confined to energy storage, insulation and thermoregulation. Now, it has come to light that adipocytes play a role in a broad range of physiological processes, possibly including lipid metabolism in pregnancy.

Scientists have identified that adipocytes secrete proteins that may contribute to insulin resistance (tumour necrosis factor) or improve insulin sensitivity (adiponectin) (Trayhurn, 2005).

Most recently, Ritterath et al. (2009) measured adiponectin levels in 32 pregnant women during and after pregnancy. It was found that triglyceride levels were lower and high-density lipoprotein levels higher in women with elevated serum adiponectin concentrations. Although adiponectin production appears to be closely related to fat metabolism, it has not yet been established how this may take place (Ritterath et al., 2009). This is certainly an area where considerably more work is needed; it is possible that adiponectin may play a much larger role in maternal metabolism than initially thought.

4.4.4   Lipid transfer to the foetus

As mentioned previously, fatty acids are mobilised from maternal fat reserves in the later stages of pregnancy. This includes the release of long-chain polyunsaturated fatty acids (LC-PUFA) that are needed for foetal growth at this stage of pregnancy. The transfer of these fatty acids is supported by the presence of lipoprotein receptors on the placenta. These allow fatty acids to pass through and diffuse into the foetal plasma (Herrera et al., 2006). Although LC-PUFA requirements are higher at this stage of pregnancy, more remains to be known about whether these could enhance peroxidation, increasing levels of oxidative stress (Herrera, 2002b).

Diabetes in Pregnancy Alters Lipid Transfer to the Foetus?

When women develop diabetes in pregnancy, insulin resistance means that lipid profile can change – levels of triglycerides typically raise and levels of LC-PUFA decline. It has not yet firmly established why such changes occur, but it is known that the quality and quantity of lipids being transferred to the foetus is different for women with gestational diabetes. Scientists have proposed that such metabolic disturbances may be linked to the higher rates of large-for-gestational-age infants and infants with macrosomia (also see Chapter 9) born to these mothers (Herrera and Ortega-Senovilla, 2010).

4.5 Protein metabolism

Changes in protein metabolism are complex and ongoing throughout pregnancy. Unlike glucose and fatty acid metabolism, amino acids are not conserved and stored in early pregnancy for utilisation later on. Therefore, protein metabolism adapts according to maternal and foetal needs. However, more often than not the body is in a state of hypoaminoacidemia meaning that, if needed, additional amino acids are most likely to be utilised from soft tissue organs (Kalhan, 2000). One way of determining protein metabolism during pregnancy is to explore findings from studies that have used nitrogen balance techniques.

4.5.1 Nitrogen retention

Nitrogen, a component of all amino acids, is widely used a marker of protein metabolism. To conserve nitrogen during pregnancy and increase protein synthesis during this time, several metabolic changes take place.

Generally, studies show that more nitrogen is retained as pregnancy progresses. For this to occur, rates of protein synthesis must be increased and less nitrogen must be excreted (decreased urea synthesis) (Duggleby and Jackson, 2002). In one Dutch study, nitrogen balance was measured over 8 days on 4 occasions: (1) before pregnancy, (2) first trimester (12 weeks), (3) second trimester (23 weeks) and (4) third trimester (34 weeks). During this time, meals were provided to keep energy and nutrient intakes constant. Scientists found that significantly less nitrogen was excreted and more retained later compared to earlier in pregnancy (Mojtahedi *et al.*, 2002).

4.5.2 Protein turnover

Some studies show that rates of protein turnover may be related to birth outcome. One study found that women with a higher lean body mass and higher rates of protein turnover 18 weeks into pregnancy had babies that were longer at birth (26% variation in length) (Duggleby and Jackson, 2001). The same authors also identified that heavier infants were born to mothers who had lower levels of amino acid turnover in pregnancy (Figure 4.3), even after adjustments were made for length of pregnancy and the infant's gender (Duggleby and Jackson, 2002). Overall, it appears that rates of amino acid oxidation vary widely between pregnant mothers and may influence pregnancy outcomes, including birth weight. This may have implications when new protein dietary recommendations are developed for pregnancy.

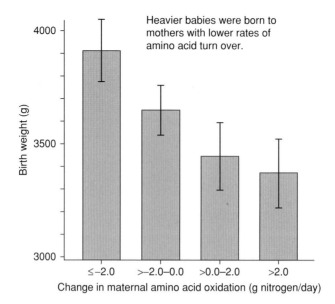

Figure 4.3 Relation between mean (±SEM) birth weight and changes in maternal amino acid oxidation from mid- to late-pregnancy. Twenty-five women were divided into four groups based on changes in amino acid oxidation: ≤-2.0 g N/day ($n = 6$), >-2.0–0.0 g N/day ($n = 9$), > 0.0–2.0 g N/day ($n = 5$) and >2.0 g N/day ($n = 5$). (Duggleby and Jackson (2002), reproduced with permission from the *American Journal of Clinical Nutrition*.)

4.5.3   Amino acid transfer to the foetus

For the foetus to grow efficiently, amino acids need to be transported across the placenta effectively. When foetal growth is restricted, this may have implications for cardiovascular health and renal function in the longer term, particularly at the population level (Geelhoed and Jaddoe, 2010).

The process of amino acid transfer to the foetus across the placenta is complex. Overall, levels of amino acids in maternal plasma are lower than in foetal plasma, causing amino acids to move against a concentration gradient. The movement of amino acids across the placenta is facilitated by a combination of transporters and exchangers. Together, they ensure that foetal cells are supplied with amino acids that will ultimately support foetal growth (Cleal and Lewis, 2008).

4.6   Calcium metabolism

Pregnancy places considerable demands on the mother to provide sufficient supplies of calcium to her developing child. Consequently, the mother must adapt her metabolic pathways to meet demands created by the foetus (Figure 4.4). In this case, calcium reserves may need to be drawn from the mother to supply the developing foetal skeleton. Potential adaptations may include

- Increasing dietary consumption of calcium
- Increasing intestinal absorption of calcium
- Decreasing renal excretion of calcium
- Mobilising and utilising calcium from the mothers' skeleton.

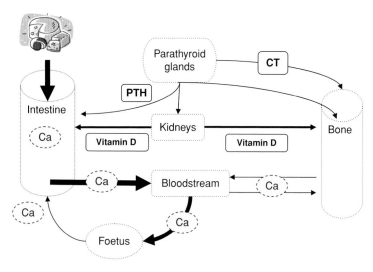

Figure 4.4 Calcium metabolism in pregnancy. Ca, calcium; CT, calcitonin; PTH, parathyroid hormone; vitamin D (1,25(OH)$_2$D), 1,25-dihydroxyvitamin D.

Despite the fact that expectant mothers may, theoretically, need the same magnitude of calcium, metabolic and endocrinological changes are not the same for every mother. This section will give a broad overview describing the changes in calcium metabolism throughout the course of pregnancy.

4.6.1   Calcium stores

Albright and Reifenstein (1948) were some of the first scientists to notice that pregnancy could lead to reduced skeletal calcium reserves and contribute to the development of osteoporosis. It is now widely known that the calcium requirements are higher during pregnancy. By the end of pregnancy, the foetus has generally accumulated around 30 g calcium. Around 80% or 340 mg/day calcium is deposited in the third trimester of pregnancy – when foetal demands are highest (Ward *et al.*, 2005). Consequently, expectant mothers need to start metabolic adaptations early in pregnancy to meet the demands of the foetus later in pregnancy.

4.6.2   Calcitropic hormones

Calcitropic hormones are a group of hormones that are involved in calcium metabolism. Generally, parathyroid hormone (PTH), 1,25-dihydroxyvitamin D (1,25(OH)$_2$D) and calcitonin (CT) are most actively involved in calcium metabolism during pregnancy. It is important that calcium metabolism is closely regulated during pregnancy to facilitate calcium deposition in the foetus, without drawing excessively on maternal reserves. Although homeostasis can be maintained to a point, there are instances when hypocalcaemia may occur in both the mother and/or foetus. Changes and functions of calcitropic hormones (and key minerals) are summated in Tables 4.3 and 4.4.

Table 4.3 Changes in calcium metabolism in pregnancy.

Factor	Levels in pregnancy
Calcitropic hormones	
1,25(OH)$_2$D (vitamin D)	Increases rapidly in the first trimester, reaching a plateau in the second and third trimester (highest levels)
Calcitonin	Levels increase in the first trimester, reaching a plateau in the second and third trimester (highest levels)
PTH	Low to low-normal from early pregnancy. Levels are highest in the first trimester, declining mid-pregnancy and rising at term.
PTH-related protein	Secretion increases steadily as pregnancy proceeds
Minerals	
Ionised calcium	Stable throughout pregnancy
Phosphate	Stable throughout pregnancy
Total calcium	*Declines over the first 5 months of pregnancy, reaching a plateau thereafter (lowest levels)*

4.6.3   Absorption and excretion

During pregnancy, intestinal absorption of calcium increases to accommodate increasing physiological requirements. Calcium binds to specific proteins (calcium-binding proteins) whose synthesis is stimulated by calcitriol, promoting intestinal absorption.

Urinary excretion of calcium may also decrease during pregnancy, although studies report conflicting findings. Most recently, Kumar *et al.* (2009) monitored mid-pregnancy calcium excretion in an Indian pregnant population. On average, 130 mg/day of calcium was excreted, just over a third of the total dietary intake (324 mg/day). Other studies have measured levels of calcium excretion amongst women with pre-eclampsia. It has been reported that levels of urinary calcium excretion are significantly lower (hypocalciuria) in women with pre-eclampsia, compared to healthy controls, and that vitamin D$_3$ and IGF-I (insulin-like growth factor-I) may be involved in its regulation (Halhali *et al.*, 2007).

Table 4.4 Function of calcitropic hormones in pregnancy.

Calcitropic hormone	Function
Parathyroid hormone (PTH)	PTH promotes bone resorption (remodelling) and helps to convert vitamin D into its active form. Levels are generally suppressed during pregnancy but increase at term.
Vitamin D (1,25(OH)$_2$D) (calcitriol)	Increases intestinal absorption of calcium (increases twofold in pregnancy).
Calcitonin (CT)	Protects against bone resorption during pregnancy. Role is not yet firmly established.
Parathyroid-related protein (PTHrP)	May help to increase levels of calcitriol and suppress PTH during pregnancy. Once again, its role is not yet firmly established.

Overall, increased intestinal absorption of calcium in pregnancy appears to be a major maternal adaptation to meet the foetal need for calcium. Increased absorption in early pregnancy may, in particular, take place to allow the maternal skeleton to store calcium for later use.

4.6.4 Skeletal calcium

Several markers can be used to measure bone turnover during pregnancy (resorption and formation). In a recent study, dietary intakes of calcium were recorded in 206 pregnant women who completed food frequency questionnaires. Urine samples were collected and bone resorption was measured in each trimester of pregnancy (using collagen as a marker). It was found that bone resorption increased as pregnancy proceeded and was higher amongst older mothers. Mothers, however, with higher calcium intakes, particularly from dairy products, had lower levels of bone resorption. Authors concluded that one glass of milk per day (around 300 mg calcium) may help to reduce bone resorption in pregnancy (Avendano-Badillo *et al.*, 2009). This may particularly be of benefit in the third trimester when calcium is most likely to be utilised from bone reserves.

4.6.5 Calcium transfer to the foetus

The foetus needs calcium to mineralise its skeleton and for other functions, such as blood coagulation. The foetal–placental unit can adapt to extract calcium from the mother's blood stream in proportions that are needed to mineralise the foetal skeleton later in pregnancy. The movement of calcium across the placenta is regulated by levels of maternal calcium and calcitropic hormones. Calcium is transported actively across the placenta and calcium-binding proteins are thought to be involved in this process. It is not clear when active transport of calcium begins in pregnancy, but it is thought to be underway by the third trimester. It is thought that PTHrP and CT may play a key role in supporting the transport of calcium to and metabolism of calcium in the foetus (Kovacs and Kronenberg, 1997).

4.7 Vitamin D metabolism

Vitamin D is a steroid hormone that can be manufactured in the skin by the action of radiation in the UVB spectrum (290–315 nm). Generally, no radiation of this length is available between the winter and early spring months in countries of lower latitudes meaning that the body relies on stores made in the summer (Roach and Benyon, 2004).

As can be seen in Figure 4.5, when exposed to radiation at the right frequency, 7-dehydrocholesterol in the skin is converted to previtamin D (precholecalciferol), which then forms cholecalciferol and is transported to the liver for storage. Dietary cholesterol (ergocalciferol and cholecalciferol) is also transported to the liver and then the kidney where hydroxylase enzymes convert vitamin D into its active form 1,25-dihydroxycholecalciferol ($1,25(OH)_2D$), also known as calcitriol (Gropper *et al.*, 2009).

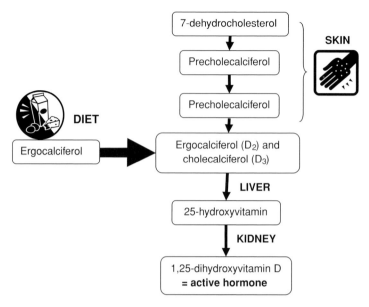

Figure 4.5 Conversion of vitamin D to the active hormone (1,25(OH)$_2$D). (SACN, 2007.)

4.7.1   Vitamin D and the placenta

Vitamin D deficiency in pregnancy correlates with an increased risk of pre-eclampsia, gestational diabetes, genitourinary infections and c-section deliveries, but most recently, there is evidence to show that the placenta also responds to vitamin D, possibly facilitating implantation, cytokine production and supporting immune function. It therefore seems that vitamin D is not only needed for maternal and infant health, but also for placenta function.

Scientific Highlight   Mothers' vitamin D status and risk of infantile rickets

Both in pregnancy and after birth, the mother provides the main source of 25(OH)D to her child. Consequently, maternal vitamin D status is an important risk factor in determining the offspring's vitamin D status and their risk of infantile rickets. At present, the optimal concentrations of 25(OH)D for good health are largely unknown, which has made defining normal ranges and biochemical cutoffs difficult (Barrett and McElduff, 2010). It is becoming increasingly apparent that current dietary recommendations, particularly for pregnant and lactating mothers, are insufficient, which means that women may be at risk of inadequate vitamin D status (Thandrayen and Pettifor, 2010). There is a clear need for studies to determine the optimal doses of vitamin D needed during and after pregnancy, particularly in terms of the doses needed to reduce the risk of infantile rickets in vulnerable populations. This research would greatly benefit policy makers in the future, helping to underpin any new dietary guidelines.

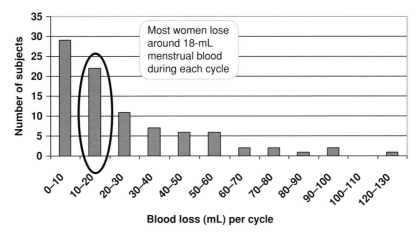

Figure 4.6   Menstrual blood loss (mL/cycle) in women aged 18–45 years. (Used with permission from Harvey *et al.* (2005), *British Journal of Nutrition.*)

4.8   Iron metabolism

In pregnancy, the body undergoes vast homeostatic changes in order to regulate iron metabolism, preventing both deficiency and overload. However, despite this, iron deficiency anaemia (IDA) remains to be a frequent occurrence with as many as 1 in 2 women being diagnosed in pregnancy (Scholl, 2005). IDA is when levels of red blood cell production fail to match rates of destruction meaning that haemogloblin levels, amongst other biochemical parameters, become reduced (Cavill *et al.*, 2006).

4.8.1   Iron stores and losses

For women to sustain an adequate iron balance during pregnancy, body iron reserves need to be at least 500 mg when a woman conceives (Milman, 2006a). Previous studies have shown that women lose around 17.6 mL menstrual blood during each cycle, which is equivalent to 0.43 mg iron per day (Harvey *et al.*, 2005; Figure 4.6). If this is not replenished from dietary sources, women may be iron deficient or have low iron stores at the start of pregnancy.

As can be seen in Table 4.5, a large proportion of iron is supplied to the foetus during pregnancy and to the placenta and umbilical cord. Haemoglobin mass also expands rapidly during pregnancy, requiring around 570 mg iron, and nearly 300 mg is lost from the skin and faecal/urinary excretions. Without including blood lost during delivery, total iron losses during pregnancy total to around 1000 mg, exceeding the iron stores of most women, even those in Western regions (Gautam *et al.*, 2008).

4.8.2   Iron absorption

Iron absorption varies according to the trimester of pregnancy. Rates of iron absorption are generally lower in the early stages of pregnancy – about 1.2 mg iron is absorbed into the bloodstream on a daily basis, when compared to rates before

Table 4.5 Iron distribution in pregnancy.

Iron losses	Iron requirements (mg)
Pregnancy	
Increase in red blood cell mass	570
Foetus/infant (3500 g)	270–370
Placenta and umbilical cord	35–100
Blood loss at delivery	100–250
Loss from skin, faeces, urine	270
Breastfeeding (6 months)	100–180

Source: Adapted from Stables and Rankin (2006), with permission.

pregnancy. Rates of absorption rise in the second trimester, to around 4.7 mg/day, and are highest in the third trimester, 5.6 mg/day. In total, the body absorbs about 3.3 mg/day more in the later stages of pregnancy when compared with non-pregnant women (Institute of Medicine, 2001). It is also important to consider that rates of iron absorption also vary between pregnant mothers, i.e. those with liberal body iron reserves absorb less iron than those with depleted reserves. Therefore, increased iron absorption may in part be because iron stores are already depleted (Milman, 2006b). On the whole, although the body works hard to adapt and upregulate rates of iron absorption, but for most mothers, there is usually a deficit of around 540 mg iron by the end of pregnancy (Fernandez-Ballart, 2000).

4.8.3   Iron utilised

As during every other phase of the life cycle, during pregnancy, the amount of iron consumed is not necessarily the proportion that is utilised. A range of factors, both dietary and host-related, can influence iron status and are shown in Table 4.6. A diet both inadequate in dietary iron and containing foods that inhibit iron absorption further places mothers at risk of developing IDA during pregnancy.

Table 4.6 Factors influencing iron absorption.

Dietary	Host-related
Enhancing	*Enhancing*
Vitamin C	Bile and pancretic secretions
Inhibitory	Gastric acid
Calcium and dairy products	High altitude (hypoxia)
Phytates	Homozygous for the C282Y mutation of the HFE gene
Other metals (zinc and copper)	Increased erythropoiesis
Alcohol	Iron-deficiency anaemia
Meat, poultry and fish	Low body stores
Eggs	Pregnancy
Polyphenols and flavonoids	*Inhibitory*
Tea and coffee	High body iron stores
Previous high intake of iron	
Rapid gastric emptying	

Source: Fairweather-Tait (2004), with permission.

In particular, the metabolism of copper and iron are closely inter-linked, although mechanisms of action need to be confirmed. Deficiencies in either of these can alter the distribution of the other mineral (Gambling *et al.*, 2008). A Chinese study compared the dietary habits of 1189 women in the third trimester who were both healthy and diagnosed with anaemia. It was concluded that low iron intakes, low intakes of iron enhancers and high intakes of iron inhibitors all contributed to the development of pregnancy IDA in this study (Ma *et al.*, 2002).

4.8.4   Markers of iron metabolism

Iron status and body iron can be monitored using several biochemical markers. However, classical indicators of iron status, for example haemoglobin levels, are not necessarily the best markers of iron status. Measuring iron levels is particularly difficult during pregnancy because inflammation, increased plasma volume and erythropoiesis (the production of new red blood cells) all influence markers of iron status (Mor, 2008).

Serum ferritin levels are regarded as one of the best indicators of iron status. A range of cutoff values in the past have been used to define iron deficiency in pregnancy, but 30 µg/L or less is thought to be most accurate (van den Broek *et al.*, 1998). Serum transferrin receptors (sTfR) are also highly regarded biomarkers – when supplies of iron are inadequate, sTfR upregulate to take up higher levels of transferrin-bound iron. Once used, sTfR are shed; therefore, elevated levels are a good indicator of IDA (Rusia *et al.*, 1999).

Other red cell indices such as zinc protoporphyrin (ZnPP), serum transferrin, mean corpuscular volume (MCV), serum iron, iron saturation, total iron binding capacity, transferrin saturation and Haptoglobin can also be used and calculated (Wish, 2006; Zimmermann, 2008). It is, however, important to consider that single parameters are of limited value and combinations of different markers of iron status are more accurate for the diagnosis of IDA (van den Broek *et al.*, 1998). Ideally, the best indicator of iron deficiency is a combination of at least three tests, with abnormal values for at least two indicating suboptimal iron status. Gibson (2005) reported that the combined use of serum ferritin (a measure of iron stores), transferrin receptors (the degree of iron deficiency after depletion of stores) and haemoglobin measurements (measure whether anaemia is present) may be one of the most accurate ways to determine iron status and to ensure that the entire spectrum of iron deficiency is covered. Some biochemical cutoffs usually used to define pregnancy iron-deficiency anaemia are summarised in Table 4.7.

4.8.5   Iron transport to the foetus

Compared with other aspects of iron metabolism, comparatively less is known about iron transport to the foetus. The few studies, however, that have looked into how iron is transferred across the placenta to the foetus indicate that this process is highly regulated (McArdle *et al.*, 2008).

Previous papers have reported that the number of transferrin receptors in the placenta can upregulate, as can the number of iron channels; facilitating the transport of iron from the mother to the child (Gambling *et al.*, 2001).

Table 4.7 Main cutoffs used to define pregnancy iron deficiency anaemia.

Biochemical markers of iron status	Cutoff used to define iron deficiency anaemia	Reference
Haemoglobin	<110 g/L	WHO, 2001; Rusia et al. 1999.
Serum ferritin	<30 µg/L	van den Broek et al. (1998)
Serum soluble transferrin receptors (sTfR)	>12.0 mg/L	Nair et al. (2004)
sTfR/ferritin ratio*	Negative values indicate a deficit of tissue iron	Zimmermann (2008)

*Calculated as [log(sTfR/ferritin ratio) − 2.8229]/0.1207.

4.8.6 Iron supplements

Iron supplements are generally recommended during pregnancy when requirements are higher and may not always be met through the diet alone. Historically, for the treatment of IDA, high-dose iron supplements have been prescribed, often up to 300 mg ferrous iron/day (Cook, 2005). However, there is accumulating evidence that these may be linked to gastrointestinal symptoms during pregnancy, including constipation and nausea (Bradley et al., 2007), increased oxidative stress and risk of gestational diabetes in pregnancy (Afkhami-Ardekani and Rashidi, 2009). In addition, compliance to iron supplementation in pregnancy is generally inadequate with only 49.7% women taking supplements continuously in the second and third trimesters (Habib et al., 2009).

More recently, studies have shown that lower dose iron supplements containing in the region of 30 mg/day can protect against iron-deficiency anaemia (in pregnancy and infancy) without yielding unfavourable side effects (Rioux and LeBlanc, 2007). RCTs have shown that supplementation with 40 mg/day (from mid-pregnancy to 8 weeks after birth) prevents iron-deficiency anaemia without causing gastrointestinal symptoms associated with higher intakes (Milman et al., 2005; Zhou et al., 2009). It is recommended that iron supplements are taken between meals or at bedtime to promote absorption (Milman, 2006b).

4.9 Folic acid versus folate

Synthetic folic acid is comprised of three parts: (1) a pteridine ring, (2) para-aminobenzoic acid (PABA) and (3) glutamic acid (Figure 4.7), all of which are needed for vitamin activity. Folic acid may also be referred to as pteroylglutamate or pteroylmonoglutamate (Gropper et al., 2009).

Folate from foods exists mainly in the form of methyl-tetrahydrofolate (methyl-THF). Metabolically, these two forms of folic acid (synthetic versus natural folates) follow slightly different metabolic pathways. Folic acid lacks coenzyme activity and must first be reduced to the metabolically active form of tetrahydrofolate. Dietary folate, however, is naturally consumed in a more readily available form that does not

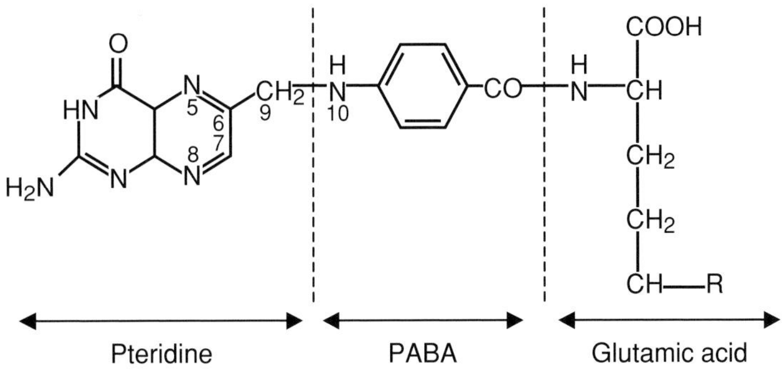

Figure 4.7 Structure of folic acid. (Adapted from Tamura and Picciano (2006), *American Journal of Clinical Nutrition,* with permission.)

need to be reduced. Although foods are a good source of folate, they do not necessarily provide the proportions needed for maternal and foetal health. Bioavailability studies have shown that methyl-THF when ingested in supplement form is as bioavailable as folic acid and is less likely to mask haematological symptoms of vitamin B_{12} deficiency (Pietrzik *et al.,* 2010).

Folic Acid or Folate?

The term 'folate' is a broad term referring to both natural and synthetic forms of the vitamin. However, officially, the term folate should only be used when the B vitamin is naturally present in food sources. The term 'folic acid' should be used when referring to supplement and fortified food sources containing the synthetic form of the vitamin (Bailey, 2000).

4.9.1 Folate metabolism

Folate plays a key role in several metabolic pathways during pregnancy, including those leading to DNA and RNA synthesis (Patterson, 2008). Folate acts as a coenzyme, facilitating the transfer of carbon to nucleic and amino acids. During periods of rapid cell division, i.e. growth of the foetus and expanding organs in pregnancy, folic acid requirements increase. This is because more folate is needed to facilitate the carbon transfer reactions and support the rapid periods of cell division that are taking place (Tamura and Picciano, 2006).

For women, folate reserves are only small. Around 10 mg is stored in the liver, which is usually used within 2–3 months (Roach and Benyon, 2004). Although there do not appear to be any formal guidelines advising women to take folic acid 3 months prior to pregnancy, from a storage perspective, women would benefit as this would help to top up their liver reserves before proceeding into pregnancy.

With regard to rates of folate turnover in pregnancy, scientists have observed that this increases in pregnancy, reaching a peak in the third trimester – when foetal growth is highest (Higgins *et al.,* 2000). It is well established that folate deficiency in early pregnancy can lead to the development of neural tube defects (NTDs), but women may also experience megaloblastic anaemia – the formation of large immature cells in pregnancy, mostly in cells that divide rapidly, i.e. red blood cells (Chandra, 2010). It therefore appears that women's folate requirements may be higher throughout the course of pregnancy, not just for the first 12 weeks. However, this is an area that is open to much debate and needs to be considered by future policy makers.

Folate/Folic Acid and Vitamin B_{12}

Metabolically, vitamin B_{12} is also needed to regulate folic acid metabolism, helping to reform tetrahydrofolate. Even if women eat plenty of folate from their diets if they have vitamin B_{12} deficiency, this can lead to secondary folate deficiency. One concern that scientists have is that folic acid, particularly from fortified foods, can mask vitamin B_{12} deficiency. Individuals most at risk of vitamin B_{12} deficiency include strict vegetarians and vegans and individuals with malabsorption problems, particularly in the elderly and *Helicobacter pylori* infection (Allen, 2008).

For women, both folate and vitamin B_{12} deficiencies can both have implications for foetal, infant and child health. Research shows that vitamin B_{12} deficiency can also increase the risk of birth defects such as NTDs and preterm deliveries although the implications of starting pregnancy with low vitamin B_{12} status is not as well researched as for other nutrients (Molloy *et al.*, 2008). In Canada, scientists have found a threefold increase in the risk of NTDs amongst mothers who have the lowest vitamin B_{12} reserves. Scientists concluded that combined fortification of foods with both folic acid and vitamin B_{12} may be a good way forward in the future (Thompson *et al.*, 2009). However, large multicenter RCTs are warranted.

4.9.2   Folate transfer to the foetus

There is not a lot of published information discussing the placental transfer of folate. Henderson et al. (1995) reported that methyl-THR, the main form of folate, found in the plasma probably binds to placenta folate receptors and then transfers folate against a concentration gradient, slowly and bidirectionally. Maternal folate status needs to be maintained at a certain threshold to ensure that plasma folate levels are high enough to ensure there can be a concentration gradient for placental transfer.

Research Highlight   Folic acid supplementation may have benefits for maternal and foetal bone turnover

A recent study has investigated whether daily folic acid supplementation in pregnancy can influence biochemical markers of bone turnover.

Scientists recruited over 100 pregnant women and randomly allocated them to two groups. In one group, women took 1 mg folic acid from the beginning of pregnancy until the end of the second trimester and the other group continued taking their daily supplement until the end of pregnancy. Groups were carefully controlled and matched and venous blood samples were taken from the mothers and umbilical cords of the newborns and then analysed for markers of bone turnover.

Results showed that daily supplementation of 1 mg folic acid had a positive impact on markers of bone turnover, particularly osteocalcin – one marker of bone formation. Findings were even more prominent when folic acid supplements were taken for the whole of pregnancy (Hossein-Nezhad *et al.*, 2010). These findings show that folic acid could have an additional role to play in pregnancy. Additional trials are now needed to establish whether these findings could be repeated.

4.10 Conclusion

In conclusion, metabolic adaptations during pregnancy are essential to ensure that the foetus grows and develops adequately. Ultimately, the foetus needs to accumulate energy stores and nutrients that are needed after birth. When metabolic pathways break down, this can have health consequences for the offspring, as scientists have seen over the last half a century with folate deficiencies and the development of NTDs. Careful dietary manipulation may help to regulate metabolic pathways and go some way towards preventing medical complications such as gestational diabetes, which are becoming an increasing occurrence in pregnancy. Health professionals are now becoming increasingly aware that dietary interventions may play a key role in the management and prevent of such metabolic disorders.

Key Messages

- Measuring energy expenditure in pregnancy poses many challenges. More follow-through studies are now needed to determine the energy needs of all three trimesters.
- In terms of carbohydrate metabolism, pregnant mothers are more sensitive to the effects of insulin in early pregnancy, but this is replaced with insulin resistance in late pregnancy. For some mothers, this may increase their chances of developing diabetes in pregnancy.
- Unlike carbohydrate and fat metabolism, protein reserves in early pregnancy are not stored for later use. Instead, metabolic pathways are adjusted to utilise protein when it is needed, increasing synthesis and decreasing excretion.
- Calcium is needed for the development of the foetal skeleton, particularly in the third trimester. Using a combination of calcitropic hormones (calcitriol, CT and PTH) regulate calcium metabolism in pregnancy.
- Research suggests that low dose iron supplements (around 30 mg/day; Rioux and LeBlanc, 2007) may help to prevent iron deficiency in pregnancy without contributing to unfavourable side effects.
- Higher rates of cell division (foetal and in the uterus and placenta) means that folate requirements are higher in pregnancy. As folate is needed in metabolic pathways involved in DNA synthesis, deficiencies may result in birth defects and megablastic anaemia, hence the need for folic acid supplementation.
- Overall, it is important that the body adjusts metabolically throughout pregnancy to ensure the foetus grows and develops appropriately and has enough energy and nutrients stores for the first few months of life.

Recommended reading

Hadden DR and McLaughlin C (2009) Normal and abnormal maternal metabolism in pregnancy. *Seminars in Fetal and Neonatal Medicine* **14**, 66–71.

Homko CJ, Sivan E, Reece EA and Boden G (1999) Fuel metabolism during pregnancy. *Seminars in Reproductive Endocrinology* **17**(2), 119–25.

Lain KY and Catalano PM (2007) Metabolic changes in pregnancy. *Clinical Obstetrics and Gynaecology* **50**(4), 938–48.

SACN (2009) *SACN Energy Requirements Working Group Draft Report*. The Stationery Office: London.

References

Afkhami-Ardekani M and Rashidi M (2009) Iron status in women and without gestational diabetes mellitus. *Journal of Diabetes and Its Complications* **23**(3), 194–8.

Albright F and Reifenstein EC (1948) *Parathyroid glands and metabolic bone disease*. Williams & Wilkins: Baltimore.

Allen LH (2008) Causes of vitamin B_{12} and folate deficiency. *Food and Nutrition Bulletin* **29**(2 Suppl), S20–34.

Avendaño-Badillo D, Hernández-Avila M, Hernández-Cadena L *et al.* (2009) High dietary calcium intake decreases bone mobilization during pregnancy in humans. *Salud Pública de México* **51**(1), S100–7.

Bailey LB (2000) New standard for dietary folate intake in pregnant women. *American Journal of Clinical Nutrition* **71**(5 Suppl), 1304S–7S.

Barrett H and McElduff A (2010) Vitamin D and pregnancy: an old problem revisited. *Best Practice & Research Clinical Endocrinology & Metabolism* **24**(4), 527–39.

Bradley CS, Kennedy CM, Turcea AM, Rao SS and Nygaard IE (2007) Constipation in pregnancy: prevalence, symptoms, and risk factors. *Obstetrics & Gynecology* **110**(6), 1351–7.

Bronstein MN, Mak RP and King JC (1995) The thermic effect of food in normal-weight and overweight pregnant women. *British Journal of Nutrition* **74**(2), 261–75.

Butte NF (2000) Carbohydrate and lipid metabolism in pregnancy: normal compared with gestational diabetes mellitus. *American Journal of Clinical Nutrition* **71**(5 Suppl), 1256S–61S.

Butte NF and King JC (2005) Energy requirements during pregnancy and lactation. *Public Health Nutrition* **8**(7A), 1010–27.

Cavill I, Auerbach M, Bailie GR *et al.* (2006) Iron and the anaemia of chronic disease: a review and strategic recommendations. *Current Medical & Research Opinion* **22**(4), 731–7.

Chandra J (2010) Megaloblastic anemia: back in focus. *Indian Journal of Pediatrics* **77**(7), 795–9.

Cleal JK and Lewis RM (2008) The mechanisms and regulation of placental amino acid transport to the human fetus. *Journal of Neuroendocrinology* **20**, 419–26.

Cook JD (2005) Diagnosis and management of iron-deficiency anaemia. *Best Practice & Research Clinical Haematology* **18**(2), 319–32.

Duggleby SL and Jackson AA (2001) Relationship of maternal protein turnover and lean body mass during pregnancy and birth length. *Clinical Science (London)* **101**(1), 65–72.

Duggleby SL and Jackson AA (2002) Higher weight at birth is related to decreased maternal amino acid oxidation during pregnancy. *American Journal of Clinical Nutrition* **76**, 852–7.

Fairweather-Tait SJ (2004) Iron nutrition in the UK: getting the balance right. *Proceedings of the Nutrition Society* **63**, 519–28.

Fernandez-Ballart JD (2000) Iron metabolism during pregnancy. *Clinical Drug Investigation* **19**(1), 9–19.

Forsum E and Lof M (2007) Energy metabolism during human pregnancy. *Annual Review of Nutrition* **27**, 277–92.

Gambling L, Andersen HS and McArdle HJ (2008) Iron and copper, and their interactions during development. *Biochemical Society Transactions* **36**(Pt 6), 1258–61.

Gambling L, Danzeisen R, Gair S *et al.* (2001) Effect of iron deficiency on placental transfer of iron and expression of iron transport proteins in vivo and in vitro. *Biochemical Journal* **356**, 883–9.

Gautam CS, Saha L, Sekhri K and Saha PK (2008) Iron deficiency in pregnancy and the rationality of iron supplements prescribed during pregnancy. *The Medscape Journal of Medicine* **10**(12), 283.

Geelhoed JJ and Jaddoe VW (2010) Early influences on cardiovascular and renal development. *European Journal of Epidemiology* **25**(10), 677–92.

Gibson RS (2005) *Principles of Nutrition Assessment*, 2nd edition. Oxford University Press: Oxford.

Gropper SS, Smith JL and Groff JL (2009) *Advanced Nutrition & Human Metabolism*. Wadsworth: Canada.

Habib F, Alabdin EH, Alenazy M and Noor R (2009) Compliance to iron supplementation during pregnancy. *Journal of Obstetrics & Gynaecology* **29**(6), 487–92.

Halhali A, Díaz L, Avila E, Ariza AC, Garabédian M and Larrea F (2007) Decreased fractional urinary calcium excretion and serum 1,25-dihydroxyvitamin D and IGF-I levels in pre-eclampsia. *The Journal of Steroid Biochemistry & Molecular Biology* **103**(3–5), 803–6.

Harvey LJ, Armah CN, Dainty JR *et al.* (2005) Impact of menstrual blood loss and diet on iron deficiency among women in the UK. *British Journal of Nutrition* **94**, 557–64.

Hay WW Jr (2006a) Placental–fetal glucose exchange and fetal glucose metabolism. *Transactions of the American Clinical & Climatological Association* **117**, 321–40.

Hay WW Jr (2006b) Recent observations on the regulation of fetal metabolism by glucose. *The Journal of Physiology* **572**(Pt 1), 17–24.

Henderson GI, Perez T, Schenker S, Mackins J and Anthony AC (1995) Maternal-to-fetal transfer of 5-methyltetrahydrofolate by the perfused human placental cotyledon: evidence for a concentrative role by placental folate receptors in fetal folate delivery. *The* Journal of Laboratory & Clinical Medicine **126**, 184–203.

Herrera E (2002a) Implications of dietary fatty acids during pregnancy on placental, fetal and postnatal development – a review. *Placenta* **23**(Suppl A), S9–19.

Herrera E (2002b) Lipid metabolism in pregnancy and its consequences in the fetus and newborn. *Endocrine* **19**(1), 43–55.

Herrera E, Amusquivar E, López-Soldado I and Ortega H (2006) Maternal lipid metabolism and placental lipid transfer. *Hormone Research* **65**(Suppl 3), 59–64.

Herrera E and Ortega-Senovilla H (2010) Disturbances in lipid metabolism in diabetic pregnancy – are these the cause of the problem? *Best Practice & Research Clinical Endocrinology & Metabolism* **24**, 515–25.

Higgins JR, Quinlivan EP, McPartlin J, Scott JM, Weir DG and Darling MR (2000) The relationship between increased folate catabolism and the increased requirement for folate in pregnancy. *British Journal of Obstetrics & Gynaecology* **107**(9), 1149–54.

Hossein-Nezhad A, Mirzaei K, Maghbooli Z, Najmafshar A and Larijani B (2010) The influence of folic acid supplementation on maternal and fetal bone turnover. *Journal of Bone & Mineral Metabolism.* [Epub ahead of print.]

Husain F, Latif SA and Uddin MM (2009) Studies on serum triacylglycerol and HDL-cholesterol in second and third trimester of pregnancy. *Mymensingh Medical Journal* **18**(1), S6–11.

Husain F, Latif S, Uddin M and Nessa A (2008) Lipid profile changes in second trimester of pregnancy. *Mymensingh Medical Journal* **17**(1), 17–21.

Institute of Medicine (2001) *Dietary Reference Intakes for Vitamin A, Vitamin K, Arsenic, Boron, Chromium, Copper, Iodine, Iron, Manganese, Molybdenum, Nickel, Silicon, Vanadium, and Zinc.* National Academy Press: Washington, DC.

Kalhan SC (2000) Protein metabolism in pregnancy. *American Journal of Clinical Nutrition* **71**(5 S), 1249S–55S.

King JC (2000) Physiology of pregnancy and nutrient metabolism. *American Journal of Clinical Nutrition* **71**(5), 1218S–25S.

Kovacs CS and Kronenberg HM (1997) Maternal–fetal calcium and bone metabolism during pregnancy, puerperium, and lactation. *Endocrine Reviews* **18**(6), 832–72.

Krishnaveni GV, Veena SR, Hill JC, Kehoe S, Karat SC and Fall CH (2010) Intra-uterine exposure to maternal diabetes is associated with higher adiposity and insulin resistance and clustering of cardiovascular risk markers in Indian children. *Diabetes Care* **33**(2), 402–4.

Kumar A, Meena M, Gyaneshwori Devi S, Gupta RK and Batra S (2009) Calcium in midpregnancy. *Archives of Gynaecology & Obstetrics* **279**(3), 315–9.

Lain KY and Catalano PM (2007) Metabolic changes in pregnancy. *Clinical Obstetrics & Gynaecology* **50**(4), 938–48.

Lázaro RM, García JJ and Pié A (2002) Insulin receptor binding to erythrocytes during normal pregnancy: an update of the method. *Analytical & Bioanalytical Chemistry* **372**(1), 148–54.

Levine JA (2005) Measurement of energy expenditure. *Public Health Nutrition* **8**(7A), 1123–32.

Lippi G, Albiero A, Montagnana M *et al.* (2007) Lipid and lipoprotein profile in physiological pregnancy. *Clinical Laboratory* **53**(3–4), 173–7.

Lof M and Forsum E (2006) Activity pattern and energy expenditure due to physical activity before and during pregnancy in healthy Swedish women. *British Journal of Nutrition* **95**(2), 296–302.

Lof M, Olausson H, Bostrom K, Janerot-Sjöberg B, Sohlstrom A and Forsum E (2005) Changes in basal metabolic rate during pregnancy in relation to changes in body weight and composition, cardiac output, insulin-like growth factor I, and thyroid hormones and in relation to fetal growth. *American Journal of Clinical Nutrition* **81**(3), 678–85.

Ma A, Chen X, Zheng M, Wang Y, Xu R and Li J (2002) Iron status and dietary intake of Chinese pregnant women with anemia in the third trimester. *Asia Pacific Journal of Clinical Nutrition* **11**(3), 171–5.

Mann JI and Cummings JH (2009) Possible implications for health of the different definitions of dietary fibre. *Nutrition, Metabolism & Cardiovascular Diseases* **19**, 226–9.

McArdle HJ, Andersen HS, Jones H and Gambling L (2008) Copper and iron transport across the placenta: regulation and interactions. *Journal of Neuroendocrinology* **20**, 427–31.

Milman N (2006a) Iron prophylaxis in pregnancy – general or individual and in which dose? *Annals of Haematology* **85**(12), 821–8.

Milman N (2006b) Iron and pregnancy – a delicate balance. *Annals of Haematology* **85**, 559–65.

Milman N, Bergholt T, Eriksen L *et al.* (2005) Iron prophylaxis during pregnancy – how much iron is needed? A randomised dose-response study of 20–80 mg ferrous iron daily in pregnant women. *Acta Obstetricia et Gynecologica Scandinavica* **84**, 238–47.

Mojtahedi M, de Groot LC, Boekholt HA and van Raaij JM (2002) Nitrogen balance of healthy Dutch women before and during pregnancy. *American Journal of Clinical Nutrition* **75**(6), 1078–83.

Molloy AM, Kirke PN, Brody LC, Scott JM and Mills JL (2008) Effects of folate and vitamin B_{12} deficiencies during pregnancy on fetal, infant, and child development. *Food & Nutrition Bulletin* **29**(2 Suppl), S101–11.

Mor G (2008) Inflammation and pregnancy: the role of toll-like receptors in trophoblast-immune interaction. *Annals of the New York Academy of Sciences* **1127**, 121–8.

Nadal A, Alonso-Magdalena P, Soriano S, Ropero AB and Quesada I (2009) The role of oestrogens in the adaptation of islets to insulin resistance. *Journal of Physiology* **587**(Pt 21), 5031–7.

Patterson D (2008) Folate metabolism and the risk of Down syndrome. *Down Syndrome Research and Practice* **12**(2), 93–6.

Pietrzik K, Bailey L and Shane B (2010) Folic acid and L-5-methyltetrahydrofolate: comparison of clinical pharmacokinetics and pharmacodynamics. *Clinical Pharmacokinetics* **49**(8), 535–48.

Rioux FM and LeBlanc CP (2007) Iron supplementation during pregnancy: what are the risks and benefits of current practices? *Applied Physiology, Nutrition & Metabolsim* **32**(2), 282–8.

Ritterath C, Rad NT, Siegmund T, Heinze T, Siebert G and Buhling KJ (2009) Adiponectin during pregnancy: correlation with fat metabolism, but not with carbohydrate metabolism. *Archives of Gynaecology & Obstetrics* **281**, 91–6.

Roach J and Benyon S (2004) *Metabolism & Nutrition*. Mosby: London.

Rusia U, Flowers C, Madan N, Agarwal N, Sood SK and Sikka M (1999) Serum transferring receptors in detection of iron deficiency in pregnancy. *Annals of Haematology* **78**, 358–63.

SACN (Scientific Advisory Committee on Nutrition) (2007) *Update on Vitamin D: Position Statement by the Scientific Advisory Committee on Nutrition*. The Stationery Office: London.

SACN (2009) *SACN Energy Requirements Working Group Draft Report*. The Stationery Office: London.

Sathyapalan T, Mellor D and Atkin SL (2010) Obesity and gestational diabetes. *Seminars in Fetal & Neonatal Medicine* **15**(2), 89–93.

Scholl TO (2005) Iron status during pregnancy: setting the stage for mother and infant. *American Journal of Clinical Nutrition* **81**, 1218S22S.

Sidebottom AC, Brown JE and Jacobs DR Jr (2001) Pregnancy-related changes in body fat. *European Journal of Obstetrics & Gynaecology and Reproductive Biology* **94**(2), 216–23.

Tamura T and Picciano MF (2006) Folate and human reproduction. *American Journal of Clinical Nutrition* **83**, 993–1016.

Thandrayen K and Pettifor JM (2010) Maternal vitamin D status: implications for the development of infantile nutritional rickets. *Endocrinology Metabolism Clinics of North America* **39**(2), 303–20.

Thompson MD, Cole DE and Ray JG (2009) Vitamin B-12 and neural tube defects: the Canadian experience. *American Journal of Clinical Nutrition* **89**(2), 697S–701S.

Trayhurn P (2005) Endocrine and signalling role of adipose tissue: new perspectives on fat. *Acta Physiologica Scandinavica* **184**(4), 285–93.

van den Broek NR, Letsky EA, White SA and Shenkin A (1998) Iron status in pregnant women: which measurements are valid? *British Journal of Haematology* **103**(3), 817–24.

Ward KA, Adams JE and Mughal MZ (2005) Bone status during adolescence, pregnancy and lactation. *Current Opinion in Obstetrics & Gynaecology* **17**(4), 435–9.

Wish JB (2006) Assessing iron status: beyond serum ferritin and transferrin saturation. *Clinical Journal of the American Society of Nephrology* **1**, S4–8.

Zhou SJ, Gibson RA, Crowther CA and Makrides M (2009) Should we lower the dose of iron when treating anaemia in pregnancy? A randomised-dose response trial. *European Journal of Clinical Nutrition* **63**(2), 183–90.

Zimmermann MB (2008) Methods to assess iron and iodine status. *British Journal of Nutrition* **99**(3), S2–9.

5 Macronutrients and Pregnancy

Summary

During pregnancy, the body adapts to provide a favourable environment for the developing child, modifying the nutritional needs of the mother. Scientific bodies advise that energy intakes only need to be amended in the third trimester of pregnancy although further work is needed to determine whether overweight/obese women should apply an extra energy increment. For macronutrients, the proportions of carbohydrate, fat and protein required for pregnancy are set at levels that are largely the same as non-pregnant women. The importance of some macronutrients, however, needs further investigation, i.e. whether low glycaemic index (GI) carbohydrates can help to improve pregnancy outcomes, particularly in the case of women who have already delivered large infants. Equally, dietary recommendations for omega-3 intakes in pregnancy have only recently been established by some organisations and now need to be communicated to health practitioners and public sectors. This chapter aims to discuss the potential roles of macronutrients in pregnancy and describe current guidelines, where these are available. Factors affecting food choices and dietary intakes will also be considered.

Learning Outcomes

- To describe why macronutrients are needed in pregnancy, the proportions in which they are needed and how this can be achieved.
- To evaluate the latest research linking macronutrient intakes to maternal, foetal and infant well-being.
- To explain how dietary intakes and diet quality may be assessed in pregnancy and discuss how social and behavioural factors can affect these.

5.1 Introduction

In Western settings, studies have shown links between the balance of macronutrients in women's diets and the size of newborns. Timing appears to play a critical role

Nutrition in the Childbearing Years, First Edition. Emma Derbyshire.
© 2011 Emma Derbyshire. Published 2011 by Blackwell Publishing Ltd.

in this – scientists believe there are critical windows in pregnancy during which maternal diets are particularly important (Moore and Davies, 2005). One example of this is the balance of energy and protein in women's diets. Evidence from past studies has shown that balanced energy and protein supplementation seems to help improve foetal growth and reduce the risk of foetal/neonatal death. However, high-protein diets alone and energy/protein restriction in overweight and obese mothers have been found to have no benefits on pregnancy outcome and could actually be harmful to infant's health (Kramer and Kakuma, 2003).

This chapter aims to further discuss the role of macronutrients in pregnancy, particularly in relation to maternal, foetal and infant health. The latest guidelines will be reviewed and suggestions given on how these can be applied in practice. Factors influencing dietary quality and food choices and methods used to assess dietary intakes will also be covered.

5.2 Food cravings and aversions

Around 61% pregnant women experience food cravings and 54% aversions at some point in pregnancy (Bayley *et al.*, 2002). The causes of food cravings are multi-faceted, but cravings for specific macronutrients, such as carbohydrate, have been linked to a physiological need to alter neurotransmitters (Yanovski, 2003). Latva-Pukkila *et al.* (2010) reported that carbohydrate intakes were higher in women experiencing nausea and vomiting in pregnancy (NVP) when compared to women without these symptoms, but more work is needed to underpin the reasons why this may be.

Food aversions are usually triggered by changes in the way food tastes and smells in pregnancy. Examples of foods that are commonly avoided in pregnancy include certain vegetables, meats, eggs, spicy foods, coffee and other stimulants (Pepper and Roberts, 2006). In a recent study, 65% women developed aversions to caffeine with intakes declining from 96 to 36 mg/day between weeks 4 and 6 of pregnancy (Christian and Brent, 2001). There are two main theories behind the symptoms of NVP in pregnancy (Table 5.1), but the prophylaxis hypotheses corresponds best with the timing of NVP and patterns of food cravings and aversions (Flaxman and Sherman, 2008).

Table 5.1 Theories behind NVP.

Theory	Explanation
The 'prophylaxis' or 'maternal and embryo protection hypothesis'	Suggests that NVP serves a beneficial function by expelling foods that may contain harmful toxins and microorganisms, triggering aversions to such foods throughout pregnancy
The 'by-product' hypothesis	Suggests that the pregnant women and the embryo are competing for nutrient reserves, resulting in food aversions and cravings

Source: Flaxman and Sherman (2008).

Research Highlight   Diabetes in pregnancy increases cravings for sweet foods

New research has shown that women with diabetes in the later stages of pregnancy (34–38 weeks) are twice as likely to crave and consume sweet foods when compared to women without diabetes (Belzer *et al.*, 2010). Scientists used food frequency questionnaires and craving surveys to determine women's food preferences during and after pregnancy and in non-pregnant controls.

Results showed that most women experienced a degree of sweet cravings in the middle of pregnancy, at around 24–28 weeks. However, women with gestational diabetes were twice as likely to experience sweet cravings on a weekly basis (12.1 versus 5.9 cravings on average a week) when compared to women with normal glucose tolerance. Women reporting more sweet cravings also had higher intakes of sweet foods and beverages. These are interesting results and show that sweet cravings may be a feature of diabetes later in pregnancy.

5.3   Energy

The total energy costs of pregnancy have been calculated to be around 80,000 kcal (from after conception to delivery). This is based on an average pregnancy weight gain of 12.5 kg (about 0.9 kg protein, 3.8 kg fat and 7.8 kg water) (Hytten and Chamberlain, 1991). These energy costs should cover the expansion of maternal and foetal tissues and rise in basal metabolism rate.

Amongst health and medical practitioners, questions have been raised about whether women need to alter their energy intakes at all in pregnancy, especially in the case of overweight/obese women. Consuming extra calories when women do not need it may be linked to permanent, long-term weight retention (Mamun *et al.*, 2010).

5.3.1   Intakes

Murphy and Abram (1993) were some of the first scientists to monitor energy intake changes in American pregnant women. These scientists found that women were well below energy recommendations both during pregnancy and when breastfeeding after birth, although these may have previously been set too high. More recently, German scientists analysed energy intakes from 32 women completing weighed food record logs at 16, 22, 30 and 36 weeks into pregnancy and 6 weeks after birth. The team of researchers found that energy and macronutrient intakes were quite similar at each of the phases of pregnancy (only carbohydrate decreased after birth) (Talai Rad *et al.*, 2009). Scientists concluded that all women had healthy babies without changing their macronutrient profile in pregnancy.

On a final note, when interpreting findings from studies that have measured energy and nutrient intakes using dietary assessment methods, it is important to consider that under-reporting can have a considerable impact on the quality of dietary data, i.e. individuals may not recall all the foods/beverages they consumed, or adapt this to please the study scientist (recall bias). Several new methods have now been compiled

Table 5.2 Accounting for under-reporting. Several methods can be used when analysing and collecting data to help account and control for under-reporting.

Method	What is it?	Reference(s)
EI: BMR ratio	EI divided by BMR*. Goldberg has derived cutoffs of 1.35 and 1.06. Ratios below these values can indicate under-reporting.	Goldberg *et al.* (1991), Prentice *et al.* (1996), Schofield *et al.* (1985)
Energy adjustment	Data could be adjusted, i.e. energy intake increased by 15%, to account for the degree to which under-reporting normally occurs.	Poslusna *et al.* (2009).
Nutrient density method	When total nutrient intakes are divided by total EI to adjust for different energy intakes.	Mirmiran (2006)
Body weight changes	In non-pregnant women, changes in body weight from the start to the end of a study can be used to monitor under-reporting.	Poslusna *et al.* (2009).

EI, energy intake; BMR, basal metabolic rate; W, weight (kg).
*For pregnant women, BMR can be calculated using traditional Schofield equations (age 10–17 years, BMR $=13.4 \times W + 692$; 18–29 years, BMR $=14.8 \times W + 487$; 30–59 years, BMR $= 8.3 \times W + 846$) and increments for pregnancy. Prentice *et al.* (1996) has reported that increments of 0.2, 0.4 and 1.1 MJ can be added to the pre-pregnancy BMR for the first, second and third trimesters respectively to derive rates of BMR at these stages.

to help scientists account for under-reporting in their studies (Table 5.2). Applying these methods will help the scientists to compile a more accurate picture of what women are really eating.

Research Highlight   Are energy intakes 10% higher in women having boys?

Birth weight data across populations has shown that baby boys are generally 100 g heavier than girls. An earlier study carried out by Tamimi *et al.* (2003) investigated whether this was because women carrying boys had higher energy intakes, or just utilised energy more efficiently than women carrying girls.

After studying birth weight data and food frequency questionnaires, scientists found that pregnant women carrying boys had energy intakes on average 10% higher than those carrying girls. Scientists concluded that women carrying boys rather than girls may have higher energy requirements and that male embryos could be more susceptible to the effects of energy restriction. Another theory put forward was that testosterone secreted by the male foetus may induce a signal that increases women's energy intakes.

Although these findings were at the time very topical and interesting, similar findings have not been replicated since. It is possible that the relationship observed in this study occurred by chance. This is a good example of how evidence from epidemiological studies should always be thoroughly evaluated before firm conclusions are made and additional research recommendations made.

Table 5.3 Energy requirements in pregnancy.

Age category	Estimated average required (kcal/day)			
	Non-pregnant (DH, 1991)	First trimester	Second trimester	Third trimester (SACN, 2009)
15–18 years	2110	No change	No change	+180
19–50 years	1940	No change	No change	+180

Energy intakes do not need to change in the first half of pregnancy.

For women living in industrialised regions, energy intakes should be increased by around 180 kcals/day in the third trimester (SACN, 2009).

For teenagers (15–18 years), energy requirements need to meet the combined effects of growth and pregnancy (i.e. 2110 kcal/day + 180 kcals/day in the third trimester) (DH, 1991).

Energy intakes beyond the needs of pregnancy may contribute to high gestational weight gain.

5.3.2   Guidelines

As more women are now entering pregnancy with body weights that exceed healthy ranges, Scientific Advisory Committee on Nutrition (SACN, 2009) consider it unlikely that women require additional energy in the first half of pregnancy. An additional intake of around 0.8 MJ/day (180 kcal/day) is advised in the third trimester, but it remains to be determined whether this is needed by all women. While this is a useful guide, it is important to consider that energy requirements are not the same for every pregnant woman. For example, pregnant teenagers need to meet the energy requirements imposed by both growth and pregnancy (Table 5.3).

5.4   Carbohydrate

The type of carbohydrate eaten in pregnancy can influence the growth of the foetus, placenta and level of weight gained in pregnancy (Clapp, 2003). For example, findings from the Australian Carbohydrate Intolerance Study (ACHOIS) showed that women eating foods with a high GI in pregnancy were more likely to have high blood sugar levels (hyperglycaemia) and experience shoulder dystocia during delivery (when the infants' shoulder becomes lodged during delivery) (Athukorala *et al.*, 2007).

In another major study, scientists are going to test whether low GI diets can help to improve the birth weight of infants born to mothers who have previously given birth to exceptionally large infants (sometimes referred to as macrosomia) (Walsh *et al.*, 2010). Women giving birth for a second time will be randomised to receive either a low GI carbohydrate diet or resume their normal diets (no intervention). Patients will then be followed up after birth and the number of large birth weight infants compared between groups. This will be a valuable study as high-GI diets have been linked to elevated maternal blood glucose levels and the delivery of large infants (McGowan and McAuliffe, 2010).

5.4.1   GI or load?

GI is normally represented as a numerical scale ranging from 0 to 100, measuring how quickly carbohydrates from foods are converted into blood sugars (glucose).

GL = GI × Amount of carbohydrate available in food (g)/100.

Example: A 90 g muffin with a GI of 50 and carbohydrate content of 50.7 g (52.3 g total carbohydrate −1.6 g dietary fibre)

= 90 × 50.7/100 = 46

The GL is therefore 46.

Figure 5.1 Calculating GL from GI data.

This scale is rather useful when studies set out to see how high and low GI diets can affect health (Esfahani *et al.*, 2009). Generally, the GI of foods is measured by calculating the area under a blood glucose response curve (Brouns *et al.*, 2005). This is usually done when a small sample of least 10 test subjects are given 50 g of a test food. Blood samples are then taken over a 2-hour time period (usually every 15 minutes) to determine how rapidly the food is converted into glucose in the bloodstream. This response is then compared against the reference food (glucose) and averaged out for the 10 test subjects. So, if the GI of cornflakes is 93, this means that eating 50 g of these produce a rise in blood sugar which is 93% as great as that produced eating the same amount of glucose, i.e. this is a high-GI food.

More recently, the glycaemic load (GL) has been developed, which also considers serving size, giving a fuller picture of the effect foods have on blood sugar levels. GL can be calculated by multiplying the GI by the amount of carbohydrate available in a food (excluding dietary fibre) and dividing by 100 (see Figure 5.1). Some examples of high and low GI/GL foods are included in Table 5.4.

Table 5.4 GI and GL values – tested in subjects with normal glucose tolerance.

Food	Serving size	GI (glucose =100%)	GL (per serving)
All-bran	30 g	38	8
Apple, raw	120 g	40	6
Baked potato	130 g	69	19
Banana, ripe	120 g	51	13
Basmati rice, boiled	150	43	18
Blueberry muffin	60 g	50	15
Cornflakes	30 g	93	23
Couscous	150 g	65	9
French baguette	30 g	57	10
Instant porridge	250 g	83	30
Muesli	30 g	67	14
Rye bread	30 g	50	7
Special K, Kellogg's	30 g	69	14
Sweetcorn, boiled	80 g	48	8
Yakult yoghurt drink	65 ml	36	3
Yoghurt, regular	200 g	36	3
Categorising GI: <55 = low, 56–69 = medium, >70 = high			
Categorising GL: <10 = low, 11–19 = medium, >20 = high			

Source: Data extracted from Mendosa (2008).

5.4.2   Guidelines

The European Food Safety Authority (EFSA, 2010a) has recently published new reference intake (RI) ranges for carbohydrates. The authority advises that adult's carbohydrate intakes should form around 45–60% of daily energy intake. Compared with UK dietary reference values set at 50% of daily energy intake (DH, 1991), the RIs allow some flexibility between individuals and population groups. Specific carbohydrate guidelines have not yet been developed for pregnant women, but this may be possible in the future as new evidence starts to emerge.

5.5   Sugar

Like any other phase of the life cycle, sugar intakes should continue to be monitored in pregnancy. Although one serving of a sugar-sweetened beverage (SSB) on a daily basis may do no harm, there is some concern that consumption of these beverages may lead to elevated blood sugar levels, extra weight gain in pregnancy and increased risk of developing gestational diabetes when consumed in excess (Moses and Brand-Miller, 2009). In turn, women who develop diabetes in pregnancy have a higher risk of developing blood pressure disorders, such as pre-eclampsia, and are more likely to deliver bigger babies and experience medical complications during delivery (Yogev and Visser, 2009).

5.5.1   Diabetes

The National Institute for Health and Clinical Excellence (NICE) advise that women with diabetes should be aware that good glycaemic control throughout pregnancy can help to improve pregnancy outcomes, reducing the risk of macrosomia, trauma during delivery (to themselves and the baby), induction of labour and caesarean section, hypoglycaemia in the newborns and perinatal death.

Women should be advised to choose, where possible, carbohydrates with a lower GI, lean proteins including oily fish and a balance of polyunsaturated and monounsaturated fats (NICE, 2008).

5.5.2   Gum disease

As mentioned previously in Chapter 3, hormonal changes can mean that pregnant women are more likely to experience dental problems, i.e. bleeding and/or infected gums. In some circumstances, when gums may become inflamed and house bacteria, high sugar intakes may help to feed and fuel the growth of these bacteria. There is some evidence that if women develop gum disease in pregnancy, there is a chance than bacteria could cross the placenta, reaching the foetus and possibly contributing to preterm deliveries (Goldie, 2003). Although the risk of this is minimal, women should adopt healthy dental routines and monitor their sugar intakes to ensure these are not too high.

5.5.3   Intakes

Sugar intakes should be monitored when planning a pregnancy. An American study of 13,475 women found that weekly consumption of 5 or more servings of SSB increased the risk of gestational diabetes by 22% (Chen *et al.*, 2009). In addition, it has been suggested that women eating high sugar diets with high body mass index may have an increased risk of neural tube defect-affected pregnancies (Shaw *et al.*, 2003). It is, however, possible that these women have a poor diet quality overall and lower intake of dietary folate. More research is now needed in the form of carefully controlled studies to see why these findings may have occurred.

5.5.4   Guidelines

As discussed above, it is well known that frequent consumption of sugary foods can increase the risk of dental caries. Equally, regular consumption of SSB may contribute to excess weight gain and there is some evidence that diets rich in added sugars may have a lower overall micronutrient density. Present data, however, is not sufficient to warrant the compilation of an upper limit intake, but some European authorities advise that individual intakes of added sugars should be less than 10% of daily energy intakes (EFSA, 2010a).

5.6   Protein

Protein is needed in pregnancy for the development of the growing child. It is needed for physical growth and cellular development of the baby as well the expansion of the placenta and maternal tissues. Extra protein is also needed to support the formation of new red blood cells and circulating proteins, especially as women's blood volume increases in pregnancy.

In particular, women should make sure that they are eating foods that provide essential amino acids (those that cannot be manufactured by the body). This includes foods such as lean meat, chicken, oily fish and dairy products. Protein is also found in whole grains and vegetables and whilst these are not high in protein, they can help contribute to total daily protein intakes.

5.6.1   Intakes

Ideally, diets should contain adequate but not excessive levels of protein. Although a certain level of protein is needed in pregnancy, high intakes in pregnancy may lead to unfavourable pregnancy outcomes. For example, one study has shown that women who consumed high-protein diets in pregnancy and delivered large infants had children with a lower ponderal index (Andreasyan *et al.*, 2007). As the ponderal index is a measure of lean body mass, the results from this study imply that high protein diets may lead to changes in infant body composition.

Equally, scientists have also followed up women who ate high-meat, low-carbohydrate diets over 30 years ago. Researchers found that women who ate more meat and fish in the second half of pregnancy had offspring with a higher systolic blood pressure in adulthood (Shiell *et al.*, 2001). Authors concluded that high-protein

Table 5.5 Some good sources of protein.

Food	Weight (g)	Protein content per portion (g)
Turkey, cooked	140	41.1
Fish, tuna salad	205	32.9
Cheese, cottage, low fat, 1% milk fat	226	28.0
Soybeans, green, cooked, boiled and drained	180	22.2
Beef, minced, 75% lean, cooked	85	21.7
Lentils, cooked, boiled, without salt	198	17.9
Beans, red kidney, boiled, without salt	177	15.4
Yoghurt, plain, low fat	227	11.9
Chickpeas, canned	240	11.9
Egg, whole, cooked, hard boiled	50	6.29
Sunflower seeds, dry, roasted	28	5.48

Source: USDA database (2010).

diets may induce a state of metabolic stress that could affect the long-term health of the offspring. It is, however, difficult to draw firm conclusions as more research is needed to understand why these study findings may have occurred.

5.6.2   Guidelines

Throughout the course of pregnancy, it has been advised that women eat around 51 g of protein each day (DH, 1991). Some foods that are good sources of protein have been included in Table 5.5. Vegetarian and vegan mothers, in particular, should make sure they are consuming enough foods that provide protein throughout their pregnancies. Pulses, seeds, soy products (tofu, textured soy protein and milk), cereals, free-range eggs and some dairy products are good examples of protein sources that can be consumed by vegetarian and vegan mothers.

Research Highlight   Does pregnancy macronutrient intakes predict offspring dietary habits 10 years later?

Using data from the Avon Longitudinal Study of Parents and Children (ALSPAC), scientists have assessed the dietary habits of over 5000 mother–child pairs and determined whether the dietary habits of women during and after pregnancy can influence the eating habits and body composition of their offspring later in life.

Dietary intakes of energy, protein, fat and carbohydrate were assessed using a food frequency questionnaire carried out 32 weeks into pregnancy and 47 months after birth. After 10 years, the diet of the offspring was measured using three 1-day food diaries (unweighted) and body composition was measured using dual-energy X-ray absorptiometry (DEXA) scanning.

After adjusting for energy, maternal intakes of fat, protein and carbohydrate in pregnancy correlated positively with the children's intakes 10 years later. Although there was no relationship between the mother's diets and adiposity in children, children with higher energy and macronutrient intakes had larger fat stores. The findings from this study suggest that the mother's diet may affect the child's diet in one of two ways: (1) by affecting the children's eating habits directly (children's dietary habits are more closely related to the mother's rather than the father's diet) or (2) by programming the offspring's appetite *in utero* by dietary habits in pregnancy. More work is needed to reinforce these theories (Brion *et al.*, 2010).

5.7 Fat

Dietary fat in pregnancy can affect pregnancy outcome, child growth, development and the short-term and long-term health of the offspring (Koletzko *et al.*, 2007). In particular, intakes of long-chain (LC) omega-3 (*n*-3) polyunsaturated fatty acids (PUFA) are important in pregnancy as these are needed to support optimal visual and cognitive development of the foetus (Koletzko *et al.*, 2008). The foetus is dependent on the maternal supply of LC *n*-3 PUFAs as it has a limited metabolic capacity to metabolise PUFAs to LC fatty acids (Singh, 2005). In particular, foetal demands for these fatty acids are highest in the third trimester when the brain is growing and accruing fat most rapidly (Cetin *et al.*, 2009).

5.7.1 Essential fatty acids

LC *n*-3 PUFAs are often referred to as 'essential fatty acids'. This is because they need to be obtained from food sources and cannot be manufactured inside the body itself (Greenberg *et al.*, 2008). Metabolically, alpha-linolenic acid (ALA) forms the foundation of the omega-3 pathway and can be converted into longer chain fatty acids, including eicosapentaenoic acid (EPA), docosapentaenoic acid (DPA) and docosahexaenoic acid (DHA). EPA, DPA and DHA are the end-products of the omega-3 pathway but are generally not synthesised in the proportions needed for good health (Doughman *et al.*, 2007). It is also important to consider that omega-6 fatty acids compete for the same enzymes involved in these pathways (Russo, 2008). This means that an excess of *n*-6 fats in the diet can inhibit the conversion of ALA to DPA, EPA and DHA (Surette, 2008). As the metabolic conversion of the essential *n*-3 fatty acids is generally insufficient, these need to be obtained from dietary and/or supplement sources.

5.7.2 Fat/trans fats intakes

Dietary intakes of fat during pregnancy are generally the same as that recommended for the general population (Koletzko *et al.*, 2007). Some evidence from animal studies using pregnant mice has found that high-fat diets up-regulate the transport of glucose (by fivefold) and amino acids (by tenfold) across the placenta, leading to foetal overgrowth and obesity (Jones *et al.*, 2009). Higher intakes of trans fatty acids in pregnancy have also been linked to reduced foetal growth and impaired development. It is thought that trans fatty acids can interfere with the metabolism of the essential *n*-3 fatty acids leading to lower levels of DHA, which is crucial for foetal brain development (Innis, 2006). Taken together, the findings from these important papers indicate that more work is needed to establish the effects these fatty acids may have on maternal and infant health.

5.7.3 Omega-3 intakes

Only a few surveys have assessed omega-3 intakes in pregnancy and these have mainly been carried out in Canada. Innis and Elias (2003) were some of the first scientists to measure LC *n*-3 PUFA intakes in pregnancy, finding that mean intakes of DHA and EPA were found to be 160 mg/day and 78 mg/day, respectively. Another study by Denomme *et al.* (2005) found that women in their second and third trimesters of pregnancy were ingesting a mean intake of 82 mg DHA/day and 90% were consuming less than 300 mg/day, and Sontrop *et al.* (2008) reported similar figures – mean EPA and DHA intakes were 85 mg/day between weeks 10 and 22 of pregnancy. There is also some evidence that ethnic-related differences in maternal omega-3 and -6 status in pregnancy due to different levels of fish consumption may lead to ethnic disparities in terms of birth outcomes (van Eijsden *et al.*, 2009), but more work is clearly needed to study this further. In essence, women appear to be getting some omega-3 fatty acids from their diets, but dietary guidelines seem to be set at much higher levels than current habitual intakes.

5.7.4 Guidelines

The EFSA recommends that fat intakes should be within a reference range of 20–35% of energy intake and intakes of trans fatty acids should be kept as low as possible (EFSA, 2010b). A summary of guidelines for LC *n*-3 PUFA during pregnancy are included in Table 5.6. As can be seen from this table, there are slight variations between organisations. EFSA (2010b) advise that an extra 100–200 mg preformed DHA should be added during pregnancy and when breastfeeding to compensate for oxidative losses of DHA in pregnancy and accumulation of DHA in the foetus/infant. On the basis of evidence from randomised clinical trials, Koletzko *et al.* (2007) have reported that intakes of up to 1 g/day DHA or 2.7 g/day *n*-3 LC PUFA have been found to be safe in pregnancy without adverse side effects.

Table 5.6 LC *n*-3 PUFA dietary guidelines for pregnancy.

Reference	How much?
EFSA (2010b)	AI of 250 mg EPA + DHA for adults +100–200 mg preformed DHA during pregnancy and lactation
ISFAAL (2004)	At least 300 mg DHA
Koletzko *et al.* (2007)	At least 200 mg/day DHA

Women can meet recommended intakes of DHA by eating 1–2 portions of fish per week (ideally, one portion should be oily fish). This level of intake rarely exceeds the tolerable intake of environmental contaminants but large predatory fish that may be a source of methylmercury should be avoided (Perinatal Lipid Intake Working Group recommendations, Koletzko *et al.*, 2007).
DHA, docosahexaenoic acid; EFSA, European Food Safety Authority; EPA, eicosapentaenoic acid; ISFAAL, International Society for the Study of Fatty Acids and Lipids.

Awareness of LC Omega-3 PUFA Risks and Benefits

Recently, Australian researchers have shown interest in women's knowledge of omega-3 fatty acids. Over 100 women were recruited from antenatal clinics and asked to complete a 27-item food safety and behaviour questionnaire.

Three-quarters of women did not receive any information about the importance of LC *n*-3 PUFA in pregnancy and only half the women were aware of issues around LC *n*-3 PUFA and health in pregnancy, i.e. knowledge about fish contamination was rather limited. Most women (28%) received information from books and magazines, followed by the family doctor (26%) and midwives (20%). Women generally had low (28%) and moderate (24%) levels of concern about LC *n*-3 PUFA and mercury, respectively (Sinikovic *et al.*, 2009). The findings from this study are important because its findings have highlighted the fact that information about the importance of omega-3 fatty acids needs to be better communicated to general practitioners and other health practitioners so that it can filter down to women having babies.

5.8   Fibre

Increasing fibre intakes in pregnancy may help to reduce weight gain, glucose intolerance, dyslipaemia, pre-eclampsia and symptoms of constipation, but few studies have determined how much fibre is consumed during pregnancy, or how this can affect health status (Buss *et al.*, 2009). It is important to consider that different definitions for dietary fibre are often used, which can make comparisons between studies and food health claims difficult (Mann and Cummings, 2009).

The new Codex definition defines total dietary fibre as 'carbohydrates polymers with ten or more monomeric units, which are not hydrolysed by the endogenous enzymes in the small intestine of humans' (WHO/FAO, 2008). This basically means that dietary fibre takes the form of LC carbohydrates (natural and synthetic) that cannot be broken down by the body. It is hoped that having a new, appropriate definition of dietary fibre can make labelling foods and setting health claims easier. Until this can be done, this makes it very difficult for the public to gauge a feel for 'how much' fibre they are eating.

5.8.1   Englyst or Southgate?

Dietary fibre may also be referred to as 'Englyst' or 'Southgate' fibre depending on the way in which it has been extracted and analysed. The Southgate method was originally developed to measure the non-starch polysaccharide (NSP), resistant starch and lignin (indigestible plant components) content of carbohydrates. Later, the Englyst method was developed from the process and involved the removal of starch from the fibre, hence the term 'non-starch' using acid hydrolysis. Englyst fibre is therefore known as indigestible fibre, or NSP that does not include starch. Englyst *et al.* (1987) thought that by defining and measuring dietary fibre as NSP, this helped the analyst to have a clear task, but retained the original concept of dietary fibre as cell wall material. NSP has therefore been a focal point of interest when referring to dietary fibre.

5.8.2 Intakes

It can be difficult for women to know how much dietary fibre they should be eating and how this can be achieved. Research has shown that even well-educated mothers do not consume enough fibre in pregnancy. In one study analysing the diets of pregnant women, those with low fibre intakes (11.6 g/day NSP) were more likely to exhbit symptoms of constipation in the third trimester of pregnancy (Derbyshire *et al.*, 2006). In other areas, such as Brazil, findings from the ECCAGE Study have shown that women's fibre intakes are higher in pregnancy – an average of 30.2 g/day (total fibre); slightly above US recommendations of 28 g/day for pregnancy. However, 50% of women expecting a baby still failed to attain these recommended levels of intake. Cereals were the largest contributor of total dietary fibre intake followed by legumes and fruits, which together provided approximately half of total fibre intake in this study (Buss *et al.*, 2009).

5.8.3 Dietary guidelines

There is a clear lack of consensus when dietary guidelines for fibre are compared between countries. Some guidelines refer to 'total fibre', others 'NSPs' (a more specific measure of fibre) and in many instances specific guidelines are lacking for pregnancy and lactation.

Currently, in the United Kingdom, it is advised that non-pregnant women consume a minimum daily intake of 12 g/day, an average of 18 g/day and maximum level of 24 g/day fibre in the form of NSP (DH, 1991). On the basis of the evidence for bowel function, the EFSA has advised that adults need to eat 25 g total fibre per day for healthy bowel movements (EFSA, 2010a). Women can increase the fibre content of their diet by integrating whole grains, fruits, vegetables, nuts and seeds on a daily basis (James *et al*, 2003). Some simple dietary changes can also help women to increase their fibre intakes (Table 5.7).

Table 5.7 Substituting low fibre with high fibre foods.

Low fibre* (g)	High fibre* (g)
Two slices white bread (0.9)	Two slices brown bread (2.3)
180 g white rice (0.2)	180 g brown rice (1.6)
30 g Cornflakes (0.9)	30 g Bran Flakes (3.9)
Sugar on cereals (Tr)	Raisins (0.2)
Apple juice (Tr)	Apple (1.8)
Two sweet biscuits (0.2–0.6)	Two wholemeal biscuits (0.8–1.8)
Sandwich biscuits (Tr)	Digestive biscuit (0.3)
Sponge cake slice (0.4)	Flapjack (2.4)

Source: Reproduced with permission (Derbyshire, 2007).
Tr, trace amount.
*Fibre content is non-starch polysaccharide.

> ## Fibre – Too Much of a Good Thing?
>
> Previous short-term studies have raised concerns that high fibre diet may lead to certain micronutrient deficiencies (James *et al.*, 2003). The theory behind this is that fibre can chelate (bind) certain nutrients, i.e. calcium, iron and zinc, reducing their bioavailability (Bennett and Cerda, 1996). However, a new cohort study comprising of 283 middle-aged women found those meeting current guidelines for NSP (up to 24.8 g NSP daily) did not reduce women's serum levels of micronutrients (Greenwood *et al.*, 2003). These are important findings and demonstrate that women may increase their fibre intakes up to these levels without it affecting their nutrient status.

5.9   Water

Water has many different roles in the body. It acts as a building material, medium for carrying nutrients and waste products, lubricant and shock absorber and plays a key role in regulating body temperature (Jéquier and Constant, 2010). Drinking adequate amounts of water in pregnancy may be beneficial to the mother, helping to alleviate some unfavourable symptoms that often accompany pregnancy.

5.9.1   Measuring hydration status

There are several ways in which hydration status can be measured. Although there is no 'gold standard', changes in body weight, heart rate and blood pressure, urine osmolality and colour and bioelectrical impedance are amongst some of the most widely used indices (Kavouras, 2002). Serum osmolality from blood samples is another way of monitoring hydration state (osmolality increases in the dehydrated state), although it has been reported that this can be regulated over a wide range of water intakes (Campbell, 2007). Further techniques are needed to measure hydration status accurately, particularly in pregnancy when physiological changes may alter some of these dimensions.

5.9.2   Links with health

The consumption of water may ease bowel habit problems, such as constipation, that can often arise in pregnancy. Eating a fibre-rich diet combined with a sufficient fluid intake may help to facilitate stool–water absorption and promote the expansion of bacterial populations forming bulky stools that can stimulate the defecation reflex (James *et al.*, 2003). Equally, drinking enough water may go some way to helping prevent urinary tract infections. Studies in the past have not been adequately designed to determine 'how much' fluid should be consumed, but it is thought that water consumption may help with the passage and eradication of bacteria (Beetz, 2003). There is also some evidence indicating that adequate hydration during pregnancy can prevent oligohydramnios (when there are smaller amounts of amniotic fluid surrounding the baby) (Ghafarnejad *et al.*, 2009).

Artificially Sweetened Soft Drinks May Increase the Risk or Pre-term Delivery

A large study of 59,334 women from the Danish National Birth Cohort has found that drinking artificially sweetened carbonated and non-carbonated soft drinks in pregnancy can increase preterm delivery risk. Preterm deliveries, i.e. delivering a baby before 37 weeks into pregnancy, are one of the most common medical complications in pregnancy and leading cause of infant morbidity and mortality (Khashu *et al.,* 2009). Although this has not been studied before on a large scale, high consumption of products containing saccharine have been found to aggregate on the foetal side of the placenta (London, 1988).

Compared to women not drinking artificially sweetened carbonated soft drinks, those drinking 4 servings or more of artificially sweetened carbonated soft drinks on a daily basis had a significantly higher risk of delivery prematurely (Halldorsson *et al.,* 2010). Despite the scale of this study, more work is needed to reinforce these initial findings.

5.9.3 Guidelines

Pregnant women have different hydration needs when compared to others in the population. As shown in Table 5.8, water requirements are around 300 mL higher in pregnancy (EFSA, 2010c). Women should drink fluids on a regular basis, even before they feel thirsty as thirst sensations usually occur when body water levels are already reduced. The British Nutrition Foundation has developed a healthy hydration model, which illustrates which fluids should be consumed on a daily basis. Ideally, water should be the main source of fluids, followed by warm beverages, milk, low calorie soft drinks, fruit juices and SSB (Figure 5.2). On a final note, moisture-rich foods can also contribute to daily water intakes (Table 5.9). It is normally assumed that the contribution of food to total water intake is 20–30%, whereas 70–80% is provided from beverage sources.

5.10 Dairy products

The UK Dairy Council's campaign promote the consumption of three servings of low-fat or fat-free milk, cheese or yoghurt. Pregnant women may benefit from getting

Table 5.8 Water requirements for women.

Reference	Source	Recommended intake 14–50 years (mL/day) (<14 years)		
		Non-pregnant	Pregnant	Lactating
EFSA (2010c)	Total water (foods + beverages)	2000	+300	+700
Benelam and Wyness (2010)	Beverages only	1200 (about 6–8 glasses)	–	–

EFSA, European Food Safety Authority; FSA, Food Standards Agency.

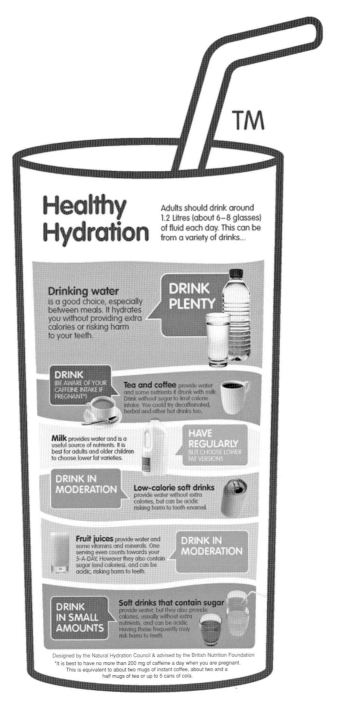

Figure 5.2 Healthy Hydration Drinking Glass Model. (Reproduced with permission from the Natural Hydration Council.)

Table 5.9 Water content of food sources.

91–100% water	80–90% water	70–79% water	Less than 69% water
Broccoli	Apple	Casseroles	Beef
Celery	Pears	Frozen yoghurt	Bread
Cucumber	Cantaloupe	Peas	Crackers
Lettuce	Carbonated drinks	Some fish	Pasta
Soup/stews	Fruit juice		Potatoes
Strawberries	Grapes		Rice
Tomatoes	Oranges		Poultry
Watermelon	Milk		

Source: FNB (2004).

their three portions of diary, although they will need to be careful with certain cheeses as discussed in Chapter 2. Dairy products provide vitamin D and calcium, which help to protect the skeletal mass of the mother and bone density of the foetus (Lowdon, 2008).

One Danish study found that women drinking more glasses of milk in pregnancy were less likely to deliver small-for-gestational-age infants. Most women drank on average 3 glasses of milk a day but those drinking more than this delivered larger infants, particularly those drinking ≥6 glasses a day. Scientists believe that cows milk provides a source of growth-promoting factors that could contribute to these increased growth rates (Olsen *et al.*, 2007). Additional work is needed to see if this relationship can be observed in other studies.

5.11   Salt

In the past, it has been thought that high salt intakes in pregnancy may contribute to high blood pressure (pre-eclampsia) in pregnancy, but there is not enough evidence to support this theory (Duley *et al.*, 2005). In fact, a certain amount of sodium is needed in pregnancy as this needs to be distributed within the extracellular fluids that expand as pregnancy proceeds – total body water increases by about 6–8 L (Davison, 1997). For the meantime, salt intakes should remain as normal but not exceed SACN (2003) guidelines of more than 6 g per day.

5.12   Application in practice

Overall, the macronutrient needs of pregnant women are not considerably different to that of non-pregnant women. On the basis of the best evidence available, most women only need to increase their energy intakes in the third trimester of pregnancy (by about 180 kcal/day; SACN, 2009). Carbohydrate intakes should remain to comprise about 45–60% daily energy intake, but women with diabetes should be advised to choose carbohydrate from low GI sources (NICE, 2008). High-quality proteins should be consumed throughout pregnancy (about 50 g/day) and include lean meat, milk, certain cheeses and cooked eggs (see Chapter 2 on food safety also) and intakes of trans fats should be kept to a minimum. To achieve recommended levels of intake for LC *n*-3 PUFA, women should be advised to eat 2 portions of fish per week (one oily) but avoid certain fish species such as shark, marlin and swordfish. At present, there is no evidence linking salt consumption to unfavourable pregnancy outcomes, but this should continue to be consumed in moderation.

5.13 Food choices

Unfortunately, not all women make the right foods choices or are aware of how their food choices should change if they are planning to have a baby. Research studying the dietary habits of 1461 mothers living in Aberdeen, Scotland, showed that women from deprived backgrounds were on average 6 years younger and more likely to have diets low in protein, fibre, alcohol interestingly and many of the vitamins and minerals (except sodium) (Figure 5.3). The diets of these women were also characterised by low intakes of fruit, vegetables, oily fish and higher in processed meat products, fried potatoes, crisps, snacks and soft drinks (Figure 5.4; Haggarty *et al.*, 2009). These findings demonstrate that deprivation in pregnancy is associated with poor quality diets, which, in turn, lead to social inequalities in terms of poor pregnancy outcomes.

Another study carried out by George *et al.* (2005) in the United States found that food choices also seem to change after birth – possibly because women are busy with their infants. Scientists found that mean daily intakes of grains, fruit and

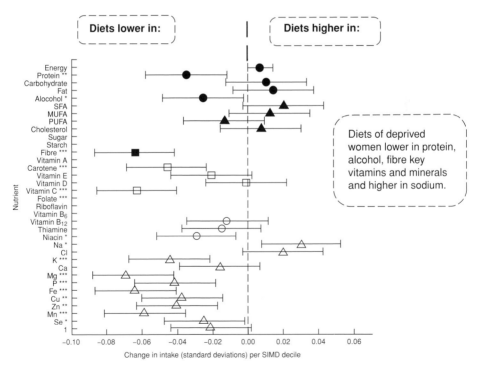

Figure 5.3 Summary of regression analysis of change in nutrient intake by Scottish Index of Multiple Deprivation (SIMD). Data are presented as standard deviations of intake per deprivation decile, with 95% CI represented by horizontal bars, to allow all nutrients to be compared in one graph. Results are shown for the major macronutrient classes (●), fats (▲), carbohydrates (■), fat-soluble vitamins (□), water-soluble vitamins (○) and for trace elements and minerals (△). The level of statistical significance for each regression is indicated beside the relevant nutrient: *$P < 0.05$, **$P < 0.01$, ***$P < 0.001$. (Reproduced with permission from the *British Journal of Nutrition*.)

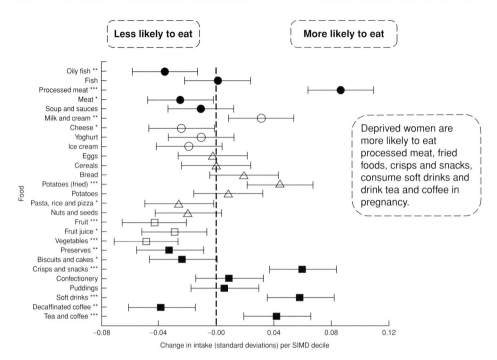

Figure 5.4 Summary of regression analysis of change in intake of food types by Scottish Index of Multiple Deprivation (SIMD). Data are presented as standard deviations of intake per deprivation decile, with 95% CI represented by horizontal bars, to allow all foods to be compared in one graph. Results are shown for the main foods (●), dairy produce (○), staples (△), fruit and vegetables (□) and for sweets and drinks (■). The level of statistical significance for each regression is indicated beside the relevant nutrient: $*P < 0.05$, $**P < 0.01$, $***P < 0.001$. (Reproduced with permission from the *British Journal of Nutrition*.)

vegetables declined after birth, whilst the percentage of energy from fat and added sugars increased. Although breastfeeding mothers made slightly better food choices, it seems that women also need to be guided after birth to help they make the right food choices to prevent excess weight retention and instil healthy eating practices in the next generation (also see Section 12.15).

5.14   Dietary assessment

As there is growing interest in the mother's diet before and during pregnancy, it is important that reliable methods are used. When obtaining dietary data, the main challenge is to obtain accurate information while limiting the time and burden on the participants. Food frequency questionnaires are a good option as these strike a fine balance, providing reliable data whilst being easy to complete (Meltzer *et al.*, 2008). A summary of different dietary assessment methods, their strengths and limitations is shown in Table 5.10. Some of the main questions to consider when assessing dietary intakes in pregnancy include (1) Which dietary method should be used? (2) Which time period should questions cover? (3) Which questions need to be included? (4) How can results be validated/piloted? and (5) How can under-reporting be accounted for?

Table 5.10   Dietary assessment methods.

Dietary assessment methods	Strengths	Limitations
Daily (24-h) recall	Relatively quick to complete. Only short-term memory is needed. Multiple 24-h recalls can be used on different days.	Under-reporting because of poor memory recall.
Diet histories	Questions can be addressed to current or past intake.	Time-consuming. Under-reporting because of poor memory recall.
Food frequency questionnaires	Focus on usual intake. Can be easily coded and analysed.	Some foods may not be included. Subjects may change their dietary habits.
Food records	A measure of current intake. Accounts for day-to-day variation.	Time-consuming. Subjects may alter their diet to what is they think is acceptable. Requires a degree of literacy.
Multiple-pass dietary interviews	Participants are prompted to recall all of the foods/beverages they have consumed. Helps to minimise omissions.	Can take a bit longer to complete (20–30 min). Those administering the interview will need some training.
Weighed inventory	Highly regarded method. Accurate estimation of dietary intakes.	Time-consuming. Food waste needs to be recorded and accounted for.

5.15   Diet quality index

Calculating diet quality in pregnancy can also be a useful predictor of maternal and infant well-being. Several studies have measured diet quality in pregnancy using a range of methods. Diet Quality Index for Pregnancy (DQI-P) scores can be calculated using eight key dietary/food categories and a point scoring system. Points are allocated depending on whether individuals are eating the recommended number of servings of grains, fruits, vegetables, fruits and their meal/snack pattern. Points are also given depending on women's folate, iron and calcium intakes as a percentage of dietary guidelines and whether her total fat intake is ≤30% energy intake.

When applied to a sample of 2063 women taking part in the American Pregnancy, Nutrition and Infection (PIN) study, researchers found that women >30 years who had graduated from high school and had no other children had the best quality diets (Bodnar and Siega-Riz, 2002). This study shows that the DQI-P is a reliable indicator of food quality, which can be used in combination with other dietary assessment tools to capture usual dietary intake. The components of the DQI-P can easily be applied to any trimester of pregnancy and adapted for public health and research purposes.

5.16   Biomarkers

Very few papers have studied the use of biochemical markers to determine nutrition status in pregnancy. As seen in the previous section, dietary assessment tools can be easy to undertake but also lead to a degree of under-reporting (Poslusna *et al.*,

2009). Moran (2007) evaluated over 40 studies that had determined the nutrition status of pregnant adolescents using nutrition biomarkers and found that many of the cutoff values used to interpret nutrition status were ill-defined, particularly for pregnancy. Clear, specific biochemical cutoffs need to be established for pregnant women, although in this paper it was identified that markers of iron status were most likely to be compromised in pregnant adolescents.

5.17   Application in practice

Research shows that social gradients exist in terms of the food choices that are made and consequently how this can impact upon pregnancy outcomes. Public health interventions are clearly needed to help women make better dietary choices so all women have the same chance of having healthy birth outcomes. This is a large challenge, but educating women early on in their school years and communicating the importance of having a 'pregnancy plan' (rather than unplanned pregnancies) may go some way to helping to achieve this. Scientists and health professionals should continue using the best dietary assessment tools they can so we can continue to get an accurate picture of what women are eating before and throughout their pregnancies.

5.18   Conclusion

Overall, this chapter has provided an insight into how women's macronutrient requirements may change in pregnancy. For most, recommendations are similar to that of non-pregnant women, but the importance of increasing LC n-3 PUFA intakes is certainly an area that needs to be better communicated in pregnancy as several studies have reported suboptimal intakes, which may impact upon the development of the infants' nervous system (Cetin and Koletzko, 2008). Further work is now needed to establish whether all women need an extra energy increment in the third trimester of pregnancy and the potential role of low GI foods, particularly in women at risk of delivering large-for-gestational-age infants.

Key Messages

- Food cravings in pregnancy may be because the mother and embryo are competing for nutrient reserves and aversions may be a natural way to prevent the mother from ingesting substances that may harm her developing child.
- Debate continues about whether all women require an extra energy increment in pregnancy. The SACN (2009) advise an extra 0.8 MJ (180 kcal/day) in the third trimester of pregnancy.
- Like any other life phase, women in pregnancy should monitor their sugar intakes, particularly those with a history or high risk of developing diabetes. Added sugars such be consumed at levels <10% daily energy intake (EFSA, 2010a).
- Daily intakes of trans fats should be kept to a minimum.
- Levels of LC n-3 PUFA should be consumed in recommended proportions of at least 200 mg/day DHA, but no more than 1 g/day DHA or 2.7 g/day LC n-3 PUFA should be ingested (Koletzko et al., 2007).

- Women should try to meet EFSA (2010a) guidelines for dietary fibre – 25 g/day – by substituting low-fibre foods for those with a high fibre content. Women should also make sure that they are consuming the right proportions of micronutrients.
- Salt intakes in pregnancy should remain a matter of personal preference.
- Women should be encouraged to drink small amounts of water and often – drinking large volumes of water at any one time may be uncomfortable for the mother. An extra 300 mL on top of the 2000 mL recommended for non-pregnant women is advised during pregnancy (EFSA, 2010c). This can be provided from both food and fluid sources.
- Measuring dietary intakes accurately in pregnancy can be challenging. Biochemical biomarkers can help to validate dietary intake data but cutoffs need to be devised specifically for pregnancy, preferably also considering the different trimesters.
- Updated guidelines for macronutrients need to be communicated to general practitioners, midwives and dieticians, so mothers can be guided to make the right food choices and achieve a favourable dietary profile.

Recommended reading

Brenna JT and Lapillonne A (2009) Background paper on fat and fatty acid requirements during pregnancy and lactation. *Annals of Nutrition and Metabolism* 55 (1–3), 97–122.

Haggarty P, Campbell DM, Duthie S *et al.* (2009) Diet and deprivation in pregnancy. *British Journal of Nutrition* 102(10), 1487–97.

NICE (National Institute of Clinical Excellence) (2008) *Diabetes in Pregnancy: Management of Diabetes and its Complications from Pre-conception to the Postnatal Period.* NICE: London.

Talai Rad N, Ritterath C, Siegmund T *et al.* (2009) Longitudinal analysis of changes in energy intake and macronutrient composition during pregnancy and 6 weeks post-partum. *Archives of Gynaecology and Obstetrics.* [Epub ahead of print.]

References

Andreasyan K, Ponsonby AL, Dwyer T *et al.* (2007) Higher maternal dietary protein intake in late pregnancy is associated with a lower infant ponderal index at birth. *European Journal of Clinical Nutrition* 61(4), 498–508.

Athukorala C, Crowther CA, Willson K *et al.*; Austrailian Carbohydrate Intolerance Study in Pregnant Women (ACHOIS) Trial Group (2007) Women with gestational diabetes mellitus in the ACHOIS trial: risk factors for shoulder dystocia. *Australian & New Zealand Journal of Obstetrics and Gynaecology* 47(1), 37–41.

Bayley TM, Dye L, Jones S, DeBono M and Hill AJ (2002) Food cravings and aversions during pregnancy: relationships with nausea and vomiting. *Appetite* 38, 45–51.

Beetz R (2003) Mild dehydration: a risk factor of urinary tract infection? *European Journal of Clinical Nutrition* 57(2), S52–8.

Belzer LM, Smulian JC, Lu SE and Tepper BJ (2010) Food cravings and intake of sweet foods in healthy pregnancy and mild gestational diabetes mellitus. A prospective study. *Appetite* 55(3), 609–15.

Benelam B and Wyness L (2010) Hydration and health: a review. *British Nutrition Foundation Nutrition Bulletin* 35, 3–25.

Bennett WG and Cerda JJ (1996) Dietary fiber: fact and fiction. *Digestive Diseases* 14, 43–58.

Bodnar LM and Siega-Riz AM (2002) A Diet Quality Index for Pregnancy detects variation in diet and differences by sociodemographic factors. *Public Health Nutrition* 5(6), 801–9.

Brion MJ, Ness AR, Rogers I *et al.* (2010) Maternal macronutrient and energy intakes in pregnancy and offspring intake at 10 y: exploring parental comparisons and prenatal effects. *American Journal of Clinical Nutrition* 91(3), 748–56.

Brouns F, Bjorck I, Frayn KN *et al.* (2005) Glycaemic index methodology. *Nutrition Research Reviews* **18**(1), 145–71.

Buss C, Nunes MA, Camey S *et al.* (2009) Dietary fibre intake of pregnant women attending general practices in southern Brazil – The ECCAGE Study. *Public Health Nutrition* **12**(9), 1392–8.

Campbell SM (2007) Hydration needs throughout the lifespan. *Journal of the American College of Nutrition* **26**(5), S585-7.

Cetin I and Koletzko B (2008) Long-chain omega-3 fatty acid supply in pregnancy and lactation. *Current Opinion in Clinical Nutrition and Metabolic Care* **11**(3), 297–302.

Cetin I, Alvino G and Cardellicchio M (2009) Long chain fatty acids and dietary fats in fetal nutrition. *Journal of Physiology* **587**(Pt 14), 3441–51.

Chen L, Hu FB, Yeung E, Willett W and Zhang C (2009) Prospective study of pre-gravid sugar-sweetened beverage consumption and the risk of gestational diabetes mellitus. *Diabetes Care* **32**(12), 2236–41.

Christian MS and Brent RL (2001) Teratogen update: evaluation of the reproductive and developmental risks of caffeine. *Teratology* **64**(1), 51–78.

Clapp JF (2003) Maternal carbohydrate intake and pregnancy outcome. *Proceedings of the Nutrition Society* **61**(1), 45–50.

Davison JM (1997) Edema in pregnancy. *Kidney International Supplement* **59**, S90–6.

Denomme J, Stark KD and Holub BJ (2005). Directly quantitated dietary (n-3) fatty acid intakes of pregnant Canadian women are lower than current dietary recommendations. *Journal of Nutrition* **135**, 206–11.

Department of Health (1991) *Dietary Reference Values for Food Energy and Nutrients for the United Kingdom*, 2nd edition. Report on Social Subjects no. 41. The Stationery Office: London.

Derbyshire E, Davies J, Costarelli V and Dettmar P (2006) Diet, physical inactivity and the prevalence of constipation throughout and after pregnancy. *Maternal & Child Nutrition* **2**(3), 127–34.

Derbyshire EJ (2007) Pregnancy: the importance of fibre and fluid. *Nursing Standard* **21**(24), 40–3.

Doughman SD, Krupanidhi S and Sanjeevi CB (2007) Omega-3 fatty acids for nutrition and medicine: considering microalgae oil as a vegetarian spurce of EPA and DHA. *Current Diabetes Reviews* **3**, 198–203.

Duley L, Henderson-Smart D and Meher S (2005) Altered dietary salt for preventing pre-eclampsia, and its complications. *Cochrane Database of Systematic Reviews* **4**, CD005548.

EFSA (European Food Standards Agency) (2010a) Scientific opinion on dietary reference values for carbohydrates and dietary fibre. *EFSA Journal* **8**(3), 1462.

EFSA (European Food Standards Agency) (2010b) Scientific opinion on dietary reference values for fats, including saturated fatty acids, polyunsaturated fatty acids, monounsaturated fatty acids, *trans* fatty acids, and cholesterol. *EFSA Journal* **8**(3), 1461.

EFSA (European Food Standards Agency) (2010c) Scientific opinion on dietary reference values for water. *EFSA Journal* **8**(3), 1459.

Englyst H, Trowell H, Southgate D and Cummings J (1987) Dietary fibre and resistant starch. *American Journal of Clinical Nutrition* **46**, 873–4.

Esfahani A, Wong JM, Mirrahimi A, Srichaikul K, Jenkins DJ and Kendall CW (2009) The glycemic index: physiological significance. *Journal of the American College of Nutrition* **28** (Suppl), 439S–45S.

Flaxman SM and Sherman PW (2008) Morning sickness: adaptive cause or nonadaptive consequence of embryo viability? *American Naturalist* **172**(1), 54–62.

FNB (Food and Nutrition Board) (2004) *Dietary Reference Intakes for Water, Potassium, Sodium, Chloride, and Sulphate*. The National Academies Press: Washington, DC.

George GC, Hanss-Nuss H, Milani TJ and Freeland-Graves JH (2005) Food choices of low-income women during pregnancy and postpartum. *Journal of the American Dietetic Association* **105**(6), 899–907.

Ghafarnejad M, Tehrani MB, Anaraki FB, Mood NI and Nasehi L (2009) Oral hydration therapy in oligohydramnios. *Journal of Obstetrics & Gynaecology Research* **35**(5), 895–900.

Goldberg GR, Black AE, Jebb SA, Cole TJ, Murgatroyd PR, Coward WA and Prentice AM (1991) Critical evaluation of energy intake data using fundamental principles of energy physiology: 1. Derivation of cut-off limits to identify under-reporting. *European Journal of Clinical Nutrition* **45**, 569–81.

Goldie MP (2003) Oral health care for pregnant and postpartum women. *International Journal of Dental Hygiene* **1**(3), 174–6.

Greenberg JA, Bell SJ and Ausdal WV (2008) Omega-3 fatty acid supplementation during pregnancy. *Reviews in Obstetrics & Gynaecology* 21(4),162–9.

Greenwood DC, Cade JE, White K, Burley VJ and Schorah CJ (2003) The impact of high non-starch polysaccharide intake on serum micronutrient concentrations in a cohort of women. *Public Health Nutrition* 7(4), 543–8.

Haggarty P, Campbell DM, Duthie S *et al.* (2009) Diet and deprivation in pregnancy. *British Journal of Nutrition* 102(10), 1487–97.

Halldorsson TI, Strøm M, Petersen SB and Olsen SF (2010) Intake of artificially sweetened soft drinks and risk of preterm delivery: a prospective cohort study in 59,334 Danish pregnant women. *American Journal of Clinical Nutrition* 92(3), 626–33.

Hytten FE and Chamberlain G (1991) *Clinical Physiology in Obstetrics*. Blackwell Scientific Publications: Oxford.

Innis SM (2006) Trans fatty intakes during pregnancy, infancy and early childhood. *Atheroscler-sclerosis Supplements* 7(2), 17–20.

Innis SM and Elias SL (2003). Intakes of essential n-6 and n-3 polyunsaturated fatty acids among pregnant Canadian women. *American Journal of Clinical Nutrition* 77, 473–8.

ISSFAL (International Society for the Study of Fatty Acids and Lipids) (2004) *Report of the Sub-Committee on Recommendations for Intake of Polyunsaturated Fatty Acids in Healthy Adults.* ISSFAL Board Meeting, Brighton.

James SL, Muir JG, Curtis SL and Ginson PR (2003) Dietary fibre: a roughage guide. *Internal Medicine Journal* 33(7), 291–6.

Jéquier E and Constant F (2010) Water as an essential nutrient: the physiological basis of hydration. *European Journal of Clinical Nutrition* 64(2), 115–23.

Jones HN, Woollett LA, Barbour N, Prasad PD, Powell TL and Jansson T (2009) High-fat diet before and during pregnancy causes marked up-regulation of placental nutrient transport and fetal overgrowth in C57/BL6 mice. *FASEB Journal* 23(1), 271–8.

Kavouras SA (2002) Assessing hydration status. *Current Opinion in Clinical Nutrition and Metabolic Care* 5(5), 519–24.

Khashu M, Narayanan M, Bhargava S and Osiovich H (2009) Perinatal outcomes associated with preterm birth at 33–36 weeks' gestation: a population-based cohort study. *Pediatrics* 123(1), 109–13.

Koletzko B, Cetin I, Brenna JT *et al.*; Perinatal Lipid Intake Working Group (2007) Dietary fat intakes for pregnant and lactating women. *British Journal of Nutrition* 98(5), 873–7.

Koletzko B, Lien E, Agostoni C *et al.*; World Association of Perinatal Medicine Dietary Guidelines Working Group (2008) The roles of long-chain polyunsaturated fatty acids in pregnancy, lactation and infancy: review of current knowledge and consensus recommendations. *Journal of Perinatal Medicine* 36(1), 5–14.

Kramer MS and Kakuma R (2003) Energy and protein intake in pregnancy. *Cochrane Database of Systematic Reviews* 4, CD000032.

Latva-Pukkila U, Isolauri E and Laitinen K (2010) Dietary and clinical impacts of nausea and vomiting during pregnancy. *Journal of Human Nutrition & Dietetics* 23(1), 69–77.

London RS (1988) Saccharin and aspartame. Are they safe to consume during pregnancy? *Journal of Reproductive Medicine* 33, 17–21.

Lowdon J (2008) Getting bone health right from the start! Pregnancy, lactation and weaning. *Journal of Family Health Care* 18(4), 137–41.

Mann JI and Cummings JH (2009) Possible implications for health of the different definitions of dietary fibre. *Nutrition, Metabolism and Cardiovascular Diseases* 19, 226–229.

Mamun AA, Kinarivala M, O'Callaghan MJ, Williams GM, Najman JM and Callaway LK (2010) Associations of excess weight gain during pregnancy with long-term maternal overweight and obesity: evidence from 21 y postpartum follow-up. *American Journal of Clinical Nutrition* 91(5), 1336–41.

McGowan CA and McAuliffe FM (2010) The influence of maternal glycaemia and dietary glycaemic index on pregnancy outcome in healthy mothers. *British Journal of Nutrition* 104(2), 153–9.

Meltzer HM, Brantsaeter AL, Ydersbond TA, Alexander J and Haugen M (2008) Methodological challenges when monitoring the diet of pregnant women in a large study: experiences from the Norweign Mother and Child Cohort Study (MoBA). *Maternal & Child Nutrition* 4(1), 14–27.

Mendosa D (2008) Revised International Table of Glycaemic Index (GI) and Glycaemic Load (GL) Values. Available at: http://www.mendosa.com/gilists.htm. (accessed March 2011.)

Mirmiran P (2006) Under-reporting of energy intake affects estimates of nutrient intakes. *Asia Pacific Journal of Clinical Nutrition* **15**, 459–64.

Moses RG and Brand-Miller JC (2009) Dietary risk factors for gestational diabetes mellitus: are sugar-sweetened soft drinks culpable or guilty by association? *Diabetes Care* **32**(12), 2314–15.

Moore VM and Davies MJ (2005) Diet during pregnancy, neonatal outcomes and later health. *Reproduction, Fertility & Development* **17**(3), 341–8.

Moran VN (2007) Nutritional status in pregnant adolescents: a systemic review of biological markers. *Maternal & Child Nutrition* **3**, 74–93.

Murphy SP and Abrams BF (1993) Changes in energy intakes during pregnancy and lactation in a national sample of US women. *American Journal of Public Health* **83**(8), 1161–3.

NICE (National Institute of Clinical Excellence) (2008) *Diabetes in Pregnancy: Management of Diabetes and its Complications from Pre-conception to the Postnatal Period.* NICE: London.

Olsen SF, Halldorsson TI, Willett WC *et al.*; NUTRIX Consortium (2007) Milk consumption during pregnancy is associated with increased infant size at birth: prospective cohort study. *American Journal of Clinical Nutrition* **86**(4), 1104–10.

Pepper GV and Roberts SC (2006) Rates of nausea and vomiting in pregnancy and dietary characteristics across populations. *Proceedings of the Royal Society B: Biological Sciences* **273**, 2675–9.

Poslusna K, Ruprich J, de Vries JHM, Jakubikova M and van't Veer P (2009) Misreporting of energy and micronutrient intake estimated by food records and 24 hour recalls, control and adjustment methods in practice. *British Journal of Nutrition* **101**, S73–85.

Prentice AM, Spaaij CJK, Goldberg GR *et al.* (1996) Energy requirements of pregnant and lactating women. *European Journal of Clinical Nutrition* **50**, S82–111.

Russo, G.L. (2008) Dietary *n*-6 and *n*-3 polyunsaturated fatty acids: from biochemistry to clinical implications in cardiovascular prevention. *Biochemical Pharmacology* **6**, 937–46.

SACN (Scientific Advisory Committee on Nutrition) (2003) *Salt and Health Report.* The Stationery Office: London.

SACN (Scientific Advisory Committee on Nutrition) (2009) *SACN Energy Requirements Working Group Draft Report.* The Stationery Office: London.

Schofield N, Schofield C and James WT (1985) Basal metabolic rate. *Human Nutrition: Clinical Nutrition* **39C**, 5–41.

Shaw GM, Quach T, Nelson V *et al.* (2003) Neural tube defects associated with maternal periconceptional dietary intake of simple sugars and glycemic index. *American Journal of Clinical Nutrition* **78**(5), 972–8.

Shiell AW, Campbell-Brown M, Haselden S, Robinson S, Godfrey KM and Barker DJ (2001) High-meat, low-carbohydrate diet in pregnancy: relation to adult blood pressure in the offspring. *Hypertension* **38**(6), 1282–8.

Singh M (2005) Essential fatty acids, DHA and human brain. *Indian Journal of Pediatrics* **72**, 239–42.

Sinikovic DS, Yeatman HR, Cameron D and Meyer BJ (2009) Women's awareness of the importance of long-chain omega-3 polyunsaturated fatty acid consumption during pregnancy: knowledge of risks, benefits and information accessibility. *Public Health Nutrition* **12**(4), 562–9.

Sontrop J, Avison WR, Evers SE *et al.* (2008). Depressive symptoms during pregnancy in relation to fish consumption and intake of *n*-3 fatty acids. *Pediatric and Perinatal Epidemiology* **22**, 389–99.

Surette ME (2008) The science behind dietary omega-3 fatty acids. *Canadian Medical Association Journal* **178**, 177–80.

Talai Rad N, Ritterath C, Siegmund T *et al.* (2009) Longitudinal analysis of changes in energy intake and macronutrient composition during pregnancy and 6 weeks post-partum. *Archives of Gynaecology & Obstetrics.* [Epub ahead of print.]

Tamimi R, Lagiou P, Mucci LA, Hsieh CC, Adami HO and Trichopoulos D (2003) Average energy intake among pregnant women carrying a boy compared with a girl. *British Medical Journal* **326**, 1245–446.

USDA (2010) National Nutrient Database for Standard Reference, Release 22. Content of selected foods per common measure, protein (g) sorted by nutrient content. Available at: http://www.ars.usda.gov/SP2UserFiles/Place/12354500/Data/SR22/nutrlist/sr22w203.pdf. (accessed March 2011.)

van Eijsden M, Hornstra G, van der Wal MF and Bonsel GJ (2009) Ethnic differences in early pregnancy maternal n-3 and n-6 fatty acid concentrations: an explorative analysis. *British Journal of Nutrition* **101**(12), 1761–8.

Walsh J, Mahony R, Foley M and Mc Auliffe F (2010) A randomised control trial of low glycaemic index carbohydrate diet versus no dietary intervention in the prevention of recurrence of macrosomia. *BMC Pregnancy Childbirth* **10**, 16.

WHO/FAO (2008) Codex Alimentarius Commission (CNFSDU). 30th session. Available at: http://www.codexalimentarius.net/web/archives.jsp?year=09. (accessed March 2011.)

Yanovski S (2003) Sugar and fat: cravings and aversions. *Journal of Nutrition* **133**(3), 835S–7S.

Yogev Y and Visser GH (2009) Obesity, gestational diabetes and pregnancy outcome. *Seminars in Fetal & Neonatal Medicine* **14**(2), 77–84.

6 Vitamins and Pregnancy

Summary

Vitamins are generally defined as organic compounds that are required by the body for good health. During pregnancy, there is a metabolic demand for high-quality nutrients, so it is important that these are obtained from the mother's diet. Both over- and underconsumption of vitamins can have health implications in pregnancy (and for the offspring), but vitamin deficiencies are generally more widespread. When vitamins deficiencies are present before and during pregnancy, this can increase the likelihood of poor pregnancy outcomes, including certain birth defects.

With careful food selection, it is possible that optimal levels of vitamins may be obtained from food sources. However, economic, social and cultural factors can mean that this is not always feasible. Consequently, some women may be more susceptible to vitamin deficiencies (particularly folate, vitamin B_{12} and vitamin D) than others. The importance of consuming adequate amounts of vitamins, how this can be achieved and the effects inadequate intakes can have on women's health and that of their offspring needs to be conveyed to women in their childbearing years.

Learning Outcomes

- To discuss the role(s) of key vitamins and explain their function(s) in pregnancy.
- To describe how under- and overconsumption of vitamins may influence maternal, foetal and infant health.
- To recognise which food sources can provide the key nutrients needed during pregnancy.
- To become aware of recommended levels of intake and upper limits (UL) of intake for key vitamins.

6.1 Introduction

It is estimated that about 30% of pregnant mothers have some form of vitamin deficiency and 75% of women would be deficient in at least one vitamin if they were to not take supplements (Kontic-Vucinic *et al.*, 2006). Vitamins are essential to maintain normal metabolic processes and regulate processes within the body. Certain vitamins are only stored in the body in small amounts, deficiencies of B

Nutrition in the Childbearing Years, First Edition. Emma Derbyshire.
© 2011 Emma Derbyshire. Published 2011 by Blackwell Publishing Ltd.

vitamins may be noticed in several days (except vitamin B_{12}) and vitamin C deficiency symptoms may become apparent within weeks. Other vitamins are stored in greater amounts, particularly the fat-soluble vitamins. Scientists have calculated that vitamin D reserves may last for up to 2 months and vitamin A stores up to 5 months (Bsoul and Terezhalmy, 2004). Clearly, every individual has different levels of vitamin stores and rates of depletion will vary depending on dietary quality and whether supplements are taken.

There are many reasons why vitamin deficiencies may occur in pregnancy. Insufficient nutrient stores, age upon conception, availability to food, level of education, individual food choices and season may all influence a women's nutritional status. For example, research in Nepal has shown that the diet quality of pregnant women is generally better in the winter months before the hot summer and monsoon seasons reduce food supplies and vitamin deficiencies (which are often multiple) become common (Jiang *et al.*, 2005).

It is important to consider that women's diet quality and health in their reproductive years can affect health in pregnancy and, in turn, the health of the next generation – leading to a cycle of poor health. This chapter aims to explain why the consumption of certain vitamins is important before and during pregnancy. Equally, implications of under- and overconsumption will also be described. This section also sets out to explain how women may adapt their diets to help them achieve dietary targets for key vitamins. Tables summarising international dietary recommendations for individual vitamins are included in the appendices.

6.2   Vitamin A

Vitamin A is a fat-soluble vitamin that is essential for the growth and differentiation of cells, which is important throughout pregnancy. In particular, vitamin A is needed for the development and maturation of foetal lungs (Strobel *et al.*, 2007). There are two forms of vitamin A: retinol (commonly found in animal foods and some fortified foods) and carotenoids (usually found in plant foods). Carotenoids are often referred to as 'provitamins' because they can be converted to retinol (the active vitamin A form) in the human body.

If the mother has inadequate vitamin A status, this means the child is also at risk of vitamin A deficiency. A clinical study in Western pregnant women with multiple births or short birth intervals found that almost one-third of women had plasma retinol levels below 1.4 μmol/L; borderline deficiency (Schulz *et al.*, 2007). There has also been some, although contradictory, evidence suggesting that vitamin A supplements may help to reduce the risk of HIV transmission from mother to child. A review of five clinical trials (7528 women) showed that there was no relationship between vitamin A supplementation before and/or after delivery and risk of mother-to-child transmission, although there were some improvements in birth weight (Kongnyuy *et al.*, 2009).

6.2.1   A note on units

Vitamin A generally circulates in its retinol form as retinyl esters in tissue secretions. In blood, tissues and milk samples, vitamin A levels are usually expressed as

Table 6.1 Converting units into retinol equivalents (RE).

1 μg retinol	= 1 RE
1 μg beta-carotene	= 0.167 μg RE
1 μg of other pro-vitamin carotenoids	= 0.084 μg RE

Source: FAO/WHO (2002).
1 RE = 3.33 IU vitamin A activity from retinol.

μmol/L or mg/dL. Values below 0.7 μmol/L have been used as a cutoff for vitamin A deficiency (Azaïs-Braesco and Pascal, 2000).

It is well known that retinol is more biologically active than carotenoids. Therefore, to express the vitamin A activity of carotenoids, the FAO/WHO (2002) recommended that retinol equivalents (RE) replace the traditional use of International Units (IU; 1 IU = 0.60 μg of beta-carotene), so comparisons can be made more easily. Table 6.1 explains how figures for retinol and beta-carotene may be converted into RE.

6.2.2 Guidelines

Women are generally discouraged from eating animal foods rich in vitamin A (such as liver and organ meats) during pregnancy because of their high vitamin A (retinol) content, which may have potential teratogenic effects, disrupting the development of the embryo or foetus (Khoury *et al.*, 1996). Subsequently, most women mainly consume vitamin A in pregnancy from plant-based sources, as carotenoids. Carotenoids are not as biologically active as retinol but their consumption should still be monitored to ensure guidelines are not exceeded (SACN, 2005). Dark green and orange/red vegetables are some of the richest sources of carotenoids as can be seen in Table 6.2.

In terms of 'how much' vitamin A is required during pregnancy, there is a lack of research quantifying the amount needed for foetal stores and maternal tissue growth. Therefore, recommendations are at best an estimation and air on the side of caution. The FAO/WHO (2002) advises that pregnant and lactating mothers

Table 6.2 Sources of carotenoids.

Green vegetables	Carotene (μg/100 g)	As retinol equivalents (RE)
Spinach (boiled)	6604	1103
Curly kale (boiled)	3375	564
Cabbage (boiled)	805	134
Mange-tout (stir-fried)	725	121
Green beans (frozen and boiled)	520	87
Orange/red vegetables		
Carrots (boiled)	13,402	2238
Sweet potato (boiled)	3960	661
Capsicum red pepper (raw)	3840	641
Mixed vegetables (frozen and boiled)	2520	421
Pumpkin (boiled)	955	159

Source: FSA (2006).
EFSA (2006) advise an upper limit of 3000 μg RE/day is applied to reduce the risk of possible teratogenic effects.

Table 6.3 Vitamin A – points for consideration.

Dietary intakes of 800/850 µg RE/day are recommended for pregnant and lactating mothers, respectively (FAO/WHO, 2002).

Vitamin A rich foods including liver, paté, faggots, haggis or any other organ meats are best avoided.

Orange and green leafy vegetables should be consumed in moderation.

Women should be advised not to take fish liver oil or single-dose vitamin A supplements.

Women should not exceed the daily tolerable upper intake level set at 3000 µg RE (EFSA, 2006).

consume no more than 800 and 850 µg RE/day respectively. The EFSA (2006) have set a daily UL of 3000 µg RE to reduce the risk of possible terotogenic effects. For Western women, there is no need to take single-dose vitamin A supplements and those purchasing over-the-counter multivitamins should make sure their vitamin A content does not exceed these guidelines (Azaïs-Braesco and Pascal, 2000). A summary of some key points for consideration are included in Table 6.3.

6.3   Thiamine (vitamin B$_1$)

Thiamine, also referred to as vitamin B$_1$, supports the role of coenzymes, particularly those involved in carbohydrate metabolism and energy production. Some studies show that women with severe nausea and vomiting in pregnancy (hyperemesis gravidarum) may be at risk of thiamine deficiency and Wernicke encephalopathy, a neurological condition that can impair memory and lead to feelings of confusion. It has therefore been advised that women with severe and/or prolonged vomiting, or symptoms of Wernicke encephalopathy may benefit from taking vitamin B$_1$ supplements (Chiossi et al., 2006). There is also some evidence to suggest that thiamine may help to reduce the risk of stillbirths (particularly in alcoholic mothers) (Bã, 2009) and improve the neuromotor maturity of the newborn (Cucó et al., 2005). Certainly, research determining the levels of consumption at which thiamine may improve pregnancy outcomes is worthy of future research.

6.3.1   Guidelines

Studies have shown that even today some women may be at risk of thiamine deficiency. After studying a group of 51 Spanish women, researchers found that one-third (26%) women consumed less thiamine than recommended and 14% showed signs of severe deficiency, which was later reflected in milk thiamine concentrations (Ortega et al., 2004). These findings show that there is still room for improvement in terms of ensuring that women are consuming enough thiamine throughout their pregnancy.

In terms of 'how much' thiamine is needed in pregnancy, the Commission of the European Communities (1993) set pregnancy guidelines at 1.0 mg/day and non-European recommendations are slightly higher at 1.4 mg/day (IoM, 2001). Fortified cereals are a particularly good source of thiamine, provided anything between 0.8 and 2.3 mg/100 g, but sunflower seeds (1.6 mg/100 g), salmon (0.25 mg/100 g) and boiled lentils (0.11 mg/100 g) are also good examples of foods that can be integrated within the daily diet to help achieve recommended levels of intake (FSA, 2006).

6.4   Riboflavin (vitamin B₂)

Riboflavin also plays an important role in carbohydrate metabolism and energy production in pregnancy. One study to date has found that riboflavin deficiency may be a possible risk factor for pre-eclampsia (Wacker *et al.*, 2000), although these findings have not be replicated in subsequent studies. Earlier studies also suggest that low birth weight infants may be deficient in riboflavin (Navarro *et al.*, 1984) and riboflavin deficiency may impair the mobilisation of iron in pregnancy (Powers and Bates, 1984). Research investigating the health benefits of this vitamin is sparse and generally confined to animal studies.

Like thiamine, dietary reference intakes (DRIs) for riboflavin are also set at 1.4 mg/day for pregnant and lactating mothers (IoM, 2001). Animal products including milk (0.23 mg/100 g), cheese (0.13–0.53 mg/100 g), yoghurt (0.22 mg/100 g), lean beef (0.10 mg/100 g) and poultry (0.18 mg/100 g) are good sources of riboflavin, as well as enriched cereals (FSA, 2006).

6.5   Niacin (vitamin B₃)

Niacin, sometimes known as vitamin B₃, may be metabolised to two active forms: (1) nicotinamide adenine dinucleotide (NAD), which may then gain an additional phosphate group forming (2) nicotinamide adenine dinucleotide phosphate (NADP). Both are involved in glycolysis (the metabolic breakdown of glucose with the release of energy), fatty acid metabolism and oxidative phosphorylation, which is the production of energy when nutrients are oxidised (Kontic-Vucinic *et al.*, 2006).

One American study found that a high percentage of mothers had niacin deficiency in the first trimester, which proceeded to get worse in later trimesters (Baker *et al.*, 2002). Since then, low maternal niacin intakes have been associated with a two- to fivefold increased risk of spina bifida (Groenen *et al.*, 2004). It is generally recommended that pregnant mothers aim to consume 18 mg niacin/day in pregnancy (IoM, 2001). Eating niacin-rich foods (wheat bran, lean chicken and turkey, oily fish and fortified cereals) may help women to achieve this.

6.6   Pantothenic acid (B₅)

Pantothenic acid (vitamin B₅) is another B vitamin that acts as a coenzyme to reactions involved in glucose and fatty acid metabolism. Generally, pantothenate is present in most food sources, particularly animal foods and green leafy vegetables (FSA, 2006), so deficiency symptoms are uncommon.

Findings in studies are often secondary outcomes, but pantothenic acid intake has been positively related to birth weight (Watson and McDonald, 2010) and birth size (birth weight, length, head circumference and placental weight) (Lagiou *et al.*, 2005).

6.7   Pyridoxine (B₆)

Pyridoxine (vitamin B₆) also helps to support the metabolism of protein, fat and carbohydrate. The vitamin acts as a coenzyme for over 100 chemical reactions within the human body (Kontic-Vucinic *et al.*, 2006). It is thought that B₆ may play a role in the prevention of pre-eclampsia and preterm birth, but evidence is lacking. There are some randomised studies suggesting that B₆ could be helpful in reducing symptoms of pregnancy-related nausea. However, there is not enough data to yet make firm recommendations (Thaver *et al.*, 2006).

DRIs for pyridoxine are set at 1.9 mg/day in pregnancy, rising to 2.0 mg/day for lactating mothers (IoM, 2001). Lean meats and wholegrains, yeast and wheat germ are a good source of vitamin B_6 (FSA, 2006). As overconsumption of vitamin B_6 may be related to neurotoxicity symptoms, the tolerable upper intake level is set at 25 mg/day for adults. Food sources do not generally pose a risk of toxicity; toxicity symptoms are usually linked to high-dose vitamin B_6 supplementation (EFSA, 2006).

6.8 Biotin

Biotin is a sulphur-containing vitamin and serves as an important coenzyme. Biotin may also affect chromatin structure and mediate the regulation of genes (Zempleni *et al.*, 2009). Research has shown that up to 50% of pregnant women may be deficient in biotin (measured using urinary markers) in early and late pregnancy (Mock *et al.*, 2002). Although more studies in different regions are needed to determine biotin status during pregnancy, a New Zealand study has recently found that biotin (as a percentage of total energy) was positively associated with infant birth weight (Watson and McDonald, 2010).

Biotin deficiency in early pregnancy is of particular concern because this is when organogenesis takes places. Biotin deficiency has been linked to the development of birth defects in mice (Mock *et al.*, 2002). Although the mechanism of action is yet to be confirmed, the proposed relationship between biotin deficiency and teratogenesis is shown in Figure 6.1. It has been proposed that reduced absorption or increased breakdown of biotin in pregnancy could lead to the depletion of reserves and reduce carboxylase enzyme activity, which in turn may lead to altered gene expression, which have teratogenic implications.

6.8.1 Guidelines

IoM (1998) DRI for biotin is 30 µg/day for non-pregnant and pregnant women and 35 µg/day for lactating mothers. A recommended safe upper levels (SUL) has not yet

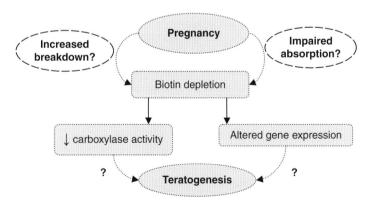

Figure 6.1 Biotin deficiency and potential teratogenesis in pregnancy. (Adapted from Mock (2009), with permission from the American Society of Nutrition.)

Table 6.4 Biotin content of selected foods.

Food and serving size (g)	Biotin/serving (μg)
Meat, fish, poultry, egg (74)	30.8
Salmon, pink, canned (63)	3.69
Pork chop, cooked (80)	3.57
Sunflower seeds, roasted (31)	2.42
Chilli (441)	2.29
Egg, whole, cooked (35)	2.02
Banana pudding (170)	1.73
Strawberries, fresh (111)	1.67
Orange juice, from concentrate (296)	1.22
Broccoli, fresh (113)	1.07

Source: Adapted from Staggs *et al.* (2004), with permission.

been established by the European Food Safety Authority (EFSA), but as biotin cannot be synthesised by the body, it is recommended that this comes from 'exogenous' sources (EFSA, 2006). The biotin content of food sources may vary depending on the method of analysis. Published values that have been determined using high performance liquid chromatography/avidin binding assay (thought to be most accurate) are shown in Table 6.4. Symptoms of biotin deficiency may include seizure, hypotonia, ataxia, dermatitis, hair loss, mental retardation, ketolactic acidosis, aciduria and birth defects (Zempleni *et al.*, 2008).

6.9   Cobalamin (B$_{12}$)

Vitamin B$_{12}$ (cyanocobalamin) is the only B vitamin to contain a mineral (cobalt) and is one of the largest and most complex of the B vitamins. Deficiency is generally defined as a serum or plasma concentration of vitamin B$_{12}$ lower than 200 pg/mL, or when serum levels of methylmalonic acid are elevated (Allen, 2009). Looking to surveys, a cutoff of >210 nmol/L has been used in the large American National Health and Nutrition Examination Survey (NHANES) as an indicator of vitamin B$_{12}$ deficiency (Pfeiffer *et al.*, 2005). Recently, researchers have shown increased interest in the role of vitamin B$_{12}$ as a measure to prevent NTDs alongside folic acid. There is now good evidence that vitamin B$_{12}$ deficiency may be associated with the development of neural tube defects (NTD) and possible cause of preterm deliveries (Molloy *et al.*, 2008). Reduced vitamin B$_{12}$ status in infancy (as a result of inadequate maternal intake and stores) may also contribute to range of neurological symptoms including irritability, failure to thrive, apathy, loss of appetite and delayed development (Dror and Allen, 2008).

6.9.1   Guidelines

At present, UK Dietary Reference Values for vitamin B$_{12}$ are only targeted at women in general (1.5 μg/day) and set at 2.0 μg/day for lactating mothers. The European Union (EU) recommends 1.6 and 1.9 μg/day vitamin B$_{12}$ for pregnant and lactating mothers, respectively (Commission of the European Communities, 1993).

Daily recommendations for non-European countries are slightly higher (2.2–2.8 µg/day) (IoM, 1998; NHMRC, 2006). Because of the lack of clearly defined adverse effects, SULs for vitamin B_{12} have not yet been established (EFSA, 2006).

Vitamin B_{12} may be found in animal foods, meat, milk, egg, fish and shellfish, although the bioavailability of the vitamin from these sources may vary considerably. The bioavailability of vitamin B_{12} from meat may range from 42% to 66% but may be less than 9% eggs sources (Watanabe, 2007). Consequently, common causes of vitamin B_{12} deficiency include a vegetarian/vegan diet, low intake of animal foods or malabsorption (possibly as a result of *Helicobacter pylori* infection) (Allen, 2009). As plant foods only contain traces of vitamin $B_{12,}$ fortified breakfast cereals are a particularly important source of vitamin B_{12} for these at risk groups (Watanabe, 2007).

Research Highlight   Vitamin B_{12} and folate status in pregnancy may affect the risk of insulin resistance in the offspring

The Pune Maternal Nutrition Study (PMNS), carried out in India, is one of the first studies to investigate the relationship between maternal nutrition and the offspring's risk of developing type 2 diabetes and cardiovascular (CV) disease.

A team of researchers have collected data from 700 mothers in relation to their anthropometric characteristics, diet, micronutrient status and levels of physical activity during pregnancy. After birth, the newborns were measured at birth and every 6 months. Once the infants were 6 years old, an assessment of insulin resistance was made, indicating the infant's risk of developing type 2 diabetes or CV disease.

Results showed that over two-third of mothers had low vitamin B_{12} status in pregnancy (defined as circulating levels <150 pmol/L) and 30% had raised homocysteine levels. In the offspring, infants born to mothers with low vitamin B_{12} status were more likely to be insulin resistant. Interestingly, the offspring of mothers with a high folate but low vitamin B_{12} status were most likely to be insulin-resistant, meaning they had a higher risk of developing diabetes of CV disease later in life (Yajnik *et al.*, 2008). Overall, the findings from this study are important because they demonstrate that the offspring needs an adequate supply of both folate/folic acid and vitamin B_{12} for good health. Further studies are needed to determine how low vitamin B_{12} concentrations are best corrected in Indian mothers.

6.10   Folate

As mentioned previously in Chapter 4, different terms are often used to define whether folate is derived from natural or synthetic sources. During pregnancy, many coenzymes rely on folate to support their function. For example, folate-containing coenzymes are needed for the conversion of homocysteine into the amino acid methionine. Research suggests that increased plasma levels of homocysteine (particularly in the third trimester of pregnancy) may be a predictor of low birth weight deliveries (Takimoto *et al.*, 2007). Homocysteine levels have also been found to be higher in women with pre-eclampsia, but the role folate may play is yet to be firmly established (Mignini *et al.*, 2005).

Table 6.5 Top ten folate-rich foods for pregnancy (per 100 g).

Food source	Folate (μg per 100 g)	Some factors affecting bioavailability
Marmite	1010	Food storage
Ovaltine (powder)	400	
Corn flakes/Special K cereals	333	Cooking methods/duration (folate has poor stability)
Wheat germ	325	
Asparagus (boiled)	173	
Horlicks (powder)	160	Food matrix
Beetroot (raw)	150	
Dark green leafy vegetables	140	Other food components
Whole grains	80	
Avocado	66	

Source: FSA (2006).
Point for consideration: Although folate can be obtained from food sources, it has low bioavailability, i.e. only small proportions are absorbed and used for metabolic processes. For this reason, women planning to have a baby should always take a folic acid supplement.

Folates are found in a wide array of foods. Yeast extract, fortified beverages and green leafy vegetables are all rich sources. Folate is also abundant in organ meats such as liver and nuts, but these are generally not recommended for consumption during pregnancy. In the United States, cereals were found to significantly contribute daily intakes amongst the 68% women who did not take supplements (Tinker *et al.*, 2010).

Lower amounts are also found in vegetables sources, as shown in Table 6.5. Generally, it can be difficult for women to consume enough folate from their diet, which is why supplementation with 400 μg folic acid is recommended before conception and during the first 12 weeks of pregnancy (COMA, 2000).

Research Highlight   800 μg/day folic acid may be more appropriate

Scientists from the University of Bonn, Germany, have carried out a study to see how long it takes women to reach recommended blood cell folate levels (>906 nmol/L; the level beyond which the risk of delivering a child with a NTD significantly decreases).

Women were given either a standard folic acid supplement (400 μ/day), 800 μg/day folic acid, or a folic acid free supplement (placebo) and took this daily over the course of 16 weeks. Blood samples, collected every 4 weeks, showed that women taking the higher dose supplement reached target blood cell folate levels within an average of 4.2 weeks, but levels were inadequate in the other groups (Brämswig *et al.*, 2009).

Findings from this study indicate that if women are to take supplements to prepare for pregnancy, they may need to start taking these more than 1 month before conception to improve their folic acid levels. Otherwise, the dose of folic acid needed to achieve optimum red blood cell levels may need to be higher than current guidelines.

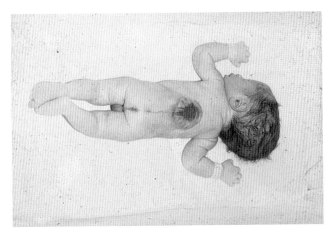

Figure 6.2 Spina bifida caused by incomplete closure of the neural tube. The risk of delivering an infant with a neural tube defect such as spina bifida can be significantly reduced if folic acid is taken before and in the early stages of pregnancy. Some studies also show that vitamin B$_{12}$ can also help to reduce the risk of NTDs. (Photograph kindly provided by E. Eliott, Consultant Paediatrician.)

6.10.1   Neural tube defects

NTDs include anencephaly, spina bifida and encepalocele (hernia of part of the brain). The neural tube is a structure that develops into the spinal column and brain during the first 28 days of pregnancy (SACN, 2006). When the neural tube does not close, this is thought to be a cause of NTDs such as spina bifida (Figure 6.2).

In the United States, fortification of flour with folic acid has been mandatory since 1998. Therefore, scientists have analysed data from the 1988–94 NHANES survey and compared this with findings from the 1999–2000 survey. It was found that mean folate intake increased by 76 µg/day after fortification (from 275 µg/day to 351 µg/day) and serum folate levels raised twofold (by 136%). After fortification, bread, rolls and crackers were the largest contributors to total folate intake (Dietrich *et al.*, 2005). Although this study did not relate findings to NTD affected pregnancy, it was found that blood folate status improved significantly after fortification. Authors, however, concluded that women of childbearing age may need to take additional folic acid supplements to reach red blood cell folate levels associated with reduced risk of NTDs.

Case Study – China, Fortification and NTD Rates

China is one region that had the highest rates of NTD in the world with 80,000–100,000 pregnancies being affected annually (Li and Qian, 1994). Because of the one child per family policy in China, improving birth outcomes was a high priority. Therefore, in 1993, as part of a NTD Prevention Programme, women preparing for marriage in China were advised to take 400 µg folic acid. After this programme was put into place, the risk of NTD reduced by 85% in Northern and 40% in Southern China and it was also thought that this programme helped to reduce the risk of cleft palate and/or lip in the region (Zhu and Ling, 2008).

Unfortunately, some women living in certain areas of China are still at risk of NTD-affected pregnancies. The folic acid status of normal women living in the Shanxi Province of China was compared to those who had delivered a child with a birth defect. Women from this area had particularly low folic acid status (14.03 nmol/L), but this was significantly lower in women who already had an infant with a birth defect (9.6 nmol/L). Overall, the findings from this study show that high rates of birth defects still exist in China and certain areas needed to be targeted in the form of health interventions and public health campaigns.

6.10.2   Cleft lip/palate

During early pregnancy, separate areas of the foetus's face develop individually and then fuse together. When some parts do not join, this may result in cleft lip (Figure 6.3), an opening in the upper lip below the nose, or cleft palate when the roof of the mouth does not join together (CLAPA, 2009).

Although the causes of cleft lip/palate remain to be firmly established, there is some evidence that folic acid supplements may help to reduce the risk of these birth defects. A large case–control study undertaken in Norway found that supplementation with at least 400 μg/day folic acid may reduce the risk of cleft lip (with or without cleft palate) by about a third (Wilcox *et al.*, 2007).

6.10.3   Guidelines

No adverse effects have been reported with the high consumption of natural folates, most concerns relate to the safety of high intakes of folic acid (particularly in relation

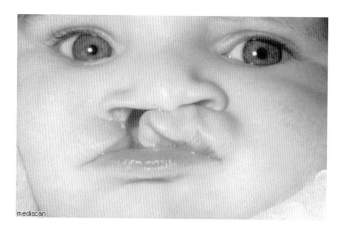

Figure 6.3 Cleft lip, sometimes known as harelip, is another example of a birth defect caused by low folic acid intakes before and in the early stages of pregnancy. Folic acid is needed for DNA synthesis and cell division. When intakes do not meet the demands of pregnancy, body structures may not fuse together as they should. Infants with cleft lip may also have cleft palate, which is when the two plates inside the roof or the mouth do not fuse completely.

to recognising symptoms of cobalamin deficiency; Carmel, 2009). The EFSA (2006) have set the UL for folic acid at 1 mg/day for women of childbearing age based on the fact that some individuals may exhibit neurological symptoms beyond this. Certainly, toxicological studies investigating health implications beyond this dose are lacking.

Otherwise, for women planning a pregnancy or in the early phases of their pregnancy (the first 12 weeks), 400 µg/day folic acid is recommended (COMA, 2000). For parents that have a NTD themselves, or previous child with a NTD, up to 5 mg/day folic acid is recommended. Women with diabetes are also recommended to take 5 mg/day folic acid before conception and 12 weeks after (SACN, 2006).

6.11   Choline

Choline is an essential nutrient needed for neurotransmitter synthesis, cell-membrane signalling, lipid transport and methyl-group metabolism (Zeisel and da Costa, 2009). In pregnancy, the demand for choline is especially high and the supply of choline is crucial. Choline consumption is particularly important during this time, because it has important roles in the foetus's brain and memory development (Zeisel, 2006) and may also help to reduce the risk of NTDs (Shaw *et al.*, 2009). Research carried out by Shaw *et al.* (2004) found that women with the lowest choline intakes had four times the risk of giving birth to a child with NTD when compared against women with the highest intakes. This was a well-designed and controlled study as scientists controlled for other factors such as body weight, race, ethnicity, education level and dietary folate/methionine intake that could also affect the data. This demonstrates that the benefits of choline were independent of folate intake from food and supplements.

6.11.1   Guidelines

Choline is found in a wide variety of foods (Figure 6.4), but egg yolks are one on the most concentrated sources of choline containing 680 mg/100 g (USDA database data). Fish, lean chicken, milk and low-fat dairy products and leafy vegetables are also good sources (Figure 6.5). In the United States, an adequate intake (AI) level of 425 mg/day has been set for non-pregnant women, 450 mg/day for pregnancy and 550 mg/day for lactating mothers, based on the amount needed to prevent liver dysfunction (IoM, 1998). Estimated average requirements (EAR), however, have not yet been established because of a clear lack of human data.

Animal studies have identified the potential implications of not consuming enough of this nutrient; research in human populations has only just begun. Indeed, the USDA is the only food database to have level of choline provided from food sources and this is crucial to be able to track the choline intakes of populations and then relate this to disease incidences. It is hoped that communicating the potential importance of choline to medical and health professionals may help to encourage further research within this important area.

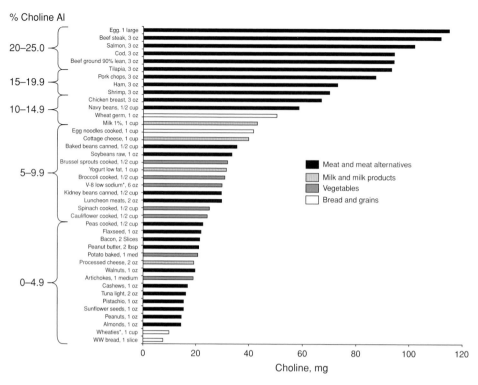

Figure 6.4   Food items with high choline levels. (Caudill (2010), with permission from Elsevier.)

Research Highlights   Can choline reverse some of the damage caused by alcohol and/or folate deficiency?

It is well known that alcohol exposure and folate deficiency in early pregnancy can have health implications for the offspring.

Now, recent animal research has shown that choline supplementation before delivery can help improve the foetus's brain development and chemistry, and even reduce the effect ethanol may have on foetus's brain development (Thomas et al., 2009). Another study using mice has shown that folate-deficient mice supplemented with choline later in their pregnancies had significantly lower levels of brain apoptosis (cell death) when compared to mice that were folate-deficient (Craciunescu et al., 2010). Overall, the findings from these animal studies may have wider implications for women and choline supplementation could be of benefit to women who drink alcohol during pregnancy and/or have low folate status. Further research in the form of human clinical trials is now needed.

6.12   Vitamin C

Vitamin C (ascorbic acid) has a wide array of actions. It is a known that antioxidant also helps to regenerate other antioxidants (vitamins A and E) and support the immune system during pregnancy (Kontic-Vucinic et al., 2006).

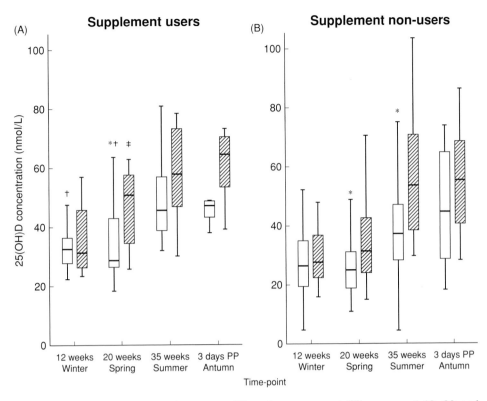

Figure 6.5 Vitamin D status of pregnant (□) and non-pregnant (▨) women at 12, 20 and 35 weeks pregnancy and 3 days after birth. Boxes represent the 5th and 95th percentiles, with the median represented by the line; whiskers at the top and bottom of the box represent the highest and lowest values excluding outliers. *$P < 0.05$. Values were significantly different from those of the pregnant non-users, †$P < 0.001$. Values were significantly different from those of the non-pregnant non-users, ‡$P < 0.05$. (Holmes *et al.* (2009), with permission from CUP.)

Some studies have shown that low vitamin C intakes may be associated with complications in pregnancy, such as pre-eclampsia, anaemia and having a small baby (Rumbold and Crowther, 2009). One of the largest studies undertaken to date is the Danish National Birth Cohort. Antioxidant intakes of over 57,000 mothers were determined using Food Frequency Questionnaires on the 25th week of pregnancy. Low intakes of vitamin C (below 70 mg/day) were associated with higher rates of pre-eclampsia, particularly when compared against mothers with higher intakes (130–170 mg/day).

In another large study of 775 mothers, those with low plasma vitamin C concentrations (<55.9 μmol/L) had a threefold increased risk of developing gestational diabetes. Authors conclude that vitamin C may influence glucose tolerance and reduce the occurrence of gestational diabetes (Zhang *et al.*, 2004). Although these are both large, well-designed studies, further research is needed to reinforce these initial findings. Subjectively, there is also some evidence that vitamin C supplementation may increase the risk of unfavourable birth outcomes, such as preterm deliveries (Steyn *et al.*, 2003). Taken together, the findings from studies looking at vitamin C status in relation to pregnancy outcomes are highly variable and more work is needed before any firm recommendations can be made.

6.12.1 Guidelines

EU recommendations are set at 55 mg/day vitamin C for pregnant and 70 mg/day for lactating mothers (Commission of the European Communities, 1993). Non-EU requirements are set at somewhat higher levels. The US RDA for vitamin C is set at 85 mg/day for pregnant and 120 mg/day for lactating mothers (IoM, 1998), based on the vitamin's role as an antioxidant as well as protection from deficiency. The tolerable upper level (TUL) has been set at 2 g/day based on gastrointestinal upset that sometimes accompanies excessive dosages (Bsoul and Terezhalmy, 2004). Further work is needed to bring these recommendations in line.

6.13 Vitamin D

Vitamin D is a steroid structured hormone that can be produced by the skin or consumed from dietary (Table 6.6) and supplement sources (Huotari and Herzig, 2008). Research carried out in UK women 12, 20 and 35 weeks into the pregnancies and 3 days postpartum has shown that 35, 44 and 16% were classified as vitamin D deficient (25(OH)D <25 nmol/L) in the three trimesters, respectively, and 96, 96 and 75% had insufficient vitamin D status (25(OH)D <50 nmol/L) (Holmes et al., 2009). Interestingly, vitamin D status improved as pregnancy proceeded, but this was probably because data was collected in the summer months. Equally, even though women taking vitamin D supplements had improved vitamin D status, insufficiencies were still apparent (Figure 6.5). Well-designed studies are needed to investigate the effects of higher doses of vitamin D supplements accounting for seasonal variation.

In turn, inadequate vitamin D status in pregnancy can have implications for foetal bone health. This has been demonstrated clearly in a study of 424 mothers taking part in the Southampton Women's Survey (United Kingdom). Researchers measured foetal bone health using high-resolution 3D ultrasound scanners and found that the femoral development was not as well established in the foetuses of women who were deficient in vitamin D (Mahon et al., 2010). Overall, the findings from this important study show that the mother's vitamin D status may affect the bone development of her infant as early as 19 weeks into pregnancy.

Table 6.6 Top ten vitamin D rich foods for pregnancy (per 100 g).

Food source	Vitamin D (per 100 g)	
	µg	IU
Pilchards (canned in tomato sauce)	14.0	560
Kippers (grilled)	9.4	376
Mackerel (grilled)	8.8	352
Salmon (steamed)	8.7	348
Sardines (canned in tomato sauce)	8.0	320
Margarine (polyunsaturated)	7.9	316
Egg (yolk)	4.9	196
Blended spread	4.1	164
Tuna (canned in oil)	3.0	120
Eggs (boiled)	1.8	72

Source: FSA (2006).
1 IU = 0.025 µg.

6.13.1 Guidelines

In terms of dietary guidelines, current recommendations are lacking for pregnant and lactating women. In a review of studies measuring vitamin D status in pregnancy, in over 50% of papers, women had inadequate vitamin D status. This is particularly the case for mothers with pigmented skin and living at northerly latitudes (Schroth et al., 2005). In the United Kingdom, recommendations for pregnant and lactating mothers are both set at 10 μg/day (400 IU) (the same as adults 65 years and over) (DH, 1991) and at 5 μg/day (200 IU); these are even lower in the United States (IoM, 1997). Research from studies to date indicate that pregnant women's vitamin D requirements are likely to fall beyond the standard 10 μg/day – requirements for pregnancy may even be as high as 150 μg (6000 IU) (Hollis, 2007). This, however, exceeds current EFSA advice to consume no more than 50 μg/day (EFSA, 2006). Therefore, consensus is clearly needed in terms of 'how much' vitamin D pregnant women need. Certainly, it seems clear that an extra increment is needed on top of adult dietary recommendations, but this remains to be established.

The Return of Rickets

There has been a long history of different strategies used to prevent rickets in the United Kingdom and indeed in other Western regions. In the 1920s, once vitamin D had been discovered, this led to the routine consumption of cod liver oil by women and children (Bivins, 2007); however, use of this later ceased once the potential teratogenic effects of high doses of vitamin A had been identified. Consequently, this has left many women living in latitudes where levels of vitamin D generated by skin synthesis are inadequate during the winter and spring months. In addition, the benefits of vitamin D supplementation to women with darker skin or cultural beliefs, which mean that skin exposure is limited, is not well imparted.

Scientists in the United States analysing cord serum as a marker of vitamin D status found that 45% of black compared with 2% white mothers were deficient in vitamin D, placing their offspring at risk of deficiency also (Bodnar et al., 2007). Clinical trials have also shown that single oral doses of vitamin D (200,000 IU) or a daily supplement (800 IU) from 27 weeks until delivery may go some way towards improving the vitamin D status of multi-ethnic women (Yu et al., 2009). However, even with supplementation, only a small percentage of women and babies were vitamin D sufficient. Further research is much needed to better determine to optimal dose, timing and method of delivery in terms of helping women to achieve optimal vitamin D status before, during and beyond pregnancy.

6.14 Vitamin E

Vitamin E is a fat-soluble vitamin and known antioxidant that is particularly important during the early phases of life (from conception to after delivery) (Debier, 2007). However, despite its widely accepted role as an antioxidant, the biological functions of vitamin E are probably the least understood of all the vitamins (Brigelius-Flohé, 2009).

Although some studies have found that inadequate intakes of vitamin E (found in vegetable oils, cereals and leafy green vegetables) may increase the risk of developing pre-eclampsia or delivering small babies, these findings are inconsistent (Rumbold and Crowther, 2009). Most studies use combinations of supplements and the effects of vitamin E alone needs to be studied further. It has also been found that high intakes of vitamin E (above 14.9 mg/day) may increase the risk of congenital heart defects in the offspring by ninefold, although the mechanisms behind this remain to be known (Smedts et al., 2009). This is worrying since US DRI is set at 15 mg/day and 19 mg/day for lactating mothers. To date, no TUL intakes for vitamin E have been set specifically for pregnant/lactating mothers. Considering the findings from this study, there is a need for these to be established. Data are insufficient at present to assert any potential role of vitamin E and pre-eclampsia risk.

6.15   Vitamin K

Vitamin K has two forms: phylloquinone (present in green leafy vegetables such as kale, spinach and broccoli) and menaquinone (normally produced by intestinal bacteria). For pregnant and lactating mothers, 90 µg phylloquinone is generally recommended and can usually be obtained from food sources (IoM, 2001).

However, in some cases, women who have experienced hyperemesis gravidarium have been deficient in vitamin K, which has been linked to foetal intracranial hemorrhage and preterm deliveries. In these instances, mothers should be carefully monitored and health practitioners may consider vitamin K prophylaxis (Eventov-Friedman et al., 2009). Inadequate maternal intakes and poor maternal–foetal transfer can place infants at high risk of vitamin K deficiency, particularly when concentrations in breast milk are also low (Booth and Al Rajabi, 2008). The American Academy of Pediatrics in 2009 reaffirmed their previous recommendation to give all infants an intramuscular injection of 0.5–1 mg vitamin K (American Academy of Pediatrics, 2003)

EFSA Vitamin and Mineral Dietary Reference Values

The EFSA has recently established dietary reference values for carbohydrates, dietary fibre, fats and water. These are a valuable contribution, providing consistently across suitable and dietary targets again which European research can be compared. The panel also aims to publish DRVs for vitamins and minerals, which will update the current Commission of the European Communities (1993) recommendations, which are commonly used as a reference point. These updated guidelines are much needed, as a wealth of important research has taken place over the last two decades and are awaited with eager anticipation.

6.16   Combined vitamin deficiencies

It is not uncommon for multiple vitamin deficiencies to co-exist, particularly when the diet is poor. An inadequate intake of animal foods is usually the main cause of multiple vitamin (and mineral) deficiencies, particularly in developing countries.

Table 6.7 Prevalence of concurrent micronutrient deficiencies (Haryana, India).

Deficiencies	Prevalence
Zinc + iron	54.9%
Zinc + magnesium + iron	25.6%
Zinc + magnesium + iron + folic acid	9.3%
Zinc + magnesium + iron + folic acid + iodine	0.8%

Source: Pathak *et al.* (2004).

Women living in wealthier regions who also avoid meat/milk consumption can also be at risk of multiple nutrient deficiencies (Allen, 2005).

In Haryana, India, the nutritional status of pregnant women (28 weeks gestation) from six villages was assessed using a combination of blood samples and nutrient intakes analysed from 24-hour recalls. Zinc, iron, magnesium, folic acid, iodine and copper deficiencies were most common, although no women were deficient in all six simultaneously. Combined vitamin deficiencies were also common and are shown in Table 6.7 (Pathak *et al.*, 2004). It has been suggested that women with iron-deficiency anaemia may also need to supplement with multiple vitamins as well. Iron-deficient Chinese pregnant mothers also have higher rates of vitamin C, folate and B$_{12}$ deficiency (Ma *et al.*, 2004).

Overall, these studies show that concurrent deficiencies are common during pregnancy. Poor diets and inadequate intakes of nutrient-dense foods combined high birth rates and short inter-pregnancy intervals may place women at particular high risk of multiple micronutrient deficiencies (Pathak *et al.*, 2004).

6.17 Supplements and pregnancy

In some situations, when recommended micronutrient intakes cannot be met through an adequate diet, supplementation may be important. It is widely acknowledged that demographic, social and economic factors all affect supplement usage (Picciano and McGuire, 2009), but when taken studies have shown that supplements can substantially contribute to total nutrient intakes.

In the Norwegian Mother and Child and Cohort Study (MoBa), the dietary and supplement habits of 40,108 women were studied in the first 4–5 months of pregnancy. Eighty-one percent reported the use of one or more dietary supplements with omega-3 fatty acids (cod liver oil/fish oil) being taken by 59% mothers. This was closely followed by folic acid supplements used by 36% women and 31% reported taking multivitamin/multimineral supplements (Haugen *et al.*, 2008). When dietary intakes were compared against recommendations, certain supplements, namely folic acid and vitamin D, significantly contributed to daily intakes, but levels of intakes were still not sufficient to reach recommended levels of intake.

6.18 Application in practice

Women should be guided to make the right food choices from early in their pregnancies, if not, ideally before conception. Nurses, midwifes and other public health practitioners can play a key role in guiding women in terms of how recommended proportions of vitamins can be obtained from food sources. Equally, eating at regular intervals and consuming a varied diet can both help to improve overall diet quality. It makes sense that nutrients should be tried to be obtained from the diet, but when this is not possible, women may consider topping up with a pregnancy-formulated multivitamin and mineral supplement.

Public health practitioners can play a key role in informing women about the benefits and importance of supplements such as folic acid, encouraging them to comply and take these on a daily basis. When women attend doctors/medical appointments before becoming pregnant or in the early stages of pregnancy, they should be prompted at every chance to make sure they are eating a balanced diet and taking appropriate supplements and complying with these, i.e. taking them on a daily basis for full benefit.

6.19 Conclusion

Pregnancy is a time when good nutrition is exceptionally important. As dietary requirements for several vitamins increase during pregnancy, these need to be met. Folate deficiency is one of the most common vitamin deficiencies worldwide and is a frequent cause of pregnancy complications and birth defects (Wolff *et al.*, 2009). Equally, women with poor vitamin B_{12} status also have up to a threefold increased risk of delivering a child with birth defects (Thompson *et al.*, 2009). From this chapter, we have also seen that other common deficiencies, such as vitamin D, may also occur during pregnancy. Ideally, the diet should be amended to satisfy requirements, but this may be difficult in some populations. Consequently, supplements and functional foods may be of benefit to some expectant mothers.

Key Messages

- Vitamins should be obtained from the diet where possible, but supplementation may be needed by some individuals and in some geographical regions.
- Dietary guidelines for pregnant mothers need to be revised, particularly in the United Kingdom, as a wealth of new information has been published since these were first established.
- Relevant increments should also be provided for separate trimesters where appropriate and recommended ULs provided for all micronutrients, which are lacking for the pregnant population.
- More research is needed to determine whether (and how) vitamins may play a role in foetal growth and development (and how they interact with each other).
- When interpreting findings from studies providing supplements, their placebo effect must be taken into consideration – some women may feel more comfortable with the belief that they are taking something that may benefit their child's health.
- There is a need to increase awareness amongst health professionals and consumers about the potential roles of vitamins B_{12}, D and choline in pregnancy, although ongoing research is needed to help formulate pregnancy-specific dietary recommendations.
- Education regarding the richest food sources of key vitamins can assist in helping expectant mothers to achieve dietary goals.
- When taking supplements, women should be encouraged to comply and take these on a daily basis for full benefit.

Recommended reading

FNB (Food and Nutrition Board) (2004) *Dietary Reference Intakes for Individuals, Elements*. The National Academies Press: Washington, DC.

Hyppönen E and Boucher BJ (2010) Avoidance of vitamin D deficiency in pregnancy in the United Kingdom: the case for a unified approach in National policy. *British Journal of Nutrition* **104**, 309–14.

SACN (Scientific Advisory Committee on Nutrition) (2007) *Update on Vitamin D. Position Statement by the Scientific Advisory Committee on Nutrition*. The Stationery Office: London.

Shaw GM, Finnell RH, Blom HJ *et al.* (2009) Choline and risk of neural tube defects in a folate-fortified population. *Epidemiology* **20**(5), 714–9.

References

Allen LH (2005) Multiple micronutrients in pregnancy and lactation: an overview. *American Journal of Clinical Nutrition* **81**(5), 1206S–12S.

Allen LH (2009) How common is vitamin B_{12} deficiency? *American Journal of Clinical Nutrition* **89**, 693S–6S.

American Academy of Pediatrics (2003) Controversies concerning vitamin K and the newborn. *Pediatrics* **112**(1), 191–2.

Azaïs-Braesco V and Pascal G (2000) Vitamin A in pregnancy: requirements and safety limits. *American Journal of Clinical Nutrition* **71**(5 Suppl), 1325S–33S.

Bâ A (2009) Alcohol and B_1 vitamin deficiency-related stillbirths. *Journal of Maternal Fetal Neonatal Medicine* **22**(5), 452–7.

Baker H, DeAngelis B, Hollard B, Gittens-Williams L and Barrett T (2002) Vitamin profile of 563 gravidas during trimesters of pregnancy. *Journal of the American College of Nutrition* **21**(1), 33–7.

Bivins R (2007) 'The English disease' or 'Asian rickets'? Medical responses to postcolonial immigration. *Bulletin of the History of Medicine* **81**, 533–68.

Bodnar LM, Simhan HN, Powers RW, Frank MP, Cooperstein E and Roberts JM (2007) High prevalence of vitamin D insufficiency in black and white pregnant women residing in the Northern United States and their neonates. *Journal of Nutrition* **137**(2), 447–52.

Booth SL and Rajabi A (2008) Determinants of vitamin K status in humans. *Vitamins & Hormones* **78**(1), 1–22.

Brämswig S, Prinz-Langenohl R, Lamers Y *et al.* (2009) Supplementation with a multivitamin containing 800 μg of folic acid shortens the time to reach the preventive red blood cell folate concentration in healthy women. *International Journal of Vitamin & Nutrition Research* **79**(2), 61–70.

Brigelius-Flohé R (2009) Vitamin E: the shrew waiting to be tamed. *Free Radical Biology & Medicine* **46**(5), 543–54.

Bsoul SA and Terezhalmy GT (2004) Vitamin C in health and disease. The *Journal of Contemporary Dental Practice* **5**(2), 1–13.

Carmel R (2009) Does high folic acid intake affect unrecognised cobalamin deficiency, and how will we know it if we see it? *American Journal of Clinical Nutrition* **90**, 1449–50.

Caudill MA (2010) Pre- and postnatal health: evidence of increased choline needs. *Journal of the American Dietetic Association* **110**, 1198–206.

Chiossi G, Neri I, Cavazzuti M, Basso G and Facchinetti F (2006) Hyperemesis gravidarium complicated by Wernicke encephalopathy: background, case report, and review of the literature. *Obstetrical & Gynaecological Survey* **61**(4), 255–68.

CLAPA (Cleft Lip and Palate Association) (2009) Understanding cleft lip and palate. Available at: http://www.clapa.com/antenatal/article/107/. (accessed March 2011.)

Commission of the European Communities (1993) *Vitamin D: In Nutrient and Energy Intakes of the European Community. Report of the Scientific Committee for Food (31st Series)*. Brussels, pp 132–9.

COMA (Committee on Medical Aspects of Food and Nutrition Policy) (2000) *Folic Acid and the Prevention of Disease*. The Stationery Office: London.

Craciunescu CN, Johnson AR and Zeisel SH (2010) Dietary choline reverses some, but not all, effects of folate deficiency on neurogenesis and apoptosis in fetal mouse brain. *Journal of Nutrition* **140**(6), 1162–6.

Cucó G, Fernandez-Ballart J, Arija V and Canals J (2005) Effect of B1, B6 and iron intake during pregnancy on neonatal behaviour. *International Journal for Vitamin & Nutrition Research* **75**(5), 320–6.

Debier C (2007) Vitamin E during pre- and postnatal periods. *Vitamins & Hormones* **76**, 357–73.

Department of Health (1991) *Dietary Reference Values for Food Energy and Nutrients for the United Kingdom*, 2nd edition. *Report on Social Subjects* no. 41. The Stationery Office: London.

Dietrich M, Brown CJ and Block G (2005) The effect of folate fortification of cereal-grain products on blood folate status, dietary folate intake, and dietary folate sources among adult non-supplement users in the United States. *Journal of the American College of Nutrition* **24**(4), 266–74.

Dror DK and Allen LH (2008) Effect of vitamin B12 deficiency on neurodevelopment in infants: current knowledge and possible mechanisms. *Nutrition Reviews* **66**(5), 250–5.

EFSA (European Food Safety Authority) (2006) Tolerable upper intake levels of vitamins and minerals by the Scientific Panel on Dietetic Products, Nutrition and Allergies (NDA) and Scientific Committee on Food (SCF). Available at: http://www.efsa.europa.eu/fr/scdocs/oldsc/upper_level_opinions_full-part33.pdf. (accessed March 2011.)

Eventov-Friedman S, Klinger G and Shinwell ES (2009) Third trimester fetal intracranial hemorrhage owing to vitamin K deficiency associated with hyperemesis gravidarium. *Journal of Pediatric Hematology & Oncology* **31**(12), 985–8.

FAO/WHO (2002) Vitamin A. In: *Human Vitamin and Mineral Requirements. Report of a Joint FAO/WHO Expert Consultation*. FAO: Rome, pp 87–1107.

FSA (Food Standards Agency) (2006) *McCance and Widdowson's, the Composition of Foods*. 6th edition. Royal Society of Chemistry: London.

Groenen PM, van Rooij IA, Peer PG, Ocké MC, Zielhuis GA and Steegers-Theunissen RP (2004) Low maternal dietary intakes of iron, magnesium, and niacin are associated with spina bifida in the offspring. *Journal of Nutrition* **134**(6), 1516–22.

Haugen M, Brantsaeter AL, Alexander J and Meltzer HM (2008) Dietary supplements contribute substantially to the total nutrient intake in pregnant Norwegian women. *Annals of Nutrition & Metabolism* **52**, 272–80.

Hollis BW (2007) Vitamin D requirement during pregnancy and lactation. *Journal of Bone and Mineral Research* **22**(2), V39–44.

Holmes VA, Barnes MS, Alexander HD, McFaul P and Wallace JMW (2009) Vitamin D deficiency and insufficiency in pregnant women: a longitudinal study. *British Journal of Nutrition* **102**, 876–81.

Huotari A and Herzig KH (2008) Vitamin D and living in northern latitudes – an endemic risk area for Vitamin D deficiency. *International Journal of Circumpolar Health* **67**, 164–78.

IoM (Institute of Medicine) (1997) *Dietary Reference Intakes for Calcium, Phosphorus, Magnesium, Vitamin D, and Fluoride*. National Academy Press: Washington, DC.

IoM (1998) *Dietary Reference Intakes for Thiamine, Riboflavin, Niacin, Vitamin B6, Folate, Vitamin B12, Pantothenic Acid, Biotin and Choline*. National Academies Press: Washington, DC.

IoM (2001) Vitamin A. In: *Dietary Reference Intakes for Vitamin A, Vitamin K, Arsenic, Boron, Chromium, Copper, Iodine, Iron, Manganese, Molybdenum, Nickel, Silicon, Vanadium and Zinc. Food and Nutrition Board, Institute of Medicine*. National Academy Press: Washington, DC, pp 82–161.

Jiang T, Christian P, Khatry SK, Wu L and West KP Jr (2005) Micronutrient deficiencies in early pregnancy are common, concurrent, and vary by season among rural Nepali pregnant women. *Journal of Nutrition* **135**(5), 1106–12.

Khoury MJ, Moore CA and Mulinare J (1996) Vitamin A and birth defects. *Lancet* **347**(8997), 322.

Kongnyuy EJ, Wiysonge CS and Shey MS (2009) A systematic review of randomized controlled trials of prenatal and postnatal vitamin A supplementation of HIV-infected women. *International Journal of Gynaecology & Obstetrics* **104**(1), 5–8.

Kontic-Vucinic O, Sulovic N and Radunovic N (2006) Micronutrients in Women's Reproductive Health: I. Vitamins. *International Journal of Fertility* **51**(3), 106–15.

Lagiou P, Mucci L, Tamimi R *et al.* (2005) Micronutrient intake during pregnancy in relation to birth size. *European Journal of Nutrition* **44**(1), 52–9.

Li Z and Qian YP (1994) *Birth defects surveillance*, 2nd edition. People's Health Press: Beijing, pp 1–3.

Ma AG, Chen XC, Wang Y, Xu RX, Zheng MC and Li JS (2004) The multiple vitamin status of Chinese pregnant women with anemia and nonanemia in the last trimester. *Journal of Nutritional Science & Vitaminology (Tokyo)* **50**(2), 87–92.

Mahon P, Harvey N, Crozier S *et al.*; The SWS Study Group (2010) Low maternal vitamin D status and fetal bone development: cohort study. *Journal of Bone Mineral Research* **25**(1), 14–9.

Mignini LE, Latthe PM, Villar J, Kilby MD, Carroli G and Khan KS (2005) Mapping the theories of pre-eclampsia: the role of homocysteine. *Obstetrics & Gynaecology* **105**(2), 411–25.

Mock DM (2009) Marginal biotin deficiency is common in normal human pregnancy and is highly teratogenic in mice. *Journal of Nutrition* **139**(1), 154–7.

Mock DM, Quirk JG and Mock NI (2002) Marginal biotin deficiency during normal pregnancy. *American Journal of Clinical Nutrition* **75**, 295–9.

Molloy AM, Kirke PN, Brody LC, Scott JM and Mills JL (2008) Effects of folate and vitamin B12 deficiencies during pregnancy on fetal, infant, and child development. *Food & Nutrition Bulletin* **29**(2 Suppl), S101–11.

Navarro J, Causse MB, Desquilbet N, Hervé F and Lallemand D (1984) The vitamin status of low birth weight infants and their mothers. *Journal of Paediatric Gastroenterology & Nutrition* **3**(5), 744–8.

NHMRC (National Health and Medical Research Council) (2006) *Nutrient Reference Values for Australia and New Zealand*. NHMRC Publications: Australia. Available at: https://www.nhmrc.gov.au. (accessed March 2011.)

Ortega RM, Martínez RM, Andrés P, Marín-Arias L and López-Sobaler AM (2004) Thiamine status during the third trimester of pregnancy and its influence on thiamine concentrations in transition and mature breast milk. *British Journal of Nutrition* **92**(1), 129–35.

Pathak P, Kapil U, Kapoor SK *et al.* (2004) Prevalence of multiple micronutrient deficiencies amongst pregnant women in a rural area of Haryana. *Indian Journal of Pediatrics* **71**(11), 1007–14.

Pfeiffer CM, Caudill SP, Gunter EW, Osterloh J, and Sampson EJ (2005) Biochemical indicators of B vitamin status in the US population after folic acid fortification: results from the National Health and Nutrition Examination Survey 1999–2000. *American Journal of Clinical Nutrition* **82**, 442–50.

Picciano MF and McGuire MK (2009) Use of dietary supplements by pregnant and lactating women in North America. *Am J Clin Nutr* **89**(2), S663–7.

Powers HJ and Bates CJ (1984) Effects of pregnancy and riboflavin deficiency on some aspects of iron metabolism in rats. *International Journal of Vitamin Nutrition Research* **54**(2–3), 179–83.

Rumbold A and Crowther CA (2009) Vitamin C supplementation in pregnancy. *The Cochrane Library* **18**(2), CD004072.

SACN (Scientific Advisory Committee on Nutrition) (2005) *Review of Dietary Advice on Vitamin A*. The Stationery Office: London.

SACN (Scientific Advisory Committee on Nutrition) (2006) *Folate and disease prevention*. The Stationery Office: London.

Schroth RJ, Lavelle CL and Moffatt ME (2005) Review of vitamin D deficiency during pregnancy: who is affected? *International Journal of Circumpolar Health* **64**(2), 112–20.

Schulz C, Engel U, Kreienberg R and Biesalski HK (2007) Vitamin A and beta-carotene supply of women with gemini or short birth intervals: a pilot study. *European Journal of Nutrition* **46**(1), 12–20.

Shaw G, Carmichael S, Yang W, Selvin S and Schaffer D (2004) Perionceptional dietary intake of choline and betaine and neural tube defects in offspring. *American Journal of Epidemiology* **160**, 102–9.

Shaw GM, Finnell RH, Blom HJ *et al.* (2009) Choline and risk of neural tube defects in a folate-fortified population. *Epidemiology* **20**(5), 714–9.

Smedts HP, de Vries JH, Rakhshandehroo M *et al.* (2009) High maternal vitamin E intake by diet or supplements is associated with congenital heart defects in the offspring. *British Journal of Obstetrics & Gynaecology* **116**(3), 416–23.

Staggs CG, Sealey WM, McCabe BJ, Teague AM and Mock DM (2004) Determination of the biotin content of select foods using accurate and sensitive HPLC/avidin binding. *Journal of Food Composition & Analysis* **17**(6), 767–76.

Steyn PS, Odendaal HJ, Schoeman J, Stander C, Fanie N and Grové D (2003) A randomised, double-blind placebo-controlled trial of ascorbic acid supplementation for the prevention of preterm labour. *Journal of Obstetrics & Gynaecology* 23(2), 150–5.

Strobel M, Tinz J and Biesalski HK (2007) The importance of beta-carotene as a source of vitamin A with special regard to pregnant and breastfeeding women. *European Journal of Nutrition* 46S(1), 1–20.

Takimoto H, Mito N, Umegaki K *et al.* (2007) Relationship between dietary folate intakes, maternal plasma total homocysteine and B-vitamins during pregnancy and fetal growth in Japan. *European Journal of Nutrition* 46, 300–6.

Thaver D, Saeed MA and Bhutta ZA (2006) Pyridoxine (vitamin B6) supplementation in pregnancy. *Cochrane Database of Systemic Reviews* 19(2), CD000179.

Thomas JD, Abou EJ and Dominguez HD (2009) Prenatal choline supplementation mitigates the adverse effects of prenatal alcohol exposure on development in rats. *Neurotoxicology & Teratology* 31(5), 303–11.

Thompson MD, Cole DEC and Ray JG (2009) Vitamin B-12 and neural tube defects: the Canadian experience. *American Journal of Clinical Nutrition* 89(suppl), 697–701S.

Tinker SC, Cogswell ME, Devine O and Berry RJ (2010) Folic acid intake among U.S. women aged 15–44 years, National Health and Nutrition Examination Survey, 2003–06. *American Journal of Preventative Medicine* 38(5), 534–42.

Wacker J, Frühauf J, Schulz M, Chiwora FM, Volz J and Becker K (2000) Riboflavin deficiency and pre-eclampsia. *Obstetrics & Gynaecology* 96(1), 38–44.

Watanabe F (2007) Vitamin B_{12} sources and bioavailability. *Experimental Biology & Medicine* 232(10), 1266–74.

Watson PE and McDonald BW (2010) The association of maternal diet and dietary supplement intake in pregnant New Zealand women with infant birthweight. *European Journal of Clinical Nutrition* 64(2), 184–93.

Wilcox AJ, Lie RT, Solvoll K *et al.* (2007) Folic acid supplements and risk of facial clefts: national population based case-control study. *British Medical Journal* 334(7591), 464.

Wolff T, Witkop CT, Miller T, Syed SB and U.S. Preventive Services Task Force (2009) Folic acid supplementation for the prevention of neural tube defects: an update of the evidence for the U.S. Preventive Services Task Force. *Annals of Internal Medicine* 150(9), 632–9.

Yajnik CS, Deshpande SS, Jackson AA *et al.* (2008) Vitamin B12 and folate concentrations during pregnancy and insulin resistance in the offspring: the Pune maternal nutrition study. *Diabetologia* 51, 29–38.

Yu CKH, Sykes L, Sethi M, Teoh TG and Robinson S (2009) Vitamin D deficiency and supplementation during pregnancy. *Clinical Endocrinology* 70, 685–90.

Zeisel SH (2006) The fetal origins of memory: the role of dietary choline in optimal brain development. *Journal of Pediatrics* 149(5 Suppl) S131–6.

Zeisel SH and da Costa KA (2009) Choline: an essential nutrient for public health. *Nutrition Reviews* 67(11), 615–23.

Zempleni J, Hassan YI and Wijeratne SS (2008) Biotin and biotinidase deficiency. *Expert Review of Endocrinology and Metabolism* 3(6), 715–24.

Zempleni J, Wijeratne SS and Hassan YI (2009) Biotin. *Biofactors* 35(1), 36–46.

Zhang C, Williams MA, Sorensen TK *et al.* (2004) Maternal plasma ascorbic acid (vitamin C) and risk of gestational diabetes mellitus. *Epidemiology* 15(5), 597–604.

Zhu L and Ling H (2008) National neural tube defects prevention program in China. *Food and Nutrition Bulletin* 29(2), S196–204.

Summary

Minerals can be defined as macro- or microminerals depending on whether they are re-quired by the body physiologically in small or large amounts. For most pregnant women, daily requirements for minerals can be met through the consumption of a balanced diet. However, there is evidence to suggest that certain minerals such as iron, iodine and se-lenium are being underconsumed by a proportion of women. Whilst the potential health benefits of consuming adequate levels of certain minerals in pregnancy is well docu-mented, i.e. iron and iodine, less is known about the potential role(s) of other minerals, such as selenium, copper and chromium. It would be useful to carry out additional studies to see if any of these understudied minerals could be of benefit to maternal/infant health. With regard to dietary recommendations for minerals, pregnancy-specific guidelines are lacking in many instances and safe upper limits, i.e. in the case of iron, may be useful in the future as new evidence begins to emerge.

Learning Outcomes

- To discuss the role(s) of key macro- and microminerals and explain their function(s) in pregnancy.
- To describe how under- and overconsumption of minerals can influence maternal and infant health.
- To recognise which food sources provide important sources of minerals and how women can reach recommended levels of intake.
- To be aware of current dietary guidelines for key minerals and their safe upper limits.

7.1   Introduction

A balanced diet, rich in essential minerals, is of pivotal importance for both maternal and infant health. Although dietary recommendations are available, it is important to consider that mineral requirements will also depend upon nutrient stores before pregnancy, socio-demographic characteristics and the health status of the mother. Women in industrialised regions generally have a wide range of food choices, whilst in less developed regions, foods consumption may depend heavily on the seasonal production of food. Subsequently, food availability impacts heavily on the nutrient

Nutrition in the Childbearing Years, First Edition. Emma Derbyshire.
© 2011 Emma Derbyshire. Published 2011 by Blackwell Publishing Ltd.

and mineral status of expectant mothers. For this reason, many supplement trials have been undertaken in developing regions. These studies have set out to establish whether both single and multiple (mineral) supplements improve maternal health and pregnancy outcomes. This chapter aims to explain the physiological role of key minerals during pregnancy, recommended levels of intake (and how these can be achieved) and will discuss and review findings from some of the largest, most pertinent studies within this area.

7.2   Macrominerals

7.2.1   Calcium

Calcium is one of the most abundant minerals in the human body. Around 99% of calcium is stored in the bones and teeth, whilst the remainder is transported in intracellular and extracellular fluid. Calcium has important biochemical and physiological roles in pregnancy, including supporting cell growth, the transmission of nerve signals and the release of brain neurotransmitters. There is some research to suggest that calcium also helps to stimulate the contraction of uterine muscles (Wray and Shmygol, 2007).

Pre-eclampsia, a blood pressure disorder in pregnancy, is a major cause of death in pregnancy and newborn babies worldwide, affecting as many as 10% of pregnant mothers (Ritchie and King, 2000). A review of 12 clinical trials found that calcium supplementation in pregnancy seems to be an effective and safe way of reducing pre-eclampsia risk, particularly in communities where women's dietary calcium intakes are inadequate. Taking up to 1 g/day calcium was found to reduce pre-eclampsia risk by as much as 50% as well as the risk of preterm deliveries (Hofmeyr *et al.*, 2010). Further studies are needed, however, to confirm whether these doses are appropriate for all women.

Guidelines

The foetus accumulates around 25–30 g calcium by the end of pregnancy (Lafond and Simoneau, 2006). Although it is important to consume a diet adequate in calcium throughout the course of pregnancy, scientists have found that it is the calcium consumed before pregnancy that is utilised from the mother's skeletal reserves (Kontic-Vucinic *et al.*, 2006).

Firstly, women should try to increase their daily dietary intakes of calcium. This can be done by substituting low calcium foods with calcium-rich alternatives (Table 7.1). Current dietary requirements for calcium in pregnancy range from 700 mg/day in the United Kingdom (DH, 1991) to 1000 mg/day in the United States (FNB, 1997) and Australasia (NHMRC, 2006). The European Food Safety Authority (EFSA) (2006) have identified that calcium intakes up to 2500 mg/day are deemed safe; no health ramifications have been documented up to this level of intake.

7.2.2   Magnesium

Magnesium is also mainly stored within the bones and is involved in over 300 essential body reactions (Kontic-Vucinic *et al.*, 2006). When compared with levels of

Table 7.1 Low calcium versus high calcium foods.

Low calcium (mg per 100 g)	High calcium (mg per 100 g)
Weetabix, dry (35)	Ready Brek, dry (1200)
White bread (177)	Granary bread (209)
Cream crackers (110)	Rye crispbread (145)
Low fat fruit yoghurt (162)	Whole milk yoghurt, plain (200)
Currants (93)	Fresh figs (230)
Lemon sole, steamed (21)	Sardines, canned in brine, drained (540)
Green salad (19)	Watercress, raw (170)
Beanburger, fried in vegetable oil (69)	Tofu, steamed (510)
Brussels sprouts, boiled (20)	Curly kale, boiled (150)
Oat-based biscuits (37)	Gingernut biscuits (130)
Eccles cake (70)	Plain scone (186)
Hot chocolate powder (411)	Horlicks powder (640)

Source: FSA (2006).

research for other minerals, only a handful of studies have investigated the potential role of magnesium in relation to maternal/foetal well-being.

Intake studies show that about two-thirds of the population do not consume adequate levels of magnesium. In pregnancy, low magnesium intakes have been linked to preterm deliveries brought about by hyperactivity (stimulation) of the uterine muscles (Durlach, 2004). When infants are born before term, this means that their magnesium reserves will be low – around 80% of the infant's magnesium stores are accrued before delivery. As magnesium is needed for neurological and visual function, this is thought to be one of the underlying causes for medical conditions such as cerebral palsy (CP) and mental retardation (Caddell *et al.*, 1999) (also see Table 7.2). Children with CP often have other related conditions or problems, such as epilepsy, learning difficulties, visual and/or hearing impairments, speech impairments, delayed growth and curvature of the spine (Figure 7.1).

Guidelines

Professor Lex Doyle, an Australian paediatrician, found that women taking 300 mg/day magnesium (Mg) either before or in the early stages of pregnancy delivered infants with a higher birth weight and larger head circumference (Doyle *et al.*, 1989). A recent systematic review by the same scientist has shown that when women at risk of preterm deliveries are treated with magnesium sulphate, this can reduce the

Table 7.2 Possible consequences of Mg deficiency.

Neurodevelopmental damage (cerebral palsy, blindness, deafness, physical disabilities)	Doyle *et al.* (2009)
Sudden infant death (SID) syndrome	Chiu *et al.* (2005)
Spina bifida	Groenen *et al.* (2004)
Uterine hyperactivity and preterm labour	Durlach (2004)
Reduced birth weight, length and/or head circumference	Doyle *et al.* (1989)

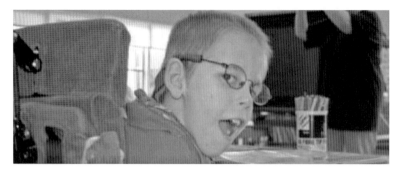

Figure 7.1 CP in childhood. Cerebral palsy is caused by damage to the brain before, during or after birth. Around 1 in 400 children in the United Kingdom are affected by cerebral palsy each year and about 1800 babies are diagnosed with the condition each year. (With permission from scope (NHS, 2010).)

risk of preterm deliveries and help to protect the foetus from neurological disorders such as CP (Doyle *et al.*, 2009).

Currently, dietary guidelines are set at similar to levels to those identified to be beneficial by Professor Lex Doyle. UK recommendations for Mg are 270 mg/day (DH, 1991) and slightly higher in the United States at 350 mg/day (FNB, 2001). Research carried out on a sample of 249 pregnant women found that women's diets were more likely to be lacking in certain nutrients before pregnancy, when compared with dietary patterns after conception. However, even after falling pregnant, 21% women were found to have diets lacking in magnesium (Pinto *et al.*, 2009). Although work by Doyle has shown that magnesium sulphate supplements can help to improve pregnancy outcomes, women should also make sure that they are eating enough magnesium-rich foods (Table 7.3).

7.2.3 Sodium

Sodium, commonly referred to as salt, is found in most foods in the form of sodium chloride. It may also take the form of sodium bicarbonate, monosodium glutamate, sodium phosphate, sodium carbonate or sodium benzoate. One gram of sodium chloride contains 390 mg (17 mmol) of sodium (SACN), 2003).

Table 7.3 Mg-rich sources (per 100 g).

Food source	Mg content (mg per 100 g)
Sunflower seeds	390
Breakfast cereals (bran flakes)	100
Dark/plain chocolate	89
Wholemeal bread	66
Lightly steamed spinach	54
Brown rice	43
Raisins	35
White fish (halibut)	29
Low fat yoghurt	16

Source: FSA (2006).

Animal studies, mainly using rats, show that high-sodium intakes often lead to side effects that are similar to manifestations observed in pre-eclampsia patients (Beauséjour *et al.*, 2003). The effects of high sodium (or salt) intakes have not been studied in detail in human pregnancies because this work is difficult to undertake. Two trials so far have set out to study whether salt restriction diets can help to reduce blood pressure and pre-eclampsia risk in pregnancy. Unfortunately, high rates of withdrawal were experienced in both of these studies, mainly because the diets were reported to be unpalatable (Duley *et al.*, 2009).

Caution should therefore be exercised when giving guidance on salt intakes in pregnancy. There is a lack of evidence linking high sodium intake to pre-eclampsia risk, but there is a clear lack of research in this area caused mainly by obstacles linked to study design.

7.3 Microminerals

7.3.1 Chromium

Chromium is needed for the metabolism of glucose, insulin and blood lipids. It is thought that chromium may help insulin to bind to cells, upregulate insulin receptors, increase insulin sensitivity and help to protect against the development of diabetes in pregnancy (Anderson, 2000).

On the basis of this theory, American scientists have carried out research to see if women's poor chromium status has a higher risk of developing diabetes in pregnancy. In this follow-through study, 425 women had their serum chromium levels measured in the first and second trimesters of pregnancy. No differences in chromium levels were observed when test results from mothers with and without diabetes were compared (Woods *et al.*, 2008). It is, however, possible that no significant findings were observed in this study because the number of women developing diabetes (25 cases) was too small and data was not collected in the third trimester of pregnancy. Gunton *et al.* (2001) reported similar results; plasma chromium levels had no effect on glucose intolerance, insulin resistance or serum lipids levels in pregnancy, but study methods (determination of chromium levels) were reported to be flawed in this study.

On the whole, contrary to belief, chromium status does not appear to reduce diabetes risk in pregnancy. It is, however, important to consider that studies so far have been inadequately designed with small sample sizes and short periods of follow-up. It is possible that higher levels of chromium are needed to have any benefit, for these reasons, well-designed clinical trials would be particularly useful.

7.3.2 Copper

Copper is a trace metal and key component of copper-containing enzymes, also known as cuproenzymes. Pregnancy is a time when women and the developing child are both vulnerable to changes in dietary supplies. Even though copper deficiencies are generally rare, dietary intakes rarely exceed recommended levels of adequate intake (Gambling *et al.*, 2008). For this reason, even marginal copper deficits during pregnancy may lead to developmental, neurological and immunological problems in the offspring (Uriu-Adams and Keen, 2005).

Table 7.4 Copper-rich food sources (per 100 g).

Food source	Copper content (mg per 100 g)
Cocoa powder	3.90
Sunflower seeds	2.27
Crab, boiled	1.77
Sesame seeds	1.46
Bran, wheat	1.34
Lentils, green and brown, whole, dried, raw	1.02
Weetabix	0.54

Source: FSA (2006).

Copper also helps with the formation of red blood cells. Deficiencies can therefore lead to anaemia and neuropenia – when there is a reduced number of neutrophils in the body (a form of white blood cell). Low copper intakes have also been linked to a condition known as 'swayback' in both mother and child. This includes symptoms of spinal cord damage (myelopathy) and reduced co-ordination (Kumar, 2006).

Guidelines

In terms of copper intakes, 1.0–1.3 mg/day is recommended in most countries (see appendices). Most healthy adults with adequate food supplies can achieve these levels of intake. Good food sources of copper include whole grain cereals, leafy green vegetables, dark chocolate and lean chicken/turkey (Table 7.4).

It is also important to consider that certain minerals when consumed from dietary and supplement sources can interact and affect the transport and absorption of each other. Iron and copper are a good example of this – copper deficiency has been found to alter iron metabolism, leading to anaemia and an accumulation of iron in the liver. Much more remains to be known about how these minerals interact with each other, (Gambling *et al.*, 2008) but it is a point that needs to be considered when assessing either copper or iron status in pregnancy.

7.3.3 Iodine

Iodine is a non-metallic trace element and an essential component of thyroid hormones. Over two billion adults worldwide have insufficient iodine intakes – iodine intakes in industrialised regions such as the United States and Australia have fallen in recent years and about 50% of European residents are iodine deficient. South Asia and sub-Saharan Africa appear to be some of the areas that are worst affected (Zimmermann, 2009).

Recent research carried out in America as part of the National Health and Nutrition Examination Survey (NHANES) found that the iodine status of pregnant women was borderline sufficient. For all women, pregnant and non-pregnant, dairy foods were a particularly important source of iodine and those consuming the lowest intakes had some of the lowest urinary iodine concentrations (UICs) (Figure 7.2). These are important study findings and show that even in countries where salt is

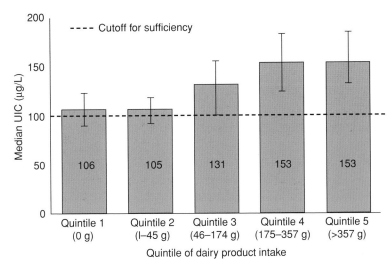

Figure 7.2 UIC of non-pregnant, non-lactating women by quintiles of previous day's dairy product intake. (Reproduced with permission (Perrine *et al.*, 2010).)

iodised, women are only borderline iodine sufficient (Perrine *et al.*, 2010). Equally, women who do not consume dairy foods regularly may be placing themselves at risk of iodine deficiency.

Goitre in pregnancy

Pregnant women have higher iodine requirements because renal clearance and foetal demands are higher during this phase of the lifecycle (Zimmermann, 2007). Levels of serum thyroid-stimulating hormone (TSH) rise and thyroxine decrease during pregnancy, making women more sensitive to iodine deficiency or related disorders (Delange, 2007). Iodine deficiency during pregnancy may cause the thyroid to underfunction and lead to the development of goitre (Glinoer, 2003), a condition when the thyroid gland is enlarged. In some severe cases, the thyroid gland of the newborn may be enlarged and in extreme cases goitre may occur.

Mental retardation

Iodine deficiency is also a major cause of preventable mental retardation. Thyroid hormones are needed for the development and maturation of the foetal brain and the nervous system of the developing child is highly sensitive to changes in the mother's thyroid status (Pemberton *et al.*, 2005).

   In areas of New Guinea and Ethiopia where iodine deficiency is prevalent, this has been found to affect the well-being of both mothers and their children. One study carried out in a rural village in Southern Ethiopia diagnosed 85% women and 33% children with goitre. UICs were <49 μg/L for all 100 participants, indicating iodine deficiency. Children, in particular, were found to have poor short-term memory, possibly caused by low iodine status *in utero* and after birth (Bogale *et al.*, 2009). It is therefore important to consider that the health implications of iodine deficiency often extend beyond goitre.

Table 7.5 WHO, UNICEF and ICCIDD recommended iodine intakes for women of childbearing age, pregnant and lactating women.

Authority	Life stage	Basis of amount	µg/day
WHO, UNICEF, ICCIDD	Pregnant/lactating mothers	–	200 µg/day
US IoM	Women ≥ 14 years	EAR	95 µg/day
	Women ≥ 14 years	RDA	150 µg/day
	Pregnancy	EAR	160 µg/day
	Pregnancy	RDA	220 µg/day
	Lactation	EAR	209 µg/day
	Lactation	RDA	290 µg/day

Source: Table adapted and reproduced with permission from Zimmerman (2007).
EAR, estimated average requirement (iodine intakes meeting the requirements of 50% healthy individuals in a particular age range); RDA, recommended dietary allowance (level of intake that will meet the needs of 97% healthy individuals).

Guidelines

The World Health Organisation (WHO), United Nations Children's Fund (UNICEF) and International Council for the Control of Iodine Deficiency (ICCIDD) (2001) recommend iodine intakes of 200 µg/day during pregnancy, and the Institute of Medicine (2001) has set guidelines at 220 µg/day, based on the bioavailability of iodine and urinary outputs (Table 7.5). Even though dietary intakes are a useful guide to a person's iodine status, UICs are a more accurate way of determining a person's iodine status.

One study analysed both the iodine intakes and UICs of 300 Spanish women in their third trimester of pregnancy. UICs were found to be significantly lower (104 µg/L) than WHO recommended cutoffs (150–249 µg/L for pregnancy) (Alvarez-Pedrerol *et al.*, 2009). Milk and iodised salt were the most important dietary sources of iodine although levels of consumption were not high enough for women to meet recommended UIC targets. Other examples of iodine-rich food sources that may help women to achieve dietary targets are included in Table 7.6.

Table 7.6 Iodine-rich sources (per 100 g).

Food source	Iodine content (µg per 100 g)
Fish paste	310
Haddock, steamed,	260
Mackerel, grilled	170
Drinking chocolate powder	165
Cod, baked	130
Jaffa cakes	48
Pasta, plain, fresh, cooked	36
Oat based biscuits	31
Whole milk, average	31
Cheddar cheese	30

Source: FSA (2006).

Iodised Salt – a Good Step Forward?

As mentioned, in certain regions worldwide, women's iodine intakes are not adequate. There are many different reasons for this, but low levels of iodine in the soil and reduced iodine content of vegetables is one of the main causes. Iodised salt is a cheap way to address this large scale public health problem and involves adding iodine-containing salts to table salt. Although this has been effective to some extent in some areas, women still have low iodine status, despite iodisation of salt.

One example of this is in the United States where salt has been iodised since the early 1920s. Research carried out by Hollowell and Haddow (2007) found that 15% of women in the childbearing years and 4–8% pregnant women had UICs less than 50 μg/L, indicating suboptimal iodine status. Scientists are now also formulating double-fortified salt (DFS), containing both iodine and iron. Research is currently taking place in regions such as Ghana, India, Morocco and Kenya to test the efficacy of this (Vinodkumar *et al.*, 2007).

7.3.4   Iron

Iron is an essential trace element and important component of body enzymes. The prevalence of iron deficiency varies globally, with South-East Asia having some of the highest rates (Table 7.7). During pregnancy, women are particularly susceptible to the onset of iron deficiency with around 1 in 2 being diagnosed with iron deficiency (Scholl, 2005), but women whose diets are largely comprised of non-haem iron foods such as cereals and millet with high phytate and low ascorbic acid/iron ratios are at particularly high risk (Nair and Iyengar, 2009).

Iron deficiency in pregnancy has been linked to preterm deliveries, reduced infant birth weight, length and iron stores (Daily and Wylie, 2008). Low iron stores during periods of infant brain growth may also have permanent effects on the cognitive function of the offspring (Lozoff, 2007). Definitions for iron deficiency are included in Table 7.8. Actual iron deficiency is usually defined as 'levels of body iron that fall below cellular levels needed for metabolic/physiological functions' (Zimmermann, 2008).

Table 7.7   Prevalence of iron-deficiency anaemia.

Region	Iron-deficiency anaemia (%)
Africa	44 (27–68)
Americas	31 (20–54)
Eastern Mediterranean	30 (0–61)
Europe	35 (12–63)
South-East Asia	45 (26–62)
Western Pacific	35 (21–48)

Source: Data extracted from WHO Statistical Information Service (2011).

Table 7.8   Different states of iron deficiency.

Deficiency states	Definition
Iron deficiency (ID)	Levels of body iron that fall below cellular levels needed for metabolic/physiological functions
Iron-deficiency anaemia	Defined as ID combined with low haemoglobin levels
Iron-deficient erythropoiesis (IDE)	When circulating levels of iron fall below the levels needed for the synthesis of red blood cells. Reduced levels of iron saturation, plasma transferrin or signs of ID in erythrocytes are all indicative of IDE

Source: Zimmermann (2008).

Guidelines

The body can to some extent regulate its own iron status. In pregnancy, transit time slows down (the length of time the food takes to pass through the body). This gives the body extra time to absorb iron and other nutrients from the foods that have been eaten. Some scientists believe, however, that this process only takes place once iron depletion has already commenced (Milman, 2006).

It is generally advised that women strive to consume 27 mg iron/day (FNB, 2001; NHMRC, 2006), but studies show that intakes are much lower than this –13.1 mg/day (Rubio *et al.*, 2009), 15.8 mg/day (Cockell *et al.*, 2009) and 15.0 mg/day (Gautam *et al.*, 2008). Incorporating iron-rich foods (Table 7.9) into the daily diet may go some way towards helping to achieve these guidelines although the bio-availability of iron from these should be considered (Gibson *et al.*, 2006).

The EFSA (2006) have not yet established a tolerable upper intake level for iron as the level of evidence is not thought to be sufficient. However, there is now justifiable concern that high-dose iron supplements may have their own health implications.

Iron supplements

High-dose iron supplements may lead to reduced compliance and unfavourable GI symptoms (Zhou *et al.*, 2009). There is also conflicting evidence about the use

Table 7.9   Iron-rich foods for pregnancy (per 100 g).

Food source	Iron (mg per 100 g)
Sesame seeds	10.4
Liquorice allsorts	8.1
Sardines	4.6
Figs (dried)	4.2
Raisins	3.8
Rye crisp bread	3.5
Tofu (steamed/fried)	3.5
Wholemeal bread	3.2
Twiglets	2.9
Lean beef	2.8

Source: FSA (2006).

> **Women with different serum ferritin levels in pregnancy require different doses of iron to prevent iron-deficiency anaemia.**
>
> Serum ferritin ≤30 µg/L = 80–100 mg ferrous iron/day
>
> Serum ferritin 31–70 µg/L = 40 mg ferrous iron/day
>
> Serum ferritin ≤70 µg/L = No need for iron supplementation

Figure 7.3 Should use of iron supplements be based on serum ferritin status? (Milman *et al.*, 2006.)

of iron-containing prenatal multivitamins. In one study, women with severe nausea and vomiting in pregnancy (NVP) were asked to discontinue iron-containing prenatal multivitamin use and just take folic acid, an adult multivitamin or children's chewable multivitamin. It was found that after the cessation of prenatal supplements containing iron, symptoms of NVP significantly improved (Gill *et al.*, 2009).

Consequently, lower-dose iron supplements or food-based approaches may be alternative ways to improve pregnancy iron status and prevent the onset of anaemia, with fewer symptoms and side effects. In terms of dose, Milman *et al.* (2006) has provided the most succinct guidelines to date recommending that the majority of women (serum levels 31–70 µg/L) take no more than 40 mg ferrous iron/day. This was an important study identifying that different women may require different doses of iron supplement to improve serum ferritin levels and prevent iron deficiency (Figure 7.3).

> ## Should We be Wary of High-Dose Iron Supplements?
>
> Traditionally, high-dose iron supplements have been used to treat iron-deficiency anaemia in pregnancy. Now there are increasing concerns that high-dose iron supplements may have their own health implications.
>
> Scientists from the University of Turin found that women taking iron supplements showed signs of insulin resistance and were more likely to develop gestational diabetes, hypertension and markers of metabolic syndrome in pregnancy (Bo *et al.*, 2009). Equally, elevated serum iron and ferritin levels have been associated with an increased risk of pre-eclampsia; serum iron and ferritin levels have been found to be significantly higher in women diagnosed with pre-eclampsia when compared with healthy controls (Siddiqui *et al.*, 2010).
>
> More trials are now needed to reconfirm these findings and underpin exactly how iron may exert its actions. This may be partly due to iron increasing levels of oxidative stress within the body (Bhatla *et al.*, 2009). Further research is now needed to define the optimum dose of iron that can be consumed on a daily basis, without side effects.

7.3.5 Manganese

Manganese is an essential trace metal found in all body tissues. It is needed for amino acid, lipid, protein and carbohydrate metabolism (Erikson *et al.*, 2007). Manganese is also a key constituent of several body enzymes, including superoxide dismutase, the main antioxidant enzymes that neutralises oxidative damage (Soldin and Aschner, 2007). Generally, manganese deficiency in adult populations is rare, but toxicity symptoms can occur (Erikson *et al.*, 2007).

Both animal and human studies have shown that excess manganese may cause neurological damage and foetuses are particularly vulnerable (Aschner *et al.*, 2005). A recent study undertaken by Zota *et al.* (2009) studied the manganese status of 470 mother–infant pairs. Maternal blood levels of manganese were 2.4 μg/dL and cord blood concentration levels 4.2 μg/dL. Birth weight increased with manganese levels up to 3.1 μg/L, and then a slight reduction in weight was observed at higher levels. The effects of elevated manganese level of birth outcomes needs to be studied in further detail (and in high exposure populations).

Guidelines

Manganese is found in a range of food sources: per 100 g of food consumed, wheatgerm (12.3 mg), rye crispbread (3.5 mg), muesli (2.6 mg) and wholemeal bread (1.8 mg) are all good sources of manganese (FSA, 2006). Subsequently, recommended intakes of 1.4 mg/day (DH, 1991) are easy to attain. High intakes of manganese have been linked to neurotoxic effects but because of the limited number of human studies, an upper limit has not been set (EFSA, 2006).

7.3.6 Selenium

Selenium is an essential trace element with important antioxidant properties. Selenium forms part of the glutathione peroxidise enzyme (an enzyme that protects against oxidative, cellular damage) (DH, 1991) and is an essential component of at least 25 selenoproteins (Pappas *et al.*, 2008). The amount of selenium in food largely depends upon the environment in which the product was grown. The selenium content of European and UK soils is low, although this varies regionally (Broadley *et al.*, 2006).

Maternal consumption of selenium may protect the offspring from oxidative stress and help regulate gene expression, although more work is needed in this area (Pappas *et al.*, 2008). Recent research has shown that glutathione peroxidise activity is reduced in the placenta of women diagnosed with pre-eclampsia, indicating that increase levels of oxidative stress may increase selenium requirements in these women (Mistry *et al.*, 2008). Some research has shown that selenium supplements (100 μg/day) when taken from the first trimester of pregnancy may help to prevent premature (pre-labour) rupture of membranes (Tara *et al.*, 2010).

Guidelines

Research has shown previously that average selenium intakes in Western mothers are around 50 μg/day (Derbyshire *et al.*, 2009). It is generally recommended that 60 μg/day selenium is consumed during pregnancy in the United States and 66 μg/day in Australia and New Zealand (NHMRC, 2006). Women may benefit from adapting their diets slightly to help them achieve these levels of intake. As can be seen in Table 7.10, lean and oily fish are both good sources of selenium.

Table 7.10 Selenium-rich foods (per 100 g).

Food source	Selenium content (μg per 100 g)
Lemon sole (steamed)	73
Sardines (canned in oil)	49
Sunflower seeds	49
Herring (grilled)	46
Lentils (boiled)	40
Plaice (steamed)	40
Kipper (grilled)	36
Mackerel (grilled)	36
Salmon (grilled)	31

Source: FSA (2006).

7.3.7 Zinc

The average adult contains 2–3 g of zinc, of which about 0.1% is replenished daily (Maret and Sandstead, 2006). Zinc is a major component of over 100 metalloenzymes involved with metabolism, oxygen uptake and transport, folate utilisation and gene expression (Kontic-Vucinic *et al.*, 2006). Observational studies suggest a link between maternal zinc deficiency and adverse pregnancy outcomes for the mother and child, but findings from studies are highly variable and more information is needed (Hess and King, 2009). In a sample of Spanish mothers, scientists found that serum zinc levels declined steadily from the first trimester of pregnancy (71.3 μg/L) to <35 weeks into pregnancy (58.5 μg/L). Authors in this study concluded that the progressive decline in serum zinc could affect the growth of the foetus and lead to birth complications (Izquierdo *et al.*, 2007).

In another study, 84 pregnant women at risk of preterm delivery were given 50 mg/day of zinc sulphate or a placebo from 12 to 16 weeks until term. The head circumference of infants born to zinc-supplemented mothers was significantly higher, but the length of gestation was unaffected (Danesh *et al.*, 2010).

Multiple Mineral Deficiencies in Developing Countries

Minerals are essential for human development and functioning of the body, but it is not uncommon for women to be deficient in several minerals at any one time. Mineral deficiencies are recognised as a major health problem in many developing countries, which can mainly be attributed to undernutrition.

One study carried out in 375 Ethiopian women analysed serum levels of key minerals using mass spectrometry (an analytical technique used to quantify how much of a nutrient is in a blood serum sample). Blood results indicated that 67%, 26%, 22% and 9% of women were deficient in zinc, magnesium, selenium and calcium, respectively. Fourteen percent of women were deficient in two minerals, 10% three minerals and 5% four minerals (Kassu *et al.*, 2008).

In summary, the findings from these studies show that women living in developing regions are often deficient in more than one mineral. Intervention measures need to be tested to see which approaches may be most effective at reducing the prevalence of these deficiencies.

Guidelines

Generally, it is recommended that women improve their dietary intakes of zinc before taking zinc supplements (Mahomed *et al.*, 2007). Dietary recommendations for zinc are set at 13 mg/day in the United Kingdom (DH, 1991) and 11 mg/day in the United States (FNB, 2001). Generally, these can be met from usual habitual intakes but guiding women to integrate foods naturally rich in zinc, such as wheatgerm (17 mg), wheat bran (16 mg), tahini paste (5.4 mg), sesame seeds (5.3 mg) and cheddar cheese (4.1 mg) (per 100 g consumed), may also help to increase habitual intakes.

Prioritising Micronutrient Needs

For many countries, there are discrepancies when vitamin and mineral dietary guidelines are compared. This can make comparisons between studies and surveys difficult and lead to different conclusions in terms of what percentage of population have low vitamin/mineral intakes.

To address this problem, the EFSA are currently in the process of formulating new vitamin and mineral guidelines. The European Micronutrients Recommendations Aligned Network (EURRECA) has carried out a scientific publication search to assess the levels of evidence available studying each of the vitamins. On the basis of their findings, they concluded that 10 key vitamins and minerals should be given priority when it comes to revising dietary guidelines – these included vitamin D, iron, folate, vitamin B_{12}, zinc, calcium, vitamin C, selenium, iodine and copper (Cavelaars *et al.,* 2010).

7.4   Application in practice

Even in the twenty-first century, it is not uncommon for women's diets to be lacking in certain minerals. Women should be guided in terms of how to make the best dietary choices and opt for nutrient-dense foods providing suitable levels of important minerals. In particular, women should be encouraged to consume foods rich in iodine and iron, since there appears to be strongest evidence for these in terms of suboptimal intakes and poor bioavailability. Particularly, in the case of iron, women should be advised about how they can improve the bioavailability of iron from their diets (the amount that's absorbed). This is especially important in low-meat consumers and vegetarian women. Drinking orange juice with non-haem iron sources such as cereals or soaking beans and lentils before their consumption are just a few examples of how this can be achieved.

7.5   Conclusion

As with vitamins, it appears that certain minerals are being underconsumed by a proportion of women. This may have implications for both maternal and infant health. However, compared to evidence for certain vitamins, such as folic acid and vitamin B_{12}, current evidence linking minerals to unfavourable pregnancy outcomes is at best patchy. It seems that iodine and iron deficiencies have been studied in most detail with good evidence linking suboptimal status for both of these minerals to poor pregnancy outcomes. Women should be guided about how these minerals can be best obtained from dietary sources.

In some regions where the prevalence of these mineral deficiencies is high, women may be guided to use appropriate doses of supplements or functional foods. On a final note, it is important to consider that the mixed roles of different vitamins and minerals and complexity of different messages creates difficult public health challenges. Messages that need to be communicated to public sectors should therefore be based on the strength of evidence available and severity of health outcomes.

Key Messages

- Micronutrients should be obtained from the diet where possible, but mineral-containing supplements may be needed by some individuals and geographical regions.
- Maternal mineral deficiencies are not uncommon and may coexist in many settings.
- Women should increase their intakes of nutrient-dense foods in order to promote vitamin and mineral adequacy.
- Taking up to 1 g/day calcium may help to reduce pre-eclampsia risk in those with high blood pressure in early pregnancy or a history of the condition (Hofmeyr and Haddow, 2007).
- There is some evidence to suggest that suboptimal magnesium status may lead to development problems in the offspring and increase the risk of medical conditions such as CP.
- There is no firm evidence linking high sodium intakes to pre-eclampsia in pregnancy, although few well-designed trials have been carried out.
- Iodine deficiency is a common problem in some areas and may be linked to thyroid problems in both the mother and child.
- Women should be encouraged to eat iron-rich foods in pregnancy and advised how the bioavailability of iron from the foods can be improved.
- Poor zinc status in pregnancy may be associated with reduced foetal growth, but more research is needed.
- In the case of some minerals, i.e. iron, tolerable upper intakes may need to be developed as new evidence starts to emerge.

Recommended reading

Christian P (2010) Micronutrients, birth weight and survival. *Annual Review of Nutrition* 30, 83–104.

FNB (Food and Nutrition Board) (2004) *Dietary Reference Intakes for Individuals, Elements.* The National Academies Press: Washington, DC.

Vinodkumar M, Rajagopalan S, Bhagwat IP *et al.* (2007) A multicenter community study on the efficacy of double-fortified salt. *Food and Nutrition Bulletin* 28(1), 100–8.

References

Alvarez-Pedrerol M, Ribas-Fitó N, García-Esteban R *et al.* (2009) Sources and iodine levels in pregnant women from an area without known iodine deficiency. *Clinical Endocrinology (Oxford)* **72**(1), 81–6.

Anderson RA (2000) Chromium in the prevention and control of diabetes. *Diabetes & Metabolism* **26**(1), 22–7.

Aschner M, Erikson KM and Dorman DC (2005) Manganese dosimetry: species differences and implications for neurotoxicity. *Critical Reviews in Toxicology* **35**(1), 1–32.

Beauséjour A, Auger K, St-Louis J and Brochu M (2003) High-sodium intake prevents pregnancy-induced decrease of blood pressure in the rat. *Americal Journal of Physiology and Heart Circulatory Physiology* **285**(1), H375–83.

Bhatla N, Kaul N, Lal N *et al.* (2009) Comparison of effect of daily versus weekly iron supplementation during pregnancy on lipid peroxidation. *Journal of Obstetrics & Gynaecology Research* **35**(3), 438–45.

Bo S, Menato G, Villois P *et al.* (2009) Iron supplementation and gestational diabetes in midpregnancy. *American Journal of Obstetrics & Gynaecology* **201**(2), 158.e1–6.

Bogale A, Abebe Y, Stoecker BJ, Abuye C, Ketema K and Hambidge KM (2009) Iodine status and cognitive function of women and their five-year-old children in rural Sidama, southern Ethiopia. *East African Journal of Public Health* **6**(3), 296–9.

Broadley MR, White PJ, Bryson RJ *et al.* (2006) Biofortification of UK food crops with selenium. *Proceedings of the Nutrition Society* **65**(2), 169–81.

Cockell KA, Miller DC and Lowell H (2009) Application of the dietary reference intakes in developing a recommendation for pregnancy iron supplements in Canada. *American Journal of Clinical Nutrition* **90**(4), 1023–8.

Caddell JL, Graziani LJ, Wiswell TE, Hsieh HC and Mansmann HC Jr (1999) The possible role of magnesium in protection of premature infants from neurological syndromes and visual impairments and a review of survival of magnesium-exposed premature infants. *Magnesium Research* **12**(3), 201–16.

Cavelaars AE, Doets EL, Dhonukshe-Rutten RA *et al.* (2010) Prioritizing micronutrients for the purpose of reviewing their requirements: a protocol developed by EURRECA. *European Journal of Clinical Nutrition* **264** (Suppl 2), S19–30.

Chiu HF, Chen CC, Tsai SS, Wu TN and Yang CY (2005) Relationship between magnesium levels in drinking water and sudden infant death syndrome. *Magnesium Research* **18**(1), 12–8.

Daily JP and Wylie BJ (2008) Iron deficiency during pregnancy: blessing or curse? *The Journal of Infectious Diseases* **198**, 157–8.

Danesh A, Janghorbani M and Mohammadi B (2010) Effects of zinc supplementation during pregnancy on pregnancy outcome in women with history of preterm delivery: a double-blind randomized, placebo-controlled trial. *Journal of Maternal, Fetal and Neonatal Medicine* **23**(5), 403–8.

Delange F (2007) Iodine requirements during pregnancy, lactation and the neonatal period and indicators of optimal iodine nutrition. *Public Health Nutrition* **10**(12A), 1571–80.

DH (Department of Health) (1991) *Dietary Reference Values for Food Energy and Nutrients for the United Kingdom*, 2nd edition. *Report on Social Subjects no. 41*. The Stationery Office: London.

Derbyshire EJ, Davies GJ, Dettmar PW and Costarelli V (2009) Habitual micronutrient intakes throughout and after pregnancy. *Journal of Maternal and Child Nutrition* **110**(11), 119–32.

Doyle LW, Crowther CA, Middleton P, Marret S and Rouse D (2009) Magnesium sulphate for women at risk of preterm birth for neuroprotection of the fetus. *Cochrane Database of Systemic Reviews* **21**(1), CD004661.

Doyle W, Crawford MA, Wynn AH and Wynn SW (1989) Maternal magnesium intake and pregnancy outcome. *Magnesium Research* **2**(3), 205–10.

Duley L, Henderson-Smart DJ and Meher S (2009) Altered dietary salt for preventing pre-eclampsia, and its complications. *Cochrane Database Systematic Reviews* **19**(4), CD005548.

Durlach J (2004) New data on the importance of gestational Mg deficiency. *Journal of the American College of Nutrition* **23**(6), 694S–700S.

EFSA (European Food Safety Authority) (2006) Tolerable upper intake levels of vitamins and minerals by the Scientific Panel on Dietetic Products, Nutrition and Allergies (NDA) and Scientific Committee on Food (SCF). Available at: http://www.efsa.europa.eu/fr/scdocs/oldsc/upper_level_opinions_full-part33.pdf. (accessed March 2011.)

Erikson KM, Thompson K, Aschner J and Aschner M (2007) Manganese neurotoxicity: a focus on the neonate. *Pharmacology & Therapeutics* **113**(2), 369–77.

FSA (Food Standards Agency) (2006) *McCance and Widdowson's, the Composition of Foods.* 6th edition. Royal Society of Chemistry: London.

FNB (Food and Nutrition Board); Institute of Medicine (1997) *Dietary Reference Intakes for Calcium, Phosphorus, Magnesium, Vitamin D and Fluoride.* National Academy Press: Washington, DC.

FNB (Food and Nutrition Board); Institute of Medicine (2001) *Dietary Reference Intakes for Vitamin A, Vitamin K, Arsenic, Boron, Chromium, Copper, Iodine, Iron, Manganese, Molybdenum, Nickel, Silicon, Vanadium and Zinc.* National Academy Press: Washington, DC.

Gaetke LM and Chow CK (2003) Copper toxicity, oxidative stress and antioxidant nutrients. *Toxicology* **189**(1–2), 147–63.

Gambling L, Andersen HS and McArdle HJ (2008) Iron and copper, and their interactions during development. *Biochemical Society Transactions* **36**(Pt 6), 1258–61.

Gautam VP, Taneja DK, Sharma N, Gupta VK and Ingle GK (2008) Dietary aspects of pregnant women in rural areas of Northern India. *Maternal and Child Nutrition* **4**(2), 86–94.

Gibson RS, Perlas L and Hotz C (2006) Improving the bioavailability of nutrients in plant foods at the household level. *Proceedings of the Nutrition Society* **65**(2), 160–8.

Gill SK, Maltepe C and Koren G (2009) The effectiveness of discontinuing iron-containing prenatal multivitamins on reducing the severity of nausea and vomiting of pregnancy. *Journal of Obstetrics & Gynaecology* **29**(1), 13–16.

Glinoer D (2003) Feto–maternal repercussions of iodine deficiency during pregnancy: an update. *Annals of Endocrinology (Paris)* **64**(1), 37–44.

Groenen PM, van Rooil IA, Peer PG, Ocke MC, Zielhuis GA and Steegers-Theunissen RP (2004) Low maternal dietary intakes of iron, magnesium, and niacin are associated with spina bifida in the offspring. *Journal of Nutrition* **134**(6), 1516–22.

Gunton JE, Hams G, Hitchman R and McElduff A (2001) Serum chromium does not predict glucose tolerance in later pregnancy. *American Journal of Clinical Nutrition* **73**(1), 99–104.

Hess SY and King JC (2009) Effects of maternal zinc supplementation on pregnancy and lactation outcomes. *Food and Nutrition Bulletin* **30**(1 Suppl), S60–78.

Hofmeyr GJ, Duley L and Atallah A (2010) Calcium supplementation during pregnancy for preventing hypertensive disorders and related problems. *Cochrane Database of Systemic Reviews* **4**(8), CD001059.

Hollowell JG and Haddow JE (2007) The prevalence of iodine deficiency in women of reproductive age in the United States of America. *Public Health Nutrition* **10**(12A), 1532–9.

Institute of Medicine (IoM) (2001) *Dietary Reference Intakes for Vitamin A, Vitamin K, Arsenic, Boron, Chromium, Copper, Iodine, Iron, Manganese, Molybdenum, Nickel, Silicon, Vanadium, and Zinc.* National Academy Press: Washington, DC.

Izquierdo Alvarez S, Castañón SG, Ruata ML *et al.* (2007) Updating of normal levels of copper, zinc and selenium in serum of pregnant women. *Journal of Trace Elements in Medicine & Biology* **21** (Suppl 1), 49–52.

Kassu A, Yabutani T, Mulu A, Tessema B and Ota F (2008) Serum zinc, copper, selenium, calcium, and magnesium levels in pregnant and non-pregnant women in Gondar, Northwest Ethiopia. *Biology Trace Element Research* **122**, 97–106.

Kontic-Vucinic O, Sulovic N and Radunovic N (2006) Micronutrients in women's reproductive health: II. Minerals and trace elements. *International Journal of Fertility* **51**(3), 116–24.

Kumar N (2006) Copper deficiency myelopathy (human swayback). *Mayo Clinic Proceedings* **81**(10), 1371–84.

Lafond J and Simoneau L (2006) Calcium homeostasis in human placenta: role of calcium-binding proteins. *International Review of Cytology* **250**, 109–74.

Lozoff B (2007) Iron deficiency and child development. *Food and Nutrition Bulletin* **28**(4S), S560–71.

Mahomed K, Bhutta Z and Middleton P (2007) Zinc supplementation for improving pregnancy and infant outcome. *Cochrane Database of Systemic Reviews* (2), CD000230.

Maret W and Sandstead HH (2006) Zinc requirements and the risks and benefits of zinc supplementation. *Journal of Trace Elements in Medicine & Biology* **20**(1), 3–18.

Milman N (2006) Iron and pregnancy – a delicate balance. *Annals of Hematology* **85**, 559–65.

Milman N, Byg KE, Bergholt T, Eriksen L and Hvas AM (2006), Body iron and individual iron prophylaxis in pregnancy – should the iron dose be adjusted according to serum ferritin? *Annals in Haematology* **85**, 567–73.

Mistry HD, Wilson V, Ramsay MM, Symonds ME and Broughton Pipkin F (2008) Reduced selenium concentrations and glutathione peroxidase activity in pre-eclamptic pregnancies. *Hypertension* **52**(5), 881–8.

Nair KM and Iyengar V (2009) Iron content, bioavailability and factors affecting iron status of Indians. *Indian Journal of Medicine Research* **130**(5), 634–45.

NHMRC (National Health and Medical Research Council) (2006) Nutrient reference values for Australia and New Zealand. NHMRC Publications: Australia. Available at: https://www.nhmrc.gov.au. (accessed December 2010.)

NHS (2010) Cerebral Palsy. Available at: http://www.nhs.uk/Conditions/Cerebral-palsy/Pages/Introduction.aspx. (accessed March 2011.)

Pappas AC, Zoidis E, Surai PF and Zervas G (2008) Selenoproteins and maternal nutrition. *Comparative Biochemistry and Physiology. Part B: Biochemistry and Molecular Biology* **151**(4), 361–72.

Pemberton HN, Franklyn JA and Kilby MD (2005) Thyroid hormones and fetal brain development. *Minerva Ginecologica* **57**(4), 367–78.

Perrine CG, Herrick K, Serdula MK and Sullivan KM (2010) Some subgroups of reproductive age women in the United States may be at risk for iodine deficiency. *Journal of Nutrition* **140**(8), 1489–94.

Pinto E, Barros H and dos Santos Silva I (2009) Dietary intake and nutritional adequacy prior to conception and during pregnancy: a follow-up study in the north of Portugal. *Public Health Nutrition* **12**(7), 922–31.

Ritchie LD and King JC (2000) Dietary calcium and pregnancy-induced hypertension: is there a relation? *American Journal of Clinical Nutrition* **71**, 1371S–4S.

Rubio C, Gutiérrez AJ, Revert C, Reguera JI, Burgos A and Hardisson A (2009) Daily dietary intake of iron, copper, zinc and manganese in a Spanish population. *International Journal of Food Science & Nutrition* **60**(7), 590–600.

SACN (Scientific Advisory Committee on Nutrition) (2003) *Salt and Health*. Published for the Food Standards Agency and the Departments of Health. The Stationery Office: London.

Scholl TO (2005) Iron status during pregnancy: setting the stage for mother and infant. *American Journal of Clinical Nutrition* **81**, 1218S–22S.

Siddiqui IA, Jaleel A, Kadri HM, Saeed WA and Tamimi W (2010) Iron status parameters in pre-eclamptic women. *Archives of Gynecology and Obstetrics* [Epub ahead of print].

Soldin OP and Aschner M (2007) Effects of manganese on thyroid hormone homeostasis: potential links. *Neurotoxicology* **28**(5), 951–6.

Tara F, Rayman MP, Boskabadi H *et al.* (2010) Selenium supplementation and premature (prelabour) rupture of membranes: a randomised double-blind placebo-controlled trial. *Journal of Obstetrics & Gynaecology* **30**(1), 30–4.

Uriu-Adams JY and Keen CL (2005) Copper, oxidative stress, and human health. *Molecular Aspects of Medicine* **26**(4–5), 268–98.

Vinodkumar M, Rajagopalan S, Bhagwat IP *et al.* (2007) A multicenter community study on the efficacy of double-fortified salt. *Food & Nutrition Bulletin* **28**(1), 100–8.

WHO SIS (World Health Organisation Statistical Information Service) (2011) Nutrition databases. Available at: http://www.who.int/nutrition/databases/en/index.html. (accessed March 2011.)

WHO, UNICEF and ICCIDD (2001) *Assessment of the Iodine Deficiency Disorders and Monitoring their Elimination* (WHO/NHD/01.1) World Health Organisation: Geneva.

Woods SE, Ghodsi V, Engel A, Miller J and James S (2008) Serum chromium and gestational diabetes. *Journal of the American Board of Family Medicine* **21**(2), 153–7.

Wray S and Shmygol A (2007) Role of the calcium store in uterine contractility. *Seminars in Cell & Developmental Biology* **18**(3), 315–20.

Zhou SJ, Gibson RA, Crowther CA and Makrides M (2009), Should we lower the dose of iron when treating anaemia in pregnancy? A randomised dose-response trial. *European Journal of Clinical Nutrition* **63**(2), 183–90.

Zimmermann MB (2007) The impact of iodised salt or iodine supplements on iodine status during pregnancy, lactation and infancy. *Public Health Nutrition* **101**(12A), 1584–95.

Zimmermann MB (2008) Methods to assess iron and iodine status. *British Journal of Nutrition* **99** (3), S2–9.

Zimmermann MB (2009) Iodine deficiency. *Endocrine Reviews* **30**(4), 376–408.

Zota AR, Ettinger AS, Bouchard M *et al.* (2009) Maternal blood manganese levels and infant birth weight. *Epidemiology* **20**(3), 367–73.

8 Diet and Pregnancy Outcome

Summary

Most women hope to deliver a happy and healthy baby. However, unfortunately this is not always the case. Although a range of factors, including social, environmental and the inheritance of genetic conditions, may affect the health of the child, scientists are becoming increasingly aware of the role that dietary and lifestyle factors can play in terms of helping to optimise the chances of delivering a healthy baby. The roles of particular vitamins and minerals have already been discussed, but there remains many unanswered questions about other dietary constituents. For example, it is well known that alcohol intake should be kept to a minimum during pregnancy but should this be consumed at all? Equally, the advice about levels of caffeine consumption can be just as confusing. There is emerging evidence about how diet in pregnancy can modulate gene expression in the offspring – but how can this be applied? Equally, women may be unsure about how taking dietary supplements could benefit their own health and that of their child. This chapter aims to evaluate the scientific evidence for such questions and form balanced, evidence-based conclusions about how specific dietary factors may influence pregnancy outcomes.

Learning Outcomes

- To describe how specific dietary factors may influence pregnancy outcomes.
- Using scientific evidence available, to assess and evaluate some common areas of confusion.
- To make evidence-based recommendations that could be used to help improve pregnancy outcome(s) in practice.

8.1 Introduction

Unfortunately, not all babies born are healthy, nor will they all have the best start in life. As will be discussed later in this chapter, poor pregnancy outcomes can take several forms. Babies born small at term have a higher risk of heart problems later in life and increased risk of lower intelligence, poor academic performance and social skills and behavioural problems (Lundgren and Tuverno, 2008), and those

---

Nutrition in the Childbearing Years, First Edition. Emma Derbyshire.
© 2011 Emma Derbyshire. Published 2011 by Blackwell Publishing Ltd.

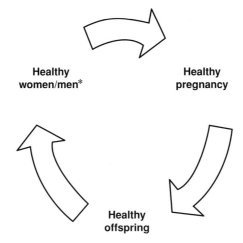

Figure 8.1 Investing in the health of women helps to improve the health of the next genera-tion. *More evidence is, however, needed to assess the effects male health status can have on pregnancy outcomes.

born larger than average have a higher risk of perinatal mortality and obesity and metabolic disorders in the long term (Galtier *et al.*, 2008).

Equally, birth defects can be fatal (when the baby does not form properly whilst developing in utero), with most occurring during the first 3 months of pregnancy. Although these can be genetic, partially genetic or of 'post-conception' origin, i.e. when the mother is exposed to agents that may be potentially teratogenic (causing birth defects). This includes dietary factors such as alcohol and iodine deficiency and also other environmental factors such as rubella and syphilis. Hundreds of thousands of babies are born worldwide with birth defects, which can be attributed to these modifiable lifestyle exposures. With clear communication strategies and government health policies, it is hoped that simple health messages, such as those presented in Figure 8.1, could help parents to realise the effects their own lifestyles can have on the next generation.

This chapter will first begin by giving a brief overview of some of the more common birth defects. It will then go on to explain how certain dietary and environmental exposures may affect pregnancy outcomes. Finally, recommendations will be given in terms of the benefits of educating the community, health professional workers, policy makers and the media about birth defects and potential opportunities for their prevention.

8.2   What is a 'healthy' baby?

A healthy baby is usually born at term (at around 37 weeks into pregnancy), has a healthy birth weight (<2500 g and >4000 g) and suitable Apgar score. Birth weight usually marks the transition from the uterine environment to a more variable external environment and is a common measure of foetal nutritional exposure in epidemiology studies. However, there are problems with using birth weight as an indicator of 'infant health' as the mother's ethnicity, body size and age may all to some degree influence this. Therefore, foetal growth restriction (when the foetus

Table 8.1 Newborn Apgar scores.

Sign	Apgar score		
	0	**1**	**2**
Colour	Blue or pale	Body pink, extremities blue	Completely pink
Heart rate	Absent	Slow ($<$100 beats/min)	$>$100 beats/min
Muscle tone	Limp	Some flexibility	Active motion
Reflex response	No response	Grimace	Cry or cough
Respiratory effort	Absent	Weak cry	Good, strong cry

Source: Stables and Rankin (2006), with permission from Elsevier.
Key: Total scores 0–2 = poor health, 3–7 = fair health and 8–10 = good health. A scoring system based on points awarded for five physiological signs.

does not achieve its potential size) is thought to be a better endpoint to determine 'pregnancy outcome' (Miles and Foxen, 2009).

8.3   A note on Apgar scores

The Apgar score was first developed by Virginia Apgar, a medical doctor in 1953. It was developed to provide a clear classification system to help categorise the health of newborn infants. Five key characteristics were selected that best described the health of the newborn child. These include (1) colour, (2) heart rate, (3) muscle tone, (4) reflex response and (5) respiration. Each of these categories can then be given a score of zero, one or two depending on whether the characteristic is present or absent and then the total scores are added (Table 8.1).

Infants with poor health generally score between 0 and 2, those in fair condition 3 and 7 and infants in good health 8 and 10. Recordings are usually taken about 1 minute after birth and are a useful initial indicator of an infant's health, which is still used today (Finster and Wood, 2005).

8.4   What is foetal growth restriction?

Foetal growth restriction is when babies fail to reach their full potential size (the acronym FGR will be used hereon). This can usually be identified when women have a sonogram and the weight, size or shape of the foetus is abnormal (Miller *et al.*, 2008).

There is much emerging information indicating that women's diets and lifestyles early in pregnancy can help to minimise the risk of FGR. A team of Spanish scientists found that women consuming a high-quality diet abundant in fruit, vegetables and wholegrains in the first trimester of pregnancy were much less likely to deliver infants with FGR. Women with the best quality diets were more likely to deliver infants that were on average 126.3 g heavier and 0.47 cm longer than those with poorer quality diets (Rodríguez-Bernal *et al.*, 2010).

8.5   Poor pregnancy outcomes

Poor pregnancy outcomes mean that the infant is not born with optimal health. This includes FGR and some of the more common birth defects such as neural tube defects

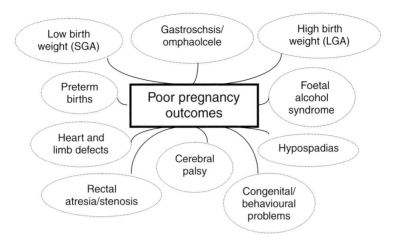

Figure 8.2 Examples of poor pregnancy outcomes. Gastroschsis is when the child's intestines protrude outside the body. Omphalocele is a similar condition to gastroschisis when the infant's intestines and/or abdominal organs protrude out through the belly button.

(NTDs) but also consists of a whole host of medical conditions that are not as well known (Figure 8.2). Women need to be aware that their diet and lifestyle both before and during the early stages of pregnancy may affect their chances of having a baby that is not healthy. There is now a wealth of information available demonstrating the significant effects a woman's lifestyle's can have on her child's quality of life.

Research Highlight   A note on ethnicity and pregnancy outcomes

Research carried out in East London, a deprived area in the United Kingdom, studied the diet quality of 165 mothers of different ethnic origins who had given birth to a low birth weight (LBW) baby (<2500 g). Across all ethnic groups, half the women did not meet dietary recommendations for folate and 88% for iron. African women had some of the highest vitamin D intakes (4.7 μg/day) and Caucasians and Asians the lowest (2.4 μg/day) (Rees *et al.,* 2005).

Overall, researchers found that women delivering LBW infants had diets that were inadequate and that nutritional deficits varied according to the mothers' ethnicity. Scientists concluded that dietary advice needs to be targeted specifically to individual ethnic groups, to improve their diet quality and pregnancy outcomes.

8.6   Sensitive windows of pregnancy

During the first trimester of pregnancy, the process of organogenesis takes place (the formation of the child's organs). It is mainly during this time that the child is most susceptible to the effects of toxic substances that may affect its development. Exposure to such substances may have short-term effects as well as implications in childhood (asthma, cancer, neurological and behavioural effects) and later in adulthood (cancer, heart disease, degenerative and behavioural conditions).

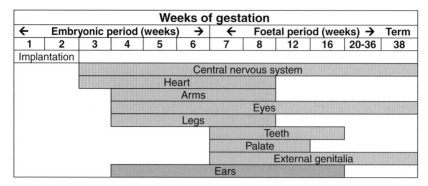

Figure 8.3   Critical windows of foetal development. (Adapted from Selevan *et al.* (2000).)

As demonstrated in Figure 8.3, different systems develop and are sensitive to teratogens at slightly different time periods. Once conception has taken place, it takes about 6–9 days for the egg to anchor to the uterus and form a blood supply to develop, linking the mother and embryo. After this, teratogens (potentially harmful substances) can pass from the mother to her developing child, affecting its development. In terms of organ systems, the central nervous system is the first to develop, followed by the cardiovascular system. The palate and genitals develop slightly later in pregnancy, but the developing child is most sensitive to factors that may affect its development between weeks 3 and 16 of pregnancy (Selevan *et al.*, 2000).

The National Birth Defects Prevention Study (NBDPS)

The NBDPS was established to identify the major causes of birth defects. When the study first began, it was known that some teratogens such as rubella and Thalidomide could cause birth defects, but the causes of more than 70% birth defects were unknown.

The NBDPS is now the largest collaborative study assessing the causes of birth defects in the United States. Data in relation to dietary, lifestyle, environmental, medical and genetic factors has been collected from 7500 mothers who have delivered infants with birth defects and compared with controls from eight states (Yoon *et al.*, 2001). This research is ongoing and by recruiting larger ethnically and geographically diverse populations, it is hoped that this research will continue to uncover important findings in the future. Some of the key findings from this research are included in this chapter.

8.7   Alcohol

Alcohol is a well-known teratogen that passes freely across the placenta to the developing child. As amniotic fluid contains less fat than plasma, the concentration of alcohol in amniotic fluid is generally higher than that in the bloodstream and may be potentially toxic to the offspring (Whitehall, 2007). The prevalence of birth defects caused by alcohol consumption in pregnancy is higher in some parts of the world when compared to others. For example, in the Western Cape Province of South Africa, over one-quarter of pregnant women have reported drinking alcohol

Table 8.2 NICE (2008) guidelines about drinking alcohol when pregnant.

1. Women planning a pregnancy and pregnant women should be advised to avoid drinking alcohol within the first three months of pregnancy. There is some evidence that this may increase the risk of miscarriage.
2. Women choosing to drink alcohol in pregnancy should be advised to drink no more than 1–2 units once or twice per week.*
3. Women should be advised that getting drunk or binge drinking (more than 5 standard drinks or 7.5 units on one occasion) may be harmful to the unborn baby.

*One unit is the equivalent to half a pint of ordinary strength lager or beer or one-shot (25 mL) spirits. One small (125 mL) glass of wine is about 1.5 units.

in pregnancy, which has been linked to high rates of foetal alcohol syndrome (FAS) in schoolchildren in this region (Viljoen *et al.*, 2003; Rosennthal *et al.*, 2005).

8.7.1 How much or not at all?

It is now well known that alcohol can be dangerous to drink in pregnancy. However, there is confusing evidence about whether pregnant women should drink alcohol at all and the maximum amount of alcohol that should be consumed. In the United Kingdom, the National Institute for Health and Clinical Excellence (NICE) is an important and independent organisation that helps to develop guidelines for health professionals. These guidelines are based on scientific evidence that is currently available and has been evaluated by medical professionals. Using this evidence, health experts advise that women should avoid drinking alcohol in early pregnancy and limit their intake after 3 months into pregnancy to no more than 1–2 units on two occasions each week (NICE, 2008; Table 8.2).

8.7.2 Foetal alcohol spectrum disorder (FASD)

Alcohol use among women of child-bearing age is one of the leading, most preventable causes of birth defects and developmental disabilities. Although most women do reduce their alcohol intakes to some extent once they are pregnant, some women may unknowingly consume large volumes of alcohol without knowing they are pregnant. It is in these instances that women are most at risk of having an alcohol-exposed pregnancy, which may lead to birth defects and developmental abnormalities in the offspring (Floyd *et al.*, 2009). If a woman drinks whilst she is pregnant, her baby is at risk of being born with FASD. This term is used to describe a series of structural, behavioural and neurocognitive impairments that can affect the child (Table 8.3).

Research Highlight   Women's attitudes and knowledge of alcohol consumption in pregnancy

A large Australian survey has now assessed the women's knowledge and attitudes about the effects drinking alcohol can have when pregnant.

Of the 1102 women surveyed, 62% heard that alcohol can affect the foetus and 55% of women were aware of the term 'FAS'. However, 16% of women did not agree that the offspring's disabilities could be lifelong (Peadon *et al.*, 2010).

On the whole, women seemed to be aware that alcohol could affect their babies' health but were less aware of what these effects could be and the fact that it could lead to lifelong disabilities and poor health for the next generation.

8.7.3   Facial abnormalities

FAS is the most clinical recognisable form of FASD because three key symptoms must be present: (1) Facial malformations, (2) impaired growth and (3) central nervous system dysfunction. As can be seen in Figure 8.4, facial characteristics include a thin upper lip, absent or elongated groove between the lip and upper nose. Maxillary hypoplasia, when the bones supporting the teeth, upper jaw and nasal cavity are underdeveloped, can also be present and the child may have extra skin on the eyelid (epicanthal folds). With regard to growth, these children may have experienced pre- and postnatal growth retardation, leading to poor brain growth and/or development. It is therefore not surprising that these children often have delayed social and mental performance (O'Leary, 2004).

8.8   Caffeine

Caffeine is a methylxanthine, a chemical structure that can pass through the placenta to the foetus, potentially leading to poor pregnancy outcomes. Despite considerable research, the evidence-base from studies is rather mixed (Table 8.4). It does, however, seem that the potential adverse effects of caffeine are stronger for the first trimester of pregnancy when compared to later in pregnancy (Adén, 2011). As mentioned previously in Chapter 2, the Food Standards Agency now advise that pregnant women consume no more than 200 mg caffeine/day, the equivalent to two cups of tea and

Table 8.3   The following major conditions are included under FASD.

Condition included under FASD	Characteristics
Foetal alcohol syndrome (FAS)	Characteristic facial abnormalities + neurological/behavioural/cognitive problems
Partial FAS (pFAS)	Characteristic facial abnormalities + one of three other complications: (1) growth retardation, (2) deficient brain growth/ abnormal development and (3) behavioural and cognitive abnormalities
Alcohol-related neurodevelopment disorder (ARND)	When alcohol exposure affects brain growth, development or there is evidence of behavioural/cognitive abnormalities
Alcohol-related birth defects (ARBD)	Characteristic facial abnormalities + other minor abnormalities, i.e. structural defects of the heart, renal system, eyes or ears linked to alcohol exposure

Source: March of Dimes Birth Defects Foundation (2006).

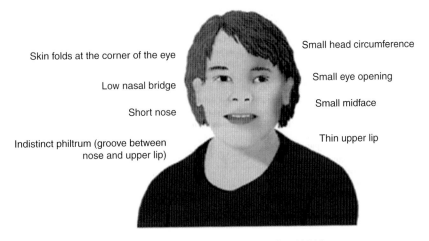

Skin folds at the corner of the eye

Low nasal bridge

Short nose

Indistinct philtrum (groove between nose and upper lip)

Small head circumference

Small eye opening

Small midface

Thin upper lip

Figure 8.4   Facial characteristics of FAS. (Warren and Foudin, 2001.)

a small bar of milk chocolate (FSA, 2008). These guidelines were reduced from 300 mg/day, originally complied in 2001 after findings from one pioneering study.

8.8.1   Caffeine and FGR

Previously, caffeine guidelines were set at 300 mg/day, but a well-designed prospective study carried out by the CARE study group (2008) found that higher caffeine intakes (over 300 mg/day) were associated with an increased risk of FGR. The study followed 2635 women throughout their pregnancy, recording total daily caffeine intakes in each trimester of pregnancy and measuring salivary caffeine levels in a sub-sample of the population. Mean caffeine consumption decreased from an average of 238 mg/day before pregnancy to 139 mg/day in the first trimester and average of 163 mg/day in the third trimester. Tea was the main source of caffeine (62%) followed by coffee (14%), cola drinks (12%), chocolate (8%) and soft drinks (2%). Other beverages including hot chocolate, energy drinks and alcoholic drinks provided the remaining sources of caffeine.

Table 8.4   Suspected food mutagens.

Suspected food mutagen	What is it?
Aflatoxin	A toxin produced by moulds that usually grow on peanuts or cereal grains.
N-nitrosamines	Compounds found in a range of foods – smoked, pickled and some fermented foods.
Heterocyclic amines	A chemical formed when meat, poultry or fish are cooked at high temperatures.
Methylmercury	A form of mercury that is highly toxic and may be absorbed into the living tissue of organisms. Consumed through the food chain (mainly from fish).
Polycyclic aromatic hydrocarbons	Produced when materials, including foods are burned. May be formed during cooking processes as smoking, grilling, roasting or frying.

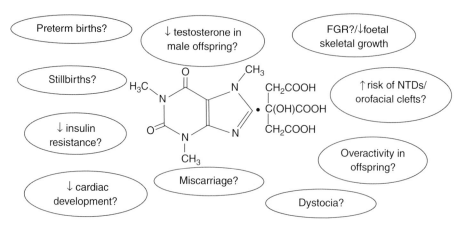

Figure 8.5 Caffeine and possible pregnancy outcomes. Further well-designed studies are needed.

After adjusting data for several confounders, caffeine consumption was found to increase the risk of FGR by around 50% at intakes of 200–299 mg/day and above and the link between the two was strongest amongst women who metabolised caffeine more quickly. On the whole, the results of this important study showed that higher intakes of caffeine increased the odds of having a child with FGR (Figure 8.5).

Research Highlight   Caffeine consumption and risk of NTDs

Animal studies have shown that caffeine consumption in pregnancy may have terato-genic effects, but findings from human studies are inconclusive.

Data from the NBDPS has now examined whether caffeine consumption in pregnancy could increase the risk of women delivering infants with NTDs, such as anencephaly, spina bifida or encephalocele (see definitions in Table 8.5). Total caffeine intakes from coffee, tea, soft drinks and chocolate were calculated the year before pregnancy in 768 mothers who delivered infants with birth defects and compared against intakes of mothers delivering healthy infants.

Table 8.5   Examples of neural tube defects – when the neural tube fails to close early in pregnancy. Taking folic acid can significantly help to cut the risk of these birth defects.

Anencephaly	When the neural tube fails to close causing the brain to only form partially. These children are usually born without part of the brain, skull and scalp and are usually born blind, deaf and unconscious.
Spina bifida	When the neural tube fails to close causing the vertebrae to not properly form. This condition often leads to paralysis, even when spina bifida can be closed by surgeons after birth.
Encephalocele	When the neural tube fails to close leading to sac-like protrusions from the brain. These are mainly filled with cerebrospinal fluid and can be removed surgically.
Hydrocephalus	When the neural tube fails to close and cerebrospinal fluid accumulates in the brain. Most infants only live for a few weeks and the fluid compression on the brain can lead to brain damage.

Study findings showed that total daily caffeine intakes were associated with an increased risk of spina bifida, but, interestingly, this did not include caffeine from tea (tea was actually found to have a protective effect). There seemed to be some findings linking caffeine intakes to anencephaly, but this varied between maternal race/ethnicity and more work is needed (Schmidt *et al.*, 2009).

Overall, these are important findings and do raise some concerns given the fact that caffeine intakes appear to be rising. Other large studies now need to replicate these methods, including more detailed information about sources of caffeine. This will then hopefully help us to understand how caffeine may exert its actions.

8.8.2   Drink or avoid caffeine?

There are a lot of mixed messages about whether caffeine should be consumed in pregnancy and in what proportions. Sensible advice based on the CARE study group (2008) findings would be to monitor caffeine intakes in pregnancy, but especially in early pregnancy (the first three months; Figure 8.6)). Women should try not to exceed FSA (2008) guidelines of no more than 200 mg/day and try to get a feel for 'how much' caffeine is in a mug of tea (about 75 mg), mug of coffee (around 100 mg; instant coffee) and bar of chocolate (about 25 mg in a 50 g bar or milk chocolate). Opting for decaf tea and coffee and herbal teas may also help to reduce total daily intakes. The American College of Obstetricians and Gynaecologists have also recently stated that moderate caffeine intakes (less than 200 mg/day) does not appear to increase the risk of miscarriage or preterm births. They also stated that

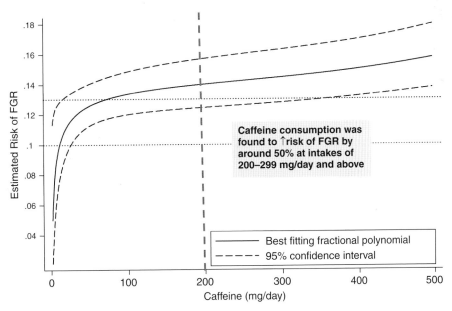

Figure 8.6   Reprinted with permission from the CARE Study Group (2008). Relation between risk of FGR and caffeine intake (mg/day) during pregnancy. The graph is restricted to <500 mg/day for clarity. Horizontal dotted lines mark national average risk of FGR (10%) and average risk in study cohort (13%).

further work is needed to study the relationship between caffeine and FGR (ACOG, 2010).

Research Highlight   A note on smoking and diet quality

A New Zealand study comprising 196 pregnant women found that food and nutrient intakes were lower in the less educated, young, those dependent on welfare and smokers. When compared with non-smokers, pregnant smokers ate around 300 kcals less each day and had a range of nutrition inadequacies. This included lower intakes of most key nutrients such as β-carotene, vitamin D, vitamin C, most B vitamins, iron and folate (just 176 μg/day) (Watson and McDonald, 2009). Although pregnancy outcomes were not reported in this study, lower energy intakes and deficits of key nutrients can have implications for pregnancy outcomes.

8.9   Dietary mutagens

Dietary mutagens are substances found in food that can cause DNA damage, either directly or through oxidative stress. Although pregnancy is a time when dietary mutagens could damage foetal DNA, it is also important to consider that foods also contain certain nutrients (antioxidants) that can help protect DNA and even alter the expression of foetal genes for the better (Goldman and Shields, 2003). For example, according to Dipple (1995), alcoholic beverages can activate the formation of *N*-nitrosamines inside the body whilst vitamin C ingestion can prevent the formation of these compounds.

In the past, animal studies have been used to show that certain food mutagens may be both mutagenic and teratogenic. It is only more recently that human studies have been carried out to investigate the effects that these components can have on the reproductive health of women. The main findings from key studies carried out to date are discussed in the next section.

8.9.1   Aflatoxins

Women mainly living in developing regions are most at risk of having a pregnancy affected by aflatoxins. In these regions, aflatoxins are commonly found in staple foods such as groundnuts, maize and seeds (Jolly *et al.*, 2006). One recent study carried out on a sample of 785 pregnant women living in Ghana studied whether women's exposure to aflatoxins had any effect on their infants' health. Scientists found that women ingesting higher levels of aflatoxins were significantly more likely to deliver low birth weight babies. This large, well carried out study indicates that the expectant mothers in such regions need to be educated about aflatoxin contamination of foods and how this could affect the health of their child (Shuaib *et al.*, 2010).

8.9.2   *N*-nitroso compounds

N-nitroso compounds (NOCs) are a family of compounds (nitrates, nitrites and nitrosamines) that can be detrimental to health. So far, animal studies have shown

Table 8.6 Top five foods most substantially contributing to nitrate, nitrite and nitrosamine intakes according to race/ethnicity.

Race/ethnicity	Main food sources
Non-Hispanic white	Skim or low fat milk, cereal, cheese, bread products and orange juice
Non-Hispanic black	Cereal, bread products, whole milk, orange juice and eggs
Hispanics	Tortillas, cereal, whole milk, orange juice and fresh apples or pears
Asian/Pacific Islanders	Rice or pasta, orange juice, cereal, skim milk and fresh apples or pears

Source: Griesenbeck *et al.* (2010).

that when consumed these compounds may be potentially carcinogenic, but the effects of it in pregnancy are largely unknown. These compounds can be made naturally inside the body (endogenously), but equally, they can also be ingested from food and water sources.

American scientists have calculated women's intakes of these compounds using data from the previously mentioned NBDPS. The ingestion of NOCs was measured using a specialised questionnaire (the Willet Food Frequency Questionnaire (FFQ). On average, women ingested 40.5 mg nitrates/day, 1.53 mg/day nitrites (3.7 mg/day total nitrites) and 0.47 µd/day of nitrosamines. This study was valuable in showing that woman's intakes and sources of NOCs (Table 8.6) varied considerably by race/ethnicity. In essence, such differences in dietary intakes of these compounds may lead to variations in reproductive outcomes and chronic diseases in women (Griesenbeck *et al.*, 2010).

Research Highlight   Can NOC exposure in pregnancy increase the risk of childhood cancers?

When the baby is developing inside the uterus, it is particularly vulnerable to certain carcinogenic compounds, such as NOCs. In turn, there is concern that ingestion of these in pregnancy may increase the risk of childhood brain tumours (CBT).

One paper has pooled the findings from studies looking at intakes of cured meats in pregnancy in relation to CBT risk in offspring. Frequent consumption of cured meats did appear to be associated with increased CBT risk. In terms of types of cured meats, regular hot dog consumption increased the risk of CBT by 33% and frequent ingestion of sausages by 44% (Huncharek and Kupelnick, 2004).

Another multicentered study collected information of the nitrate/nitrite content of tap water across five countries where they were CBT cases and compared this to the quality of tap water in areas where mothers had healthy children. CBT risk in this study did not appear to be related to higher nitrate levels in water, but scientists found that nitrites may have some effect (Mueller *et al.*, 2004). The findings from both of these studies are intriguing, but further work is needed to form definitive conclusions.

8.9.3   Heterocyclic amines

Heterocyclic amines are a group of mutagenic compounds that are found in cooked meats, particularly when cooked at high temperatures and slightly burnt. These compounds have been found to cause tumours in animal studies and epidemiology studies have linked their consumption to certain cancers, i.e. breast, colorectum and prostate cancer (Zheng and Lee, 2009). Few studies, however, looked into the effects heterocyclic amines could have in pregnancy. Although this research is yet to be carried out on large samples of pregnant mothers, it makes sense that women should consume meat that is cooked thoroughly but not overdone or burnt.

8.9.4   Methylmercury

Although fish may be a source of essential fatty acids, certain types can also be a source of methylmercury. Methylmercury (MeHg) is a fat-soluble molecule that passes easily through cell membranes and is readily taken up by aquatic organisms. All forms of mercury entering the aquatic environment, from industrial waste, or geological sources can be converted into methylmercury by microorganisms and then concentrated in fish and other aquatic species. Scientists from the Scientific Advisory Committee on Nutrition (SACN) and Committee on Toxicity (CoT) (2004) advise that larger fish, higher up in the food chain, such as shark, swordfish and marlin, have some of the highest levels of MeHg and should be avoided in pregnancy (SACN/CoT, 2004).

Effect in pregnancy

The developing brain and central nervous system of the foetus are sensitive to the effects of MeHg. Animal studies and some human studies (although findings are slightly controversial) have shown that high exposure may cause mental retardation, cerebral palsy, seizures and other developmental disabilities (Myers and Davidson, 2000). The SACN/CoT (2004) suggest that a MeHg intake of 3.3 μg/kg of body-weight a week may be used as a guideline to protect against some of these effects. As a one weekly 140 g portion of shark, swordfish or marlin would result in a dietary MeHg exposure above these levels, it is recommended that women who are pregnant or likely to become pregnant within one year avoid the consumption of these fish species.

Research Highlight   Can antioxidants protect against the effects of methylmercury?

One animal study carried out on female rats has shown that MeHg may not be as dangerous as once thought. It is thought that the harmful effects of MeHg can be reversed, even after birth if the child is exposed to a healthy environment and nutritious diet (Al-Ardhi and Al-Ani, 2008). This theory is, however, based largely on one animal study.

In this research, Canadian scientists put adult female rats on a control diet or fed them extra selenium, vitamin E, or both for 4 weeks before exposing them to MeHg. Treatment with MeHg and additional nutrients was then continued for the rest of pregnancy. Tissue mercury concentration did not vary between pups, but those born to mothers who were fed the diets highest in antioxidants had accelerated development, i.e. faster eye opening and response times (Beyrouty and Chan, 2006). This is a useful study, but one that needs further clarification. Researchers from this study believe that antioxidants could help to reduce the harmful effects of MeHg if ingested in sufficient amounts during pregnancy. Human studies are needed to determine what level of intake this is likely to be.

8.9.5   Polycyclic aromatic hydrocarbons

Polycyclic aromatic hydrocarbons (PAHs) are a group of over 100 different chemicals, formed when materials (including foods) are burnt. PAHs may be formed when foods are processed and cooked, i.e. when food are smoked, grilled, roasted or fried. The amount of PAH produced during cooking rises with increased fat content, longer exposure to flames and proximity to the heat source (EFSA, 2008). Overall, it has been estimated that the diet may provide around 3 μg/day of PAHs, while a regular smoker make be exposed to 2–5 μg PAH a day per pack of cigarettes smoked (Lioy and Greenberg, 1990; Waldman *et al.*, 1991). The diet can therefore be a significant source of PAHs.

PAHs and pregnancy

It can be difficult to quantify 'how much' PAHs are ingested or exposure to these. For this reason, benzo(a)pyrene (BaP) is often used as an additional marker of PAH exposure and can be used to analyse the health effects of PAH found in foods. Although animal research and a few studies in adult populations have assessed the effects of these compounds on health, only one large study seems to have studied this in detail in pregnant women.

European scientists have now measured intakes of both BaP and PAH in a large sample of 657 pregnant women recruited in their first trimester. The main dietary sources of these compounds were determined using a 101 item FFQ and other factors also accounted for using a general health and lifestyle questionnaire. Non-smokers were exposed to 0.18 μg/day BaP and 8.75 μg/day of PAHs from dietary sources. The main sources of PAH intake were processed and cured meats, cereals, potatoes and shellfish. Smokers were also found to have poorer quality diets and higher intakes of processed meats and shellfish, causing them to have the highest intakes of these compounds overall (0.20 μg/day BaP and 10.2 μg/day PAH) (Duarte-Salles *et al.*, 2010). Overall, these findings show that European pregnant mothers who smoke and have poor quality diets have high intakes of PAHs. In turn, this may not only affect their future health, but that of their offspring. Some studies have shown that PAHs are related to adverse reproductive outcomes, including LBW babies, preterm deliveries, reduced head circumference and lower scores on neurodevelopment tests in childhood (Choi *et al.*, 2006; Perera *et al.*, 2006). More research is now needed to underpin the development of safe levels of intake for these compounds.

8.10   Pesticides

A large volume of published studies have shown that pesticide exposure in pregnancy could have implications for maternal and infant health, especially in the first 3–8 weeks in the first trimester of pregnancy when the neural tube is forming. This particularly applies to women living in agricultural areas where pesticides are being applied. In 2007, one study in North Carolina found that the wives of farmers who were mixing or applying pesticides or helping to repair pesticide application equipment throughout their pregnancies had a higher risk of developing gestational diabetes (Saldana *et al.*, 2007). Authors concluded that certain herbicides and insecticides may increase the risk of diabetes in pregnancy. The cause of action now remains to be established.

8.10.1   Childhood behaviour

Some pesticides, such as organochlorides, can also pass across the placenta, which may affect the health of the developing foetus. Animal studies have shown that some of these chemicals can affect the development of the central nervous system and brain of the offspring when exposed inside the womb (Eskenazi *et al.*, 2008). A few human studies have shown that exposure to organochlorides in pregnancy may lead to behavioural problems such as reduced attention scores in infancy (Sagiv *et al.*, 2008) and attention deficit hyperactivity disorder in childhood (Sagiv *et al.*, 2010). Unfortunately, the number of studies in this area are quite scant and often limited in terms of study design. The long-term effects of pesticides in pregnancy and later in childhood do appear to be worthy of further investigation.

8.10.2   Exposure to pesticides

Studies have shown that women working in agricultural environments may be at the highest risk if they are pregnant and exposed to certain pesticides. Generally, the amount of pesticides we ingest from foods is minimal and can be reduced even further if we wash and/or peel fruits and vegetables. At present, there is no evidence to suggest that organic foods are better nutritionally or could lead to improved pregnancy outcomes. In terms of handling pesticides, most studies have only shown there may be risk where women are exposed to these chemicals for prolonged periods of time.

8.11   Hypospadias

Hypospadia is a male birth defect when the urethral opening is located on the underside of the penis. In boys, the urethra develops between weeks 7 and 16 of pregnancy and it is during this time, the foetus may be most vulnerable to certain foods and chemicals that can disrupt the balance of hormones within the woman's body (Baskin and Ebbers, 2006).

Data from large epidemiologic surveys show that the prevalence of hyospadias has risen from the 1970s up to present day. Recent evidence from one large Danish follow-through study monitored changes in the prevalence over a 29-year period.

The prevalence of hypospadia was found to increase from 0.24% in 1977 to 0.52% in 2005; an annual increase in prevalence of 2.40% which was unrelated to maternal age (Lund *et al.*, 2009).

8.11.1   What are the causes?

Although this birth defect can be rectified surgically the causes of hypospadias are generally unknown. Certain endocrine disruptors, foods and chemicals that can alter the balance of hormones in the mothers' body in early pregnancy have been implicated.

Scientists carrying out the Avon Longitudinal Study of Parents and Children (ALSPAC) in the United Kingdom found that 51 children born to 7928 mothers developed hypospadias. Smoking and alcohol intakes had no effect on the risk of hypospadias, but women who were vegetarian or supplemented their diet with iron in the first trimester of pregnancy were more likely to deliver infants with hypospadia (North and Golding, 2000). The findings from vegetarian mothers are easiest to explain as vegetarians have higher intakes of phytoestrogens from soy foods, which could have affected the development of male reproductive tract. However, the link between iron supplements and hypospadia is more difficult to disentangle.

One meta-analysis paper of nine key studies has looked whether pesticide exposure in pregnancy can affect the risk of male babies being born with hypospadia. Scientists found that women working with pesticides had a slight increased risk of delivering boys with hypospadias (Rocheleau *et al.*, 2009). Further large epidemiological studies would be helpful in terms of identifying the most common causes of hypospadia and how the risk of these birth defects can be reduced.

Research Highlight   Dietary factors and risk of hypospadia

Scientists have suggested that certain dietary factors may increase hypospadia risk but this has not been studied in great detail.

In Sweden and Denmark, scientists have now compared the diets of 292 mothers with babies with hypospadias to the diets of 427 control mothers using a questionnaire. Results showed that diets lacking in fish and meat increased the risk of hypospadias by almost fourfold. Equally, boys born to obese mothers (BMI ≥ 30) had a twofold increased risk of hypospadias when compared to the sons of healthy-weight mothers (BMI 21–24). Hypertension in pregnancy and the absence of nausea in early pregnancy was also associated with a 2.0-fold and 1.8-fold increased risk of hypospadia, respectively (Akre *et al.*, 2008). This was a well-designed study that builds on the findings of other studies and has identified some important risk factors for hypospadias.

8.12   Nutrigenomics

An optimal diet during pregnancy is fundamentally important for maternal and infant well-being. However, research now suggests that nutrient imbalances during pregnancy may result in alterations in foetal gene expression which could affect the long-term health of the offspring. Nutrigenomics is the study of how dietary

Table 8.7   Nutrigenomics versus nutrigenetics.

Nutrigenomics	The study of how dietary components interact with the human genome resulting in changes in the proteome and metabolome.
Nutrigenetics	The understanding of how different individual's genes respond differently to dietary components. Ultimately, this may lead to the development of nutraceuticals based on individual's genetic makeup that will help to promote health.
Other terms	
Genome	The entire set of hereditary instructions. An individual's complete set of genetic information.
Metabolome	Metabolic products that are a result of the expression of certain genes, i.e. cholesterol levels.
Proteome	Proteins with defined functions, i.e. insulin. The function of such proteins may be altered by changes in gene expression.

components can interact with an individual's genes and the way they are expressed, often leading to physical changes. Nutrigenetics is the way in which different individuals respond differently to different dietary components (Table 8.7). This area of work, in particular, provides opportunities for scientists to develop foods and nutraceuticals that could target specific health conditions, leading to 'personalised nutrition' (Subbiah, 2006).

The Human Genome Project

The Human Genome Project was completed in 2003. The project was coordinated by the US Department of Energy but the National Institute of Health and Wellcome Trust was also partners with this project.

   The project encoded all of the genes in the human body (about 20,000–25,000) and listed all of the base pairs and their sequences, making up each strand of DNA. From this, scientists have established databases that can now provide a wealth of information about genetic diseases. Even though the Human Genome Project is now complete, it will take years to continue analysing and organising data – new findings are continuously being uncovered. A project of this size and capacity also needs to address the ethical implications that may arise, i.e. as a result of this project, it will be possible to diagnose a whole host of new chronic genetic diseases.

   To overcome such problems, in 2008, the US government put the Genetic Information Nondiscrimination Act in place. This new act will hopefully help to go some way to prevent the improper use of genetic information, i.e. in health insurance and employment (Erwin, 2009). This is a good move forward and no doubt new policies will continue to be developed in the future in scientific and medical practices.

8.12.1   Diet and gene expression

There is increasing evidence that diet in pregnancy can influence the expression of the offspring's genes (also known as epigenetics). Scientists are continuously uncovering

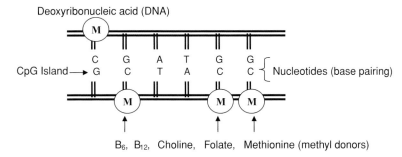

Figure 8.7 Maternal nutrition and gene expression. Methylation usually takes place around the CpG Islands. Donation of methyl (M) CH₃ groups reduces expression of genes that predispose towards disease. C, cytosine; G, guanine; A, Adenine; T, thymine. (Reproduced with permission from Derbyshire (2007).)

new findings about this field of work. One way in which the maternal diet may control the expression of the child's genes is through a process known as methylation.

In brief, methylation takes place at the molecular level when DNA can either pick up or lose methyl (CH$_3$) groups. These methyl groups can, in turn, control levels of gene expression (whether a gene expresses its trait weakly or prominently). Usually, methylation is concentrated around CpG (cytosine–phosphate–guanine) regions, also known as CpG Islands, or promoter regions within DNA (Figure 8.7). Low levels of methylation (hypomethylation) are thought to result in high levels of gene expression, predisposing towards disease. High levels of methylation (hypermethylation) are associated with the silencing of gene expression and reduced risk of disease development (Maloney and Rees, 2005).

8.12.2 Foods as methyl donors

Research suggests that epigenic inheritance is very sensitive to environmental changes, including dietary factors (Friso and Choi, 2002). It is thought that a maternal diet rich in methyl donors may help suppress the expression of harmful genes and improve the outcome of the offspring (Maloney and Rees, 2005). Methyl donors are molecules or nutrients that transfer methyl groups to DNA. B vitamins (B$_6$ and B$_{12}$, choline and folate) and amino acids such as methionine are all examples of methyl donors. The Food and Nutrition Board (2004) recommends that 13 mg of methionine are consumed per kg of body weight. Examples of nutrients that may act as methyl donors are included in Table 8.8.

8.13 Foetal origins of adult disease

Methylation is one example of how the diet in pregnancy may have the potential to influence the expression of the child's genes. However, the theory that diet in pregnancy may influence the likelihood of disease development in the offspring is not new. The foetal origins' hypothesis, an important theory proposing that inadequate maternal nutrition and a low infant birth weight can predispose towards disease later in life and was first founded by Professor David Barker in 1995. Using data from birth records stored in library archives, it was identified that adults diagnosed

Table 8.8 Food sources rich in methyl donors.

Nutrient	Food sources (per 100 g)	Recommended intake during pregnancy*
B$_6$ (Pyridoxine)	Roast chicken (0.5 mg), grilled halibut (0.4 mg), smoked mackerel (0.5 mg) and baked potato (0.5 mg)	1.9 mg/day
B$_{12}$ (Cyanocobalamin)	Parmesan (3.3 µg), eggs (2.5 µg), cheddar cheese (2.4 µg), special K cereals (1.7 µg) and semi-skimmed milk (0.9 µg)	2.6 µmg/day
Choline	Eggs (251 mg), wheatgerm (152 mg), bacon (125 mg) and dried soybeans (116 mg)	450 mg/day
Folate	Special K (333 µg), sultana bran (250 µg), boiled kale (86 µg), boiled spinach (81 µg), soft cheese (47 µg) and lentils (30 µg)	600 µg/day
Methionine	Eggs (1477 mg), brazil nuts (1008 mg), lean beef (925 mg) and roast turkey (893 mg)	13 mg/kg body weight

*Food and Nutrition Board (2004) dietary recommendations.

with cardiovascular disease were more likely to have been LBW (<2500 g) when they were born (Barker, 2003).

Since then a considerable amount of literature has been published, documenting that smaller, undernourished babies (not including premature infants) have an increased risk of developing other diseases in later life. This now not only includes cardiovascular disease but also extends to diabetes and hypertension, especially when small infants experience accelerated weight gain from 3 to 11 years of age (Barker *et al.*, 2002). Women can to some extent buffer the supply of nutrients to the foetus by utilising their own nutrient reserves. However, when there are chronic food shortages, this natural mechanism cannot yield the levels of nutrients needed for foetal growth. In these cases, when nutrients supplies cannot meet foetal demands, FGR can occur and babies may be born smaller than average. As mentioned earlier in this chapter, scientists are now particularly interested in deciphering the exact time periods or 'sensitive windows' of pregnancy when the foetus may be most susceptible to the effects of undernutrition or deficits of certain nutrients (Lumey *et al.*, 2007). This is discussed further in the next research highlight.

Research Highlight   Learning from the Dutch famine

The 'Dutch Hunger Winter' (1944–45) is a good example of the application of the Barker hypothesis. At the end of World War II, Germany imposed a food embargo in Western Holland, a period when many pregnant mothers were malnourished. Exposure to this famine meant that this was a period of time when mothers delivered smaller infants with restricted growth.

The health of these mothers and their infants has now been followed up and shows that maternal famine exposure during pregnancy can lead to chronic diseases later in life. The effects, however, later in life depend according to the phase of pregnancy when women were exposed to the famine. Rates of coronary heart disease, raised blood lipids, altered clotting and higher rates of obesity have been found amongst those exposed to famine early in pregnancy. Exposure to famine mid-pregnancy has been linked to diseases of the airways and exposure to famine later in pregnancy to glucose intolerance later in adulthood (Figure 8.8; Painter *et al.*, 2005). Overall, these findings build on the basic Barker hypothesis and demonstrate that maternal undernutrition during gestation has important effects on health in later life, but that the timing of the nutritional insult can determine which organ system is affected.

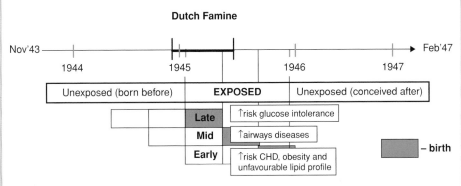

Figure 8.8   The Dutch famine birth cohort and timing of exposure. (With permission from Elsevier.)

8.14   Supplements

Emphasis must always be placed on the importance of a good-quality diet, but given the limitations of the twenty-first century lifestyle and the fact that foods today are not always a rich sources of important minerals (i.e. iron and selenium) appropriately formulated nutritional supplements, rather than single nutrient supplements, may be a good way to ensure that women achieve recommended levels of nutrients for this life-phase (Glenville, 2006).

A wealth of research has investigated the separate roles of individual vitamin and mineral supplements in relation to pregnancy outcomes, i.e. folic acid and the prevention of NTDs, as well as the potential benefits of multivitamin and mineral supplements. But how can supplements improve pregnancy outcomes? What is the evidence-base? And do women comply and take these? These are just some of the few questions that the next section aims to address.

8.14.1   Pregnancy outcomes

When it comes to studying supplement use and pregnancy outcomes more, well-designed studies following women through from early in their pregnancies (if not

Table 8.9 Some key studies – supplement use and pregnancy outcomes.

Study	Supplement and dose	Effect on pregnancy outcome
Alwan *et al.* (2010)	N/A observational study	Regular multivitamin–mineral supplementation was not related to size at birth. Supplementation in the third trimester was associated with preterm delivery.
Hauth *et al.* (2010)	1000 mg vitamin C and 400 IU (256 mg) vitamin E from 9–16 weeks pregnancy until delivery	Taking vitamins C and E did not ↓ risk of spontaneous, preterm births.
Harper *et al.* (2010)	Women with a history of preterm birth received an omega 3 (1.2 g EPA and 0.8 g DHA) or placebo supplement from mid-pregnancy until delivery	Taking the omega-3 supplement had no effect on the number of preterm deliveries.
Bánhidy *et al.* (2010)	N/A case–control study	Higher rates of preterm deliveries were observed in anaemic women who did not take iron supplements in pregnancy.
Kupka *et al.* (2008)	Women given 200 µg/day selenium or a placebo from 12–27 weeks pregnancy until delivery	Selenium supplements did not affect HIV progression but may have helped to ↑child survival.

Search terms used in Medline: 'supplements' and 'pregnancy outcomes'.

before) are needed. A sample of key studies that have looked at supplement use and pregnancy outcomes is included in Table 8.9. As can be seen, one study found that supplement use in the third trimester of pregnancy in well-nourished mothers actually increased the risk of preterm deliveries (Alwan *et al.*, 2010). Other studies have shown weak or no relationships between certain nutrients and pregnancy outcomes. More remains to be known about possible interactions between micronutrients and their metabolism, whether there is any benefit of continuing to take supplements in the third trimester of pregnancy and if well-nourished mothers can 'further benefit' from taking additional nutrients or if this could have potential adverse effects. In the meantime, women should be advised to continue taking folic acid before and in the first 12 weeks of pregnancy and 'high-risk' groups, i.e. Asian mothers, may need to seek guidance in terms of whether vitamin D supplements are needed (NICE, 2008).

Research Highlight   Can multiple-micronutrient supplements improve nutrient status in pregnancy and birth outcomes?

Scientists have now studied whether multiple-micronutrient supplements can help to improve women's nutritional status and pregnancy outcomes in a sample of 402 socially deprived pregnant mothers.

Women recruited from East London, United Kingdom, were randomised and asked to take a supplement containing 20 mg iron and 400 µg folic acid daily from the first trimester of pregnancy until delivery, or a placebo. Blood samples were taken to assess nutrient status at baseline and at 26 and 34 weeks into pregnancy and birth outcomes recorded.

Researchers found that 13% women were anaemic at the start of the study, 72% has low vitamin D status, 12% thiamine deficiency and 5% folate deficiency. When assessed in mid-pregnancy and late pregnancy, women taking the active micronutrient supplement had improved haemoglobin, ferritin, folate and vitamin D status when compared with controls. Unfortunately, more women in the control group also delivered small-for-gestational-age infants (Brough *et al.*, 2010).

Taken together, the results from this important study suggest that supplements can play a key role in terms of helping to improve women's nutrient status and reduce the risk of women delivering small infants. Although this study provided some important findings, it is important to recognise the fact that only 39% of the 402 women completed the study. Therefore, larger studies are now needed to reinforce these findings.

8.14.2   Are women taking supplements?

Although the health benefits of certain supplements taken before and during pregnancy are well known, there is one problem – compliance. Women may not comply and take supplements on a regular basis for a variety of reasons. Sometimes, tablet-based supplements, such as iron (ferrous sulphate), can cause unpleasant side effects including nausea and constipation. Habib *et al.*, (2009) in a study of 308 pregnant women reported that 49.7% used supplements in the second and third trimester of pregnancy and 38.3% only used them partially. Haemoglobin levels only improved amongst women taking iron supplements on a regular basis.

Interestingly, one study carried out in China randomised pregnant women to take folic acid, iron-folic acid or a micronutrient supplement containing 15 key vitamins and minerals. Women were asked to take their allocated supplement daily throughout pregnancy until delivery. Less than 4% women withdrew from the study because of side effects and most supplements were taken on more than 90% of the days in which they were provided. Researchers concluded that frequent contact with trained health workers may have helped to remind women to take their supplements, improving compliance figures in this research (Zeng *et al.*, 2009).

8.14.3   International use

Pregnant women in developing regions, in particular, may underconsume a range of vitamins and minerals. Therefore, multivitamin-mineral supplements may be considered an attractive option by international agencies. Supplements are cheap, easy to administer and can be distributed through national antenatal programmes although they are often not subject to the same safety standards as prescription medications (Dunlop *et al.*, 2008).

Currently, women in developing country settings have been advised to take iron–folic acid supplements to help improve their pregnancy outcomes. However, scientists have also carried out research to see whether women could further benefit if these were replaced with micronutrient supplements. Overall, evidence is mixed but one paper evaluated the findings from 12 randomised controlled trials in these regions and found that supplements containing multiple micronutrients led to small increases in birth weight and reduced the prevalence of LBW deliveries by about 10% (Fall *et al.*, 2009). Whether these small benefits outweigh the costs of prescribing these supplements is a matter that requires further contemplation.

8.15   Application in practice

From a practical point of view, women should be encouraged to eat a balanced, healthy diet throughout her reproductive years, providing adequate intakes of macronutrients and a broad range of micronutrients. In particular, women should take care not to exceed most recent guidelines for alcohol (no more than 1–2 units on two occasions/week for first trimester) and caffeine (no more than 200 mg/day), which need to be communicated clearly and consistently. Women also need to get a realistic 'feel' for what these guidelines are in everyday measures, i.e. two mugs of tea and a bar of milk chocolate.

With regard to other exposures such as aflatoxins, nitrates, PAHs, methylmercury, there is evidence that these may have some effects on the health of the offspring but only when levels of exposure/intake are high. Nurses need to be aware that under nutrition during pregnancy can impact upon the child's long-term health status and although the field of nutrigenomics is still in its early phases, a diet rich methyl donors i.e. B vitamins may help to regulate gene expression and prevent disease in adulthood. More remains to be known about the role of supplements with regard to whether these help to improve pregnancy outcomes, but the evidence-base for folic acid is strong. Therefore, women should continue to take 400 µg/day folic acid before and early in pregnancy for now until more evidence for high supplement doses become available.

8.16   Conclusion

Public health strategies are needed to improve the health of women, which subsequently will help to improve their health of their children. Optimising women's diets, managing infections and guiding them to good health is an approach that is both feasible and affordable, even for financially constrained health systems. On the whole, adequate dietary advice and guiding women about the effects certain exposures could have on their own health and that of the baby seems to be a promising strategy in terms of preventing chronic disease risk in future generations. On a final note, more work is now needed to disentangle the separate effects of these dietary and lifestyle factors so that important, clear and consistent health messages can be imparted.

Key Messages

- Nurses may wish to explain to patients that healthy diet before and throughout pregnancy can help to optimise the infant's health not only in the short-term but also in the longer term.

- Although caffeine does not need to be cut out of the diet completely, pregnant women should consume no more than 200 mg caffeine a day. Where possible, women planning a pregnancy should be made aware of these recommendations and given advice about what constitutes 200 mg/day.
- Alcohol is not advised in the first three months of pregnancy and no more than 1–2 units twice a week should be consumed after this period (if at all).
- Advice of caffeine and alcohol intake in pregnancy should be given in conjunction with other recommendations during pregnancy to minimise the risk of adverse pregnancy outcomes as much as possible.
- Nurses and health practitioners may wish to keep up-to-date with the field of nutrigenomics.
- Presently, there is no national recommendation to take multivitamin and mineral supplements at any stage of pregnancy. Although these are readily available over the counter and heavily promoted to expectant mothers, women should be advised about when these should be taken and in what doses.
- Further research is needed so that scientists can weigh the possible benefits and harms associated with supplement use in pregnancy. It is possible that the type of supplement taken should be focused more towards the individual needs of women.

Recommended reading

Langley-Evans SC (2004) *Fetal Nutrition and Adult Disease: Programming of Chronic Disease Through Fetal Exposure to Undernutrition*. CABI Publishing: Wallingford, UK.
SACN (Scientific Advisory Committee on Nutrition) (2010) *The SACN Subgroup on Maternal and Child Nutrition (SMCN): The Influence of Maternal, Fetal and Child Nutrition on the Development on Chronic Disease in Later Life*. The Stationery Office: London.
Spencer N (2003) *Weighing the Evidence – How is Birthweight Determined?* Radcliffe Medical Press: Oxon, UK.

References

ACOG (American College of Obstetricians and Gynecologists) (2010) ACOG Committee opinion no. 462: moderate caffeine consumption during pregnancy. *Obstetrics & Gynaecology* **116** (2 Pt 1), 467–8.
Adèn U (2011) Methylxanthines during pregnancy and early postnatal life. *Handbook of Experimental Pharmacology* **200**, 373–89.
Akre O, Boyd HA, Ahlgren M et al. (2008) Maternal and gestational risk factors for hypospadias. *Environmental Health Perspectives* **116**(8), 1071–6.
Al-Ardhi FM and Al-Ani MR (2008) Maternal fish consumption and prenatal methylmercury exposure: a review. *Nutrition and Health* **19**(4), 289–97.
Alwan NA, Greenwood DC, Simpson NAB, McArdle HJ and Cade JE (2010) The relationship between dietary supplement use in late pregnancy and birth outcomes: a cohort study in British women. *British Journal of Obstetrics & Gynaecology* **117**, 821–9.
Bánhidy F, Acs N, Puhó EH and Czeizel AE (2010) Iron deficiency anemia: pregnancy outcomes with or without iron supplementation. *Nutrition* **27**(1), 65–72.
Barker D (2003) *The Best Start in Life: How a Woman's Diet Can Protect Her Child from Disease in Later Life*. Century Publishing: London.
Barker DJ, Eriksson JG, Forsén T and Osmond C (2002) Fetal origins of adult disease: strength of effects and biological basis. *International Journal of Epidemiology* **31**(6), 1235–9.
Baskin LS and Ebbers MB (2006) Hypospadias: anatomy, etiology, and technique. *Journal of Pediatric Surgery* **41**(3), 463–72.

Beyrouty P and Chan HM (2006) Co-consumption of selenium and vitamin E altered the reproductive and developmental toxicity of methylmercury in rats. *Neurotoxicology and Teratology* **28**, 49–58.

Brough L, Rees GA, Crawford MA, Morton RH and Dorman EK (2010) Effect of multiple-micronutrient supplementation on maternal nutrient status, infant birth weight and gestational age at birth in a low-income, multi-ethnic population. *British Journal of Nutrition* **104**(3), 437–45.

CARE Study Group (2008) Maternal caffeine intake during pregnancy and risk of fetal growth restriction: a large prospective observational study. *British Medical Journal* **337**, 23–32.

Choi H, Jedrychowski W, Spengler J *et al.* (2006) International studies of prenatal exposure to polycyclic aromatic hydrocarbons and hydrocarbons and fetal growth. *Environmental Health Perspectives* **114**(11), 1744–50.

Derbyshire EJ (2007) Maternal nutrition and gene expression. *British Journal of Nursing* **16**(13), 738–40.

Dipple A (1995) DNA adducts of chemical carcinogens. *Carcinogenesis* **16**, 437–41.

Duarte-Salles T, Mendez MA, Pessoa V *et al.* (2010) Smoking during pregnancy is associated with higher dietary intake of polycyclic aromatic hydrocarbons and poor diet quality. *Public Health Nutrition* (**12**), 2034–43.

Dunlop AL, Gardiner PM, Shellhaas CS, Menard MK and McDiarmid MA (2008) The clinical content of preconception care: the use of medications and supplements among women of reproductive age. *American Journal of Obstetrics & Gynaecology* **199**(6 Suppl 2), S367–72.

EFSA (European Food Safety Authority) (2008) Scientific opinion of the panel on contaminants in the food chain on a request from the European commission of polycyclic aromatic hydrocarbons in food. *EFSA Journal* **724**, 1–114.

Erwin C (2009) Behind the Genetic Information Nondiscrimination Act of 2008. *American Journal of Nursing* **109**(12), 46–8.

Eskenazi B, Rosas LG, Marks AP *et al.* (2008) Pesticide toxicity and the developing brain. *Basic & Clinical Pharmacology & Toxicology* **102**(2), 228–36.

Fall CH, Fisher DJ, Osmond C, Margetts BM; Maternal Micronutrient Supplementation Study Group (2009) Multiple micronutrient supplementation during pregnancy in low-income countries: a meta-analysis of effects on birth size and length of gestation. *Food and Nutrition Bulletin* **30**(4 Suppl), S533–46.

Finster M and Wood M (2005) The Apgar score has survived the test of time. *Anesthiology* **102**(4), 855–7.

Floyd RL, Weber MK, Denny C and O'Connor MJ (2009) Prevention of fetal alcohol spectrum disorders. *Developmental Disabilities* **15**, 193–9.

Friso S and Choi SW (2002) Gene–nutrient interactions and DNA methylation. *American Society for Nutritional Sciences* **132**, 2382S–7S.

FSA (Food Standards Agency) (2008) Food Standards Agency publishes new caffeine advice for pregnant women. Available at: http://www.food.gov.uk/news/pressreleases/2008/nov/caffeineadvice. (accessed March 2011.)

Food and Nutrition Board (2004) *Dietary Reference Intakes Table*. The National Academies Press: Washington, DC.

Galtier F, Raingeard I, Renard E, Boulot P and Bringer J (2008) Optimising the outcome of pregnancy in obese women: from pregestational to long-term management. *Diabetes & Metabolism* **24**(1), 19–25.

Glenville M (2006) Nutritional supplements in pregnancy: commercial push or evidence based? *Current Opinions in Obstetrics & Gynaecology* **18**(6), 642–7.

Goldman R and Shields PG (2003) Food mutagens. *Journal of Nutrition* **133**(3), 965S–73S.

Griesenbeck JS, Brender JD, Sharkey JR *et al.*; National Birth Defects Prevention Study (2010) Maternal characteristics associated with the dietary intake of nitrates, nitrites, and nitrosamines in women of child-bearing age: a cross-sectional study. *Environmental Health* **9**, 10.

Habib F, Alabdin EH, Alenazy M and Nooh R (2009) Compliance to iron supplementation during pregnancy. *Journal of Obstetrics & Gynaecology* **29**(6), 487–92.

Harper M, Thom E, Klebanoff MA *et al.* (2010) Omega-3 fatty acid supplementation to prevent recurrent preterm birth: a randomized controlled trial. *Obstetrics & Gynaecology* **115**(2 Pt 1), 234–42.

Hauth JC, Clifton RG, Roberts JM *et al.* (2010) Vitamin C and E supplementation to prevent spontaneous preterm birth: a randomized controlled trial. *Obstetrics & Gynaecology* **116**(3), 653–8.

Huncharek M and Kupelnick B (2004) A meta-analysis of maternal cured meat consumption during pregnancy and the risk of childhood brain tumours. *Neuroepidemiology* **23**(1–2), 78–84.

Jolly P, Jiang Y, Ellis W *et al.* (2006) Determinants of aflatoxin levels in Ghanaians: sociodemographic factors, knowledge of aflatoxin and food handling and consumption practices. *International Journal of Hygiene & Environmental Health* **209**(4), 345–58.

Kupka R, Mugusi F, Aboud S *et al.* (2008) Randomized, double-blind, placebo-controlled trial of selenium supplements among HIV-infected pregnant women in Tanzania: effects on maternal and child outcomes. *American Journal of Clinical Nutrition* **87**(6), 1802–8.

Lioy PJ and Greenberg A (1990) Factors associated with human exposures to polycyclic aromatic hydrocarbons. *Toxicology & Industrial Health* **6**, 209–23.

Lumey LH, Stein AD, Kahn HS *et al.* (2007) Cohort profile: the Dutch Hunger Winter families study. *International Journal of Epidemiology* **36**(6), 1196–204.

Lund L, Engebjerg MC, Pedersen L, Ehrenstein V, Nørgaard M and Sørensen HT (2009) Prevalence of hypospadias in Danish boys: a longitudinal study, 1977–2005. *European Urology* **55**(5), 1022–6. Epub 2009 Jan 13.

Lundgren EM and Tuverno T (2008) Effects of being born small for gestational age on long-term intellectual performance. *Best Practice & Research. Clinical Endocrinology & Metabolism* **22**(3), 477–88.

Maloney CA and Rees WD (2005) Gene-nutrient interactions during fetal development. *Society for Reproduction and Fertility* **130**, 401–10.

March of Dimes Birth Defects Foundation (2006) March of Dimes Global Report on Birth Defects: the hidden toll of dying and disabled children. Available at: http://www.marchofdimes.com/downloads/Birth_Defects_Report-PF.pdf (accessed April 2011).

Miles L and Foxen R (2009) New guidelines on caffeine in pregnancy. *British Nutrition Foundation Nutrition Bulletin* **34**, 203–6.

Miller J, Turan S and Baschat AA (2008) Fetal growth restriction. *Seminars in Perinatology* **32**(4), 274–80.

Mueller BA, Nielsen SS, Preston-Martin S, *et al.* (2004) Household water source and the risk of childhood brain tumours: results of the SEARCH International Brain Tumor Study. *International Journal of Epidemiology* **33**(6), 1209–16.

Myers GJ and Davidson PW (2000) Does methylmercury have a role in causing developmental disabilities in children? *Environmental Health Perspectives* **108**(Suppl 3), 413–20.

NICE (National Institute for Clinical Excellence) (2008) *Antenatal Care: Routine Care for the Healthy Pregnant Woman.* NICE: London.

North K and Golding J (2000) A maternal vegetarian diet in pregnancy is associated with hypospadias. The ALSPAC Study Team. Avon Longitudinal Study of Pregnancy and Childhood. *British Journal of Urology International* **85**(1), 107–13.

O'Leary CM (2004) Fetal alcohol syndrome: diagnosis, epidemiology, and developmental outcomes. *Journal of Paediatrics & Child Health* **40**(1–2), 2–7.

Painter RC, Roseboom TJ and Bleker OP (2005) Prenatal exposure to the Dutch famine and disease in later life: an overview. *ReproductiveToxicology* **20**(3), 345–52.

Peadon E, Payne J, Henley N *et al.* (2010) Women's knowledge and attitudes regarding alcohol consumption in pregnancy: a national survey. *BMC Public Health* **10**, 510.

Perera FP, Rauh V, Whyatt RM *et al.* (2006) Effect of prenatal exposure to airborne polycyclic aromatic hydrocarbons on neurodevelopment in the first 3 years of life among inner-city children. *Environmental Health Perspectives* **114**(8), 1287–92.

Rees GA, Doyle W, Srivastava A, Brooke ZM, Crawford MW and Costeloe KL (2005) The nutrient intakes of mothers of low birth weight babies – a comparison of ethnic groups in East London, UK. *Maternal and Child Nutrition* **1**, 91–9.

Rocheleau CM, Romitti PA and Dennis LK (2009) Pesticides and hypospadias: a meta-analysis. *Journal of Pediatric Urology* **5**(1), 17–24.

Rodríguez-Bernal CL, Rebagliato M, Iñiguez C *et al.* (2010) Diet quality in early pregnancy and its effects on fetal growth outcomes: the Infancia y Medio Ambiente (Childhood and Environment) Mother and Child Cohort Study in Spain. *American Journal of Clinical Nutrition* **91**(6), 1659–66.

Rosennthal J, Christianson AL and Cordero J (2005) Fetal alcohol syndrome prevention in South African and other low-resource countries. *American Journal of Public Health* **95**, 1099–101.

Sagiv SK, Nugent JK, Brazelton TB *et al*. (2008) Prenatal organochlorine exposure and measures of behavior in infancy using the Neonatal Behavioral Assessment Scale (NBAS). *Environmental Health Perspectives* **116**(5), 666–73.

Sagiv SK, Thurston SW, Bellinger DC, Tolbert PE, Altshul LM and Korrick SA (2010) Prenatal organochlorine exposure and behaviors associated with attention deficit hyperactivity disorder in school-aged children. *American Journal of Epidemiology* **171**(5), 593–601.

Saldana TM, Basso O, Hoppin JA *et al*. (2007) Pesticide exposure and self-reported gestational diabetes mellitus in the Agricultural Health Study. *Diabetes Care* **30**(3), 529–34.

Schmidt RJ, Romitti PA, Burns TL, Browne ML, Druschel CM, Olney RS; National Birth Defects Prevention Study (2009) Maternal caffeine consumption and risk of neural tube defects. *Birth Defects Research. Part A: Clinical and Molecular Teratology* **85**(11), 879–89.

Scientific Advisory Committee on Nutrition/Committee on Nutrition/Committee on Toxicity (SACN/CoT) (2004), *Advice on Fish Consumption: Benefits and Risks*, The Stationery Office: London.

Selevan SG, Kimmel CA and Mendola P (2000) Identifying critical windows of exposure for children's health. *Environmental Health Perspectives* **108**(3), 451–5.

Shuaib FM, Jolly PE, Ehiri JE *et al*. (2010) Association between birth outcomes and aflatoxin B1 biomarker blood levels in pregnant women in Kumasi, Ghana. *Tropical Medicine & International Health* **15**(2), 160–7.

Stables D and Rankin J (2006) *Physiology in Childbearing*. Elsevier: London.

Subbiah MTR (2006) Nutrigenetics and nutraceuticals: the next wave riding on personalised medicine. *Translational Research* (2), 55–61.

Viljoen D, Craig P, Hymbaugh K, Boyle C and Blount S (2003) Fetal alcohol syndrome – South Africa, 2001. *Morbidity & Mortality Weekly Report* **52**, 660–2.

Waldman JM, Lioy PJ, Greenberg A and Butler JP (1991) Analysis of human exposure to benzo(a)pyrene via inhalation and food ingestion in the Total Human Environmental Exposure Study (THEES). *Journal of Exposure Science Analysis & Environmental Epidemiology* **1**, 193–225.

Warren KR and Foudin LL (2001) Alcohol-related birth defects – the past, present, and future. *Alcohol Research & Health* **25**(3), 153–8.

Watson PE and McDonald BW (2009) Major influences on nutrient intakes in pregnant New Zealand women. *Maternal and Child Health Journal* **13**, 695–706.

Whitehall JS (2007) National guidelines on alcohol use during pregnancy: a dissenting option. *Medical Journal of Australia* **186**(1), 35–7.

Yoon PW, Rasmussen SA, Lynberg MC *et al*. (2001) The National Birth Defects Prevention Study. *Public Health Reports* **116**(Suppl 1), 32–40.

Zeng L, Yan H, Cheng Y, Dang S and Dibley MJ (2009) Adherence and costs of micronutrient supplementation in pregnancy in a double-blind, randomised, controlled trial in western China. *Food and Nutrition Bulletin* **30**(4 Suppl), S480–7.

Zheng W and Lee SA (2009) Well-done meat intake, heterocyclic amine exposure, and cancer risk. *Nutrition & Cancer* **61**(4), 437–46.

9 Weight Gain in Pregnancy

Summary

It is important that women are aware of 'how much' weight to gain during pregnancy. Failure to gain weight within recommended guidelines (11.5–16 kg for women with a normal pre-pregnancy weight) may affect the short- and long-term health of both mother and child. Inadequate levels of weight gain may increase the risk of miscarriage, premature delivery and delivering small-for-gestational-age (SGA)/low birth weight babies. Equally, surplus weight gain can increase the risk of developing gestational diabetes, pre-eclampsia, delivering by elective surgery and giving birth to large-for-gestational-age (LGA) infants, or infants with congenital abnormalities. Government agencies and healthcare providers need to express the importance of attaining a healthy body weight upon conception. Women need to be guided about 'how much' weight to gain throughout the course of pregnancy and how this can be achieved safely. Clinicians, dieticians and nutritionists can play a key role in helping to disseminate this important information to women of childbearing age and pregnant mothers.

Learning Outcomes

- To understand the importance of a healthy body weight before pregnancy.
- To be aware of the components of gestational weight gain (GWG).
- To recognise health implications associated with excess and inadequate GWG.
- To be familiar with pregnancy weight gain guidelines and the application of these in practice.

9.1 Introduction

Although normal birth outcomes are possible when pregnancy weight gain is not within the recommended ranges, clinical complications are more likely to occur when this is the case. When a high or low body weight before pregnancy is coupled with unsuitable levels of weight gain, the risk of an unfavourable pregnancy outcome increases further.

Increasing proportions of women in their childbearing years are now falling into the overweight or obese weight categories. Over one-third of pregnant women are affected by obesity (Mills *et al.*, 2010) and obesity is now penetrating developing

---

Nutrition in the Childbearing Years, First Edition. Emma Derbyshire.
© 2011 Emma Derbyshire. Published 2011 by Blackwell Publishing Ltd.

regions (particularly urban areas) and rates are likely to rise further over the next two decades (Prentice, 2006). In turn, with the rise in obesity rates worldwide, medical complications often overspill into pregnancy.

Equally, at the other end of the weight spectrum, higher percentages of women are becoming more concerned about the amount of weight that they will put on and retain after their pregnancy. Although the body can adapt to some extent, this too can have health implications for the mother and child even though these may not always be noticeable from the outset.

On the whole, this section of the book aims to explain the importance of achieving a 'healthy' body weight before even becoming pregnant, the importance of gaining the right 'proportions' of weight once pregnancy and how high and low pregnancy weight gains can affect the health of mother and child. Rates of weight loss after birth will be touched on in this chapter but also be discussed later in Chapter 11.

9.2   Body weight before pregnancy

9.2.1   Overweight

Women who are overweight or obese when they conceive are more likely to experience medical and/or delivery complications when compared with healthy weight women. There is now strong evidence that body weight before pregnancy can affect the mothers' health and pregnancy outcome. In relation to the mother's health, one of the largest studies today (1.4 million women) showed that risk of pre-eclampsia in pregnancy nearly doubled with each $5–7$ kg/m^2 increase in pre-pregnancy body mass index (BMI), even when women with hypertension, diabetes or multiple pregnancies were excluded from the study (O'Brien et al., 2003). Women with a high BMI before becoming pregnant also have a significantly higher risk of developing hyperglycaemia and diabetes in pregnancy. This has been clearly demonstrated in a review and meta-analysis paper showing that for every 1 kg/m^2 increase in BMI, the risk of developing diabetes in pregnancy increased by 0.92% (Torloni et al., 2008).

With respect to the short-term and long-term health of the offspring, overweight/obesity before pregnancy may increase the chances of delivering a child with certain birth defects. Rates of neural tube defects (NTDs), spina bifida, cardiovascular anomalies, cleft lip and palate, anorectal atresia, hydrocephaly and limb anomalies have been reported to be higher in women with higher body weights before becoming pregnant (Stothard et al., 2009). Maternal body weight before pregnancy can also have a long-term persisting effect on the adiposity of the child. A UK study following a sample of 219 children found that mothers with a higher BMI before pregnancy were more likely to have children with higher levels of fat mass (FM) at 9 years of age (Gale et al., 2007).

Overall, the evidence linking overweight/obesity before pregnancy to higher chances of medical complications in pregnancy and reduced life quality and health of the next generation is strong. Helping women to plan their pregnancies and get their body weight into healthy ranges before becoming pregnant could help to reduce stresses on the health services and play a significant role in helping to get the child's health off to the best possible start.

9.2.2 Underweight

There are a whole host of reasons why a woman may be underweight when she conceives. In less developed regions, food shortages are obviously one contributory factor, but for Western women, increasing social pressures may be to blame. Modern lifestyles, i.e. being busy, eating on the go, very active lifestyles or equally displacing food calories with smoking, can also mean that women have lower body weights when they fall pregnant.

Relating this to scientific evidence, American scientists have studied the health ramifications of this in some detail. One study using data from 437,403 mothers–infant pairs in Missouri found that 'severely thin' mothers (BMI less than 15.9) had the highest risk of delivering preterm infants, compared to those that were moderately thin or a healthy bodyweight (Salihu *et al.*, 2009a). Underweight mothers were also more likely to deliver low, very low birth weight or small-for-gestational-age (SGA) infants, and the lower the body weight before pregnancy, the higher the risk of this (Salihu *et al.*, 2009b). Equally, the odds of delivering an infant with congenital anomalities including heart and genital defects and hypospadias has been found to be significantly higher in underweight (BMI $\leq$ 18.5) mothers (Rankin *et al.*, 2010). Overall, women need to be made aware that there are also risks tied to being underweight before falling pregnant. This also has separate issues, i.e. lower levels of nutrient stores such as iron and calcium and dietary intakes of important essential fatty acids are also likely to be lower in these women. As mentioned previously, if women could be encouraged to plan their pregnancies, health practitioners could help guide women to improve their diet quality, get their body weight into appropriate ranges and consider the use of a daily multivitamin/mineral supplement before falling pregnant.

Research Highlight   Low body weight in Japanese women leads to the delivery of smaller babies

Japanese women are some of the slimmest in the world and a further decline in BMI has been observed in all age groups over the last two decades (MoHLW, 2008). There are many possible reasons for this but social pressures and body image awareness, i.e. the desire to be thin, are the most likely causes.

Using antenatal records, scientists from Shiga University compared the mothers' weight before pregnancy to markers of infant health. Researchers found that women with a BMI of less than 21 kg/m^2 before pregnancy had increased odds of delivering an infant that was SGA. Equally, women gaining just 9 kg weight or less throughout the course of their pregnancy were 1.8 times more likely to deliver a SGA infant than women putting on 9–12 kg in weight (Watanabe *et al.*, 2010).

These findings clearly show that achieving a healthy BMI range before becoming pregnant, combined with suitable levels of pregnancy weight gain, could play a key role in helping to reduce rates of SGA infants in women with low body weights. SGA infants are generally not as well developed as other babies, which could increase their risk of certain diseases later in life.

Table 9.1   Rates of weight gain in pregnancy.

Pre-pregnancy BMI	BMI category	Rates of weight gain in second and third trimester (range in brackets)	
		(kg/week)	(lb/week)
<18.5 kg/m²	Underweight	0.51 (0.44–0.58)	1 (1–1.3)
18.5–24.9 kg/m²	Normal weight	0.42 (0.35–0.50)	1 (0.8–1)
25.0–29.9 kg/m²	Overweight	0.28 (0.23–0.33)	0.6 (0.5–0.7)
≥30.0 kg/m²	Obese	0.22 (0.17–0.27)	0.5 (0.4–0.6)

Source: Adapted from Rasmussen and Yaktine (2009), with permission.

9.3   Weight gain – how much and when?

Hytten and Leith (1971) were some of the first scientists to derive figures for weekly rates of pregnancy weight gain. It was estimated that rates of pregnancy weight are generally lowest in the first trimester (around 0.36 kg, or 0.8 lb per week), increase in the second trimester to about 0.45 kg (1.0 lb) per week and then reduce slightly in the third trimester to around 0.36–0.41 kg (0.8–0.9 lb) per week.

Although these estimated rates of weight gain were useful markers of comparison, it is important to consider that these usual levels of pregnancy weight gain were for women nearly 40 years ago. It is important to consider that our access to food, food choices and lifestyles have changed considerably since then and the amounts/rates of weight gain are not what they once were. For this very reason, the Institute of Medicine has now developed new rates of pregnancy weight gain that are specific to individual weight categories (Rasmussen and Yaktine, 2009). As can be seen in Table 9.1, estimated rates of weight gain are higher for underweight mothers and lower for overweight mothers. Recommended rates of pregnancy weight gain are also combined for second and third trimesters. Women gaining levels of weight within these ranges have been found to have fewer preterm and SGA deliveries, less pre-eclampsia and non-elective caesarean deliveries, although some overweight and obese mothers have been found to have unfavourable pregnancy outcomes (Beyerlein *et al.*, 2010). No figures are given for the first trimester because data is lacking; it is difficult to recruit and study women in this phase of pregnancy.

Women's knowledge and beliefs about pregnancy weight gain

Many women gain weight during their childbearing years, which is often caused by weight retained after pregnancy. In addition, women from certain racial/ethnic groups (i.e. black and Hispanic mothers) may gain more weight than needed during pregnancy and retain higher levels after birth. There are several possible explanations for this; one may be a lack of knowledge about recommended levels of weight gain, whilst the other may be different cultural beliefs and perceptions about weight gain and pregnancy.

Research carried out on a small sample of ethnically diverse mothers found that more women were more concerned about 'insufficient' levels of pregnancy weight gain. Concerns about excess pregnancy weight gain were not as widespread or well known. Women had minimal knowledge about appropriate levels of pregnancy weight or how these could be achieved. Most women presumed that they would return to their pre-pregnancy weight, even with excessive pregnancy weight gains (Groth and Kearney, 2009). Although clear weight gain reference ranges have been developed, it seems that ethnic minority women are not aware of these. Equally, the health and medical complications linked to high pregnancy weight gains clearly need to be expressed.

9.4   Components of weight gain

The proportion of total weight gained throughout pregnancy is also referred to as GWG. Generally, scientists have calculated that the average woman should gain around 12.5 kg throughout her pregnancy (Hytten and Chamberlain, 1991). Recommendations have now been updated and should ideally fall between 11.5 and 16 kg for women with a 'normal' body weight (BMI 18.5–24.9) before pregnancy (Rasmussen and Yaktine, 2009).

In terms of components of pregnancy weight, the net weight of the foetus is normally around 3.4 kg by 40 weeks into pregnancy (about 27% of weight gain). The remaining weight mainly takes the form of water, which is mainly distributed within the foetus, as extracellular fluid and amniotic fluid. Some fluid is also retained within the uterus, placenta and mammary glands (Hytten and Chamberlain, 1991). The main components and proportions of GWG are shown in Table 9.2. It should be remembered that although these are useful benchmarks, they are not likely to be the same for every pregnant woman.

9.5   Proportions of pregnancy weight gain

As mentioned previously, it is recommended that women should aim to gain around 12.5 kg during pregnancy (or between 11.5 and 16 kg). Studies have shown that overweight or obese women generally gain lower levels of weight during pregnancy

Table 9.2   Components of pregnancy weight gain.

Component	Pregnancy weight gain (kg)			
	10 weeks	20 weeks	30 weeks	40 weeks
Foetus	0.005	0.3	1.5	3.4
Placenta	0.02	0.17	0.43	0.65
Amniotic fluid	0.03	0.35	0.75	0.80
Uterus	0.14	0.32	0.60	0.97
Mammary gland	0.045	0.18	0.36	0.41
Blood	0.10	0.60	1.3	1.45
Extracellular fluid	–	0.50	1.52	4.70
Total weight gain (kg)	*0.34*	*2.4*	*6.5*	*12.4*

Source: Hytten and Chamberlain (1991).

Table 9.3   Proportions of pregnancy weight gain for different populations.

Population group	Usual level of weight gain
The average, normal weight women	10–16.7 kg
Pregnant adolescent	14.6–18.0 kg
Overweight/obese women	9.1–7.4 kg
Twin pregnancy	15–22 kg

Source: Rasmussen and Yaktine (2009).

whilst pregnant adolescents appear to be most at risk in terms of gaining excess weight when pregnant. For mothers expecting twin births, weight gain may be between 15 and 22 kg (although more studies are needed to investigate this further). Additional research is also needed to study proportions of weight gain in mothers expecting multiple births, i.e. more than two babies. Average GWGs for different populations are presented in Table 9.3.

When considering levels of GWG, it is important to understand that different studies may use different definitions and cutoffs to determine levels of pregnancy weight gain. For example, it needs to be defined when the first and final weight measurements should be taken, gestational age needs to be confirmed accurately and it should be determined whether foetal weight should be included in the measurement or not (Amorim *et al.*, 2008). Confirmation of these 'gray areas' would ultimately ease comparisons between studies.

9.6   Measuring body composition in pregnancy

Maternal body composition adapts and changes throughout the course of pregnancy. FM, fat free mass (FFM) and total body water (TBW) measures are usually derived from body composition studies and can be used to predict maternal health status and pregnancy outcome. There are a host of ways in which body composition data can be collected in pregnancy, some being better than others (Table 9.4). For example, some methods can determine where body fat is distributed, i.e. central or peripheral distribution of fat, i.e. skinfold thickness and dual-energy X-ray absorptiometry (DEXA) scans, whereas others can further determine whether fat stores are located in the abdominal between organs (visceral) or underneath the skin, i.e. computed tomography and magnetic resonance imaging (McCarthy *et al.*, 2004).

Research Highlight   Parity may affect body composition changes in pregnancy

Very few studies have followed women through longitudinally throughout their pregnancies and assessed changes in body weight and composition using highly regarded methods (as summarised in Table 9.4). Equally, the effects of parity (whether women already have a child or not) and its effects on body composition has not been studied in detail.

Using bioelectrical impedance methods, body composition changes in pregnancy were determined at 14–20 weeks, after 35 weeks, 6–8 months after birth and compared between women having their first child and those having another pregnancy. All women gained weight and body fat as pregnancy progressed, but more women having their first child gained more weight (12 kg[+]) and retained more fat when followed up after birth (To and Wong, 2009). There are many possible explanations for this, which need to be explored in more detail. Researchers in this study concluded that women having their first child may, physiologically, have an exaggerated response to pregnancy.

9.6.1 Pregnant adolescents

The body composition of pregnant adolescents very much depends on whether they are from developing or developed regions. A study carried out in Jamaica found that when compared with mature mothers, younger pregnant girls had lower levels of fat and FFM at their first antenatal appointment and 35 weeks into pregnancy. However, their increment gain determined using skinfold thickness measurements was higher when compared with mature mothers (Thame *et al.*, 2007). Although only marginal, an extra 0.98 kg fat mass was also retained in the adolescent mothers compared with older women (Thame *et al.*, 2010).

Table 9.4 Body composition methods.

Body composition method	Description
Air-displacement plethysmography (ADP)	When air is displaced to determined body volume and then calculations used to derive levels of FM.
Bio-impedance analysis (BIA)	When a low level electrical current is pass through tissues and levels of resistance measured ($\uparrow$resistance = $\uparrow$body fat).
Computed tomography (CT)	Gives a cross-sectional image of body profile and composition. A very accurate and highly regarded method.
Dual-energy X-ray absorptiometry (DEXA)	When X-rays are used to measure levels of FM, FFM and bone density.
Hydrodensitometry (underwater weighing)	When water is displaced to determined body volume and then calculations used to derive levels of FM.
Magnetic resonance imaging (MRI)	Gives a cross-sectional image of body profile and composition. A very accurate and highly regarded method.
Skinfold thickness	When calipers are used to measure levels of fat beneath the skin.
Total body potassium (TBK)	An indicator of FFM.
Ultrasound (USS)	When high frequency sound waves can be used to obtain body composition images.
Waist–hip ratio	When the hip circumference is measured at its largest point and waist circumference around the belly button.

Source: McCarthy *et al.* (2004).

In developed regions, however, body composition changes do not appear to be as controlled or favourable. In the United States, 1849 young girls aged 9–10 years of mixed race enrolled to take part in a cohort study and were followed up 10 years later when body weight and composition changes were recorded. On the whole, levels of body fat and waist circumference (central adiposity) were much higher amongst the girls who had teenage/early adulthood pregnancies when compared to girls who had not had a teenage pregnancy (Gunderson *et al.*, 2009). These are important findings and demonstrate that levels of weight gain seem to be amplified amongst Western adolescent mothers. In turn, this can contribute to life-long weight gain, which can affect the health and well-being of young women later in their life.

Research Highlight   Greater levels of weight gain may help to support foetal growth in teenagers?

There is a lot of contradictory evidence about the levels of weight gain in pregnant adolescents and obesity risk. One viewpoint is that excess weight gained in teenage pregnancies can lead to weight retention, contributing to the obesity epidemic. The other theory supported by latest research is that higher levels of pregnancy weight gain and insulin-like growth factor in growing teenagers may help to support foetal growth whilst preventing the mother's own growth from being restricted (Jones *et al.*, 2010). These findings make sense; pregnant teenagers may have higher energy requirements and need extra 'weight' to fuel both themselves and foetal growth. However, optimal thresholds should ideally be formulated to prevent excessive weight gains. This is clearly a complex area for which evidence needs to be thoroughly evaluated and studied in more detail.

9.6.2   Ethnicity

Only few studies seem to have investigated the effects ethnicity can have on body composition changes in pregnancy. As previously mentioned, Gunderson *et al.* (2009) have studied this to some extent in the United States. Adolescent black girls were more likely to have high levels of central adiposity 10 years later when compared with white girls. This is possibly because fewer white girls became pregnant in the study, skewing the data slightly.

9.6.3   Diabetes

It seems likely that women who develop diabetes in pregnancy may have a different body profile when compared with women with normal glucose tolerance. One Spanish study used bioelectrical impedance to compare the body composition of 79 women (24–32 weeks into pregnancy) with, without and at risk of developing diabetes in pregnancy, which was diagnosed using a glucose tolerance test. Fat mass was found to be significantly higher in women with diabetes and pre-gestational diabetes compared to those with normal glucose tolerance (Moreno Martinez *et al.*, 2009).

9.6.4   Pre-eclampsia risk

Some studies suggest there may be a link between women's body composition and risk of developing blood pressure disorders such as pre-eclampsia in pregnancy. Research comprising 204 women found that those with a history of pre-eclampsia had higher levels of abdominal fat, which is also a risk factor for heart disease (Berends *et al.*, 2009). Another study using bioelectric impedance found that the average level of fat mass was higher (27 kg) in women experiencing hypertension in pregnancy when compared to mothers with normal blood pressure (their fat mass was 20 kg) (Levario-Carrillo *et al.*, 2006). Alongside this, women experiencing hypertension in pregnancy may have difficulties in returning to their pre-pregnancy weight and have metabolic chances (elevated low-density lipoprotein cholesterol and fasting glucose) that could be permanent (Suntio *et al.*, 2010). More research is needed but, taken together, the findings from these studies indicate that body shape and level of body fat could be used as a possible marker of pre-eclampsia risk.

Research Highlight   Is gut microbiota linked to weight gain in pregnancy?

Some studies have shown that the composition of microbiota (flora) in the gut may be another risk factor for obesity, possibly because certain gut bacteria may harvest energy from food more efficiently than others. This theory has now been extended and studied in pregnancy.

Scientists have found that levels of *bacteroides* and *staphylococcus* bacteria are higher in overweight when compared with healthy weight pregnant women and levels of these bacteria increase from the first trimester of pregnancy (Collado *et al.*, 2008). Equally, higher levels of these bacteria have been linked to altered metabolic profiles (Santacruz *et al.*, 2010) and even the microbial composition of the infants born to overweight mothers (Collado *et al.*, 2010). Considerably, more work is needed to disentangle how gut flora changes in pregnancy, how it exerts its actions and how this can have implications for maternal and infant health.

9.7   High pregnancy weight gain

9.7.1   Maternal health

Pregnancy is a time when many women relax their normal eating habits and see this as a window of opportunity to enjoy themselves. Some new pregnancy weight gain guidelines have been developed, but in reality, pregnancy weight gains are often higher than these (Rasmussen and Yaktine, 2009). Some previous studies have compared patterns of pregnancy weight gain against original IoM (1990) guidelines. One study using data from over 20,000 infants and their mothers reported that weight gain was more likely to exceed original IoM guidelines (Table 9.5) than fall below them; 43% of women gained weight above and 20% below the recommendations (Stotland *et al.*, 2006).

Table 9.5   IoM (1990) original weight gain guidelines.

Pre-pregnancy BMI	BMI category	Total weight gain for singleton pregnancies	
		(kg/week)	(lb/week)
<19.8 kg/m^2	Underweight	13–18	28–40
19.8–26 kg/m^2	Healthy	11–16	25–35
26.1–29 kg/m^2	Overweight	7–11	15–5
>29 kg/m^2	Obese	7	15

Source: IoM (1990) guidelines for weight gain during pregnancy.

Women with a healthy body weight before pregnancy but gaining excess weight during pregnancy are also more likely to develop high blood pressure in pregnancy, experience longer labours and use epidurals (Crane *et al.*, 2009). Equally, findings from 'Project Viva', a European study of nearly 2000 mothers and their children found that women gaining excess pregnancy weight were more likely to have impaired glucose tolerance (Herring *et al.*, 2009), which, in turn, has been related to an elevated risk of cardiovascular disease in the mother later in life (Retnakaran and Shah, 2009). In terms of mode of delivery, the risk of delivering via caesarean section has been found to rise from 18.2% in women with a healthy body weight to 40.6% in women who are morbidly obese (Mantakas and Farrell, 2010).

9.7.2   A note on extreme obesity

Women's body weights are increasingly falling even beyond that traditional BMI cutoffs for overweight and obese. 'Extreme' obesity may be defined as a BMI of 50 or higher and is now a common occurrence amongst women living in more industrial regions (around 1 in 1000 women in the United Kingdom now fall within this weight category). Extremely obese women have been found to experience higher rates of pre-eclampsia, gestational diabetes, preterm deliveries, complications with general anaesthesia and are much more likely to have to deliver by c-section when compared to normal weight women (Knight *et al.*, 2010). The Institute of Medicine have now compiled weight gain guidelines for such women, advising 5–9 kg (11–20 lbs) for all obese women (Bodnar *et al.*, 2010). It is possible that these may be modified in the future depending on the severity of obesity as more evidence becomes available.

Overall, rises in extreme obesity mean there is an urgent need to try and address this problem pre-conceptionally. Basic equipment may not be in place medically for these women and risk of medical and delivery complications with no doubt considerably higher. The Institute of Medicine and National Research Council have now published a call for 'a radical change in the care provided to women of childbearing age' particularly in terms of a clear need for individual medical care both before, during and after pregnancy to help women attain a healthy weight, gain within the guidelines, and return to a healthy weight (Rasmussen *et al.*, 2010). This is certainly an approach that is also needed in other countries, such as the United Kingdom.

Table 9.6 Implications of high maternal weight gain.

Maternal health – increased risk of

Caesarean section
Gestational diabetes mellitus
Hyperglycaemia
Hypertension
Perineal tears
Post-partum haemorrhage
Preterm labour
Epidural use
Longer labours
Pre-eclampsia

Infant health – increased risk of
Child adiposity
Early neonatal death
High birth weight (large for gestational age)
Intrauterine death
Macrosomia/excessive foetal growth
Neural tube defects

9.7.3 Infant health

Pregravid obesity and high pregnancy weight gains can also affect the immediate and long-term health of the child (Table 9.6). Risk of excessive foetal growth is higher when women have higher levels of weight gain during pregnancy, with women gaining over 46 lbs (20.9 kg) having the highest risk of excessive foetal growth (Dietz *et al.*, 2009). Some scientists have found that pregnancy weight gains of 6.7–11.2 kg (15–25 lbs) in overweight and obese women, and less than 6.7 kg (15 lbs) in morbidly obese women helped to ease delivery and improve pregnancy outcome (Crane *et al.*, 2009).

High pregnancy weight gains (>18 kg) have also been associated with reduced infant Apgar scores, seizures, hypoglycaemia and meconium aspiration syndrome (when the newborn inhales a mixture of meconium and amniotic fluid) (Stotland *et al.*, 2006) and foetal insulin resistance (Catalano *et al.*, 2009). Unfortunately, the risk of intrauterine foetal death and stillbirth is also higher amongst obese mothers and those gaining excessive weight in pregnancy (Arendas *et al.*, 2008). Although we are only able to touch lightly on a few key studies in this section, there is a wealth of evidence linking high levels of pregnancy weight gain to adverse health outcomes in both mothers and their children.

9.7.4 A note on macrosomia

Women gaining higher levels of weight during pregnancy are more likely to deliver larger infants (over 4000 g), also known a macrosomia or 'big baby syndrome' (Figure 9.1) and retain weight themselves (for up to 3 years after birth) (Viswanathan *et al.*, 2008). Delivering larger infants can also be problematic and time-consuming from a medical perspective. Vaginal delivery of a macrosomic foetus requires considerable attention and clinicians must be prepared to deliver via caesarean section and for complications such as shoulder dystocia (when one of the babies shoulders

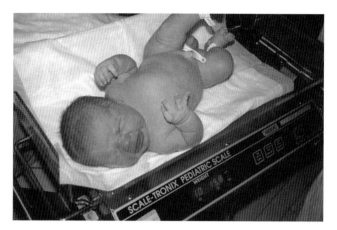

Figure 9.1 An infant with macrosomia. This is sometimes known as 'big baby syndrome' and is when infants are born exceptionally large (usually weight over 4500 g).

become stuck behind the pelvic bone) and newborn asphyxia (failure to breathe after delivery) (Henriksen, 2008). Additional health implications associated with high levels of pregnancy weight gain are summated in Table 9.6.

9.7.5 A note on NTDs

Finally, maternal obesity also appears to be a risk factor for congenital abnormalities and NTDs (Shaw *et al.*, 2000). A meta-analysis paper comprising findings from 12 studies found that the odds of having a NTD-affected pregnancy increased significantly amongst overweight, obese and severely obese women (Rasmussen *et al.*, 2008), whilst other papers have reported that women with a BMI of 30 are twice as likely to have a child with an NTD compared with healthy weight women (Scialli *et al.*, 2006).

The Society of Obstetrics and Gynaecology of Canada advise that patients with health risks such as epilepsy, insulin-dependent diabetes, family history of NTDs, belonging to a high-risk ethnic group, e.g. Sikh or a BMI >35 kg/m^2, should increase their intakes of folate-rich foods and take a daily supplement with multivitamins and 5 mg folic acid from 3 months before conception until 10–12 weeks. After this period, i.e. from 12 weeks after conception until 4–6 weeks after birth (or as long as breastfeeding continues), women should be encouraged to take a multivitamin containing 0.4–1.0 mg folic acid (Wilson *et al.*, 2007).

Why is the risk of NTDs higher in heavier women?

The causes of NTDs in overweight and obese women are not yet firmly established, but several explanations have been put forward. Firstly, babies born to these mothers are not necessarily small or undernourished. This indicates that women's diet quality, i.e. energy-rich but nutrient (folate/folic acid) poor, may be one risk factor. In addition, rates of foetal growth are generally higher in these mothers, which may push up folic acid requirements.

Another theory now supported with research is that both obesity and diabetes can lead to a sustained state of hyperglycaemia and hyperinsulinemia (elevated glucose and insulin levels), which can increase NTD risk. This has been reflected in work carried out at Boston University. Scientists found that 25% women delivering NTD-affected infants had diets with a high glycaemic index and 4% a high glycaemic load when compared to controls (Yazdy *et al.*, 2010). This is an important study providing further evidence that hyperglycaemia may lie within the pathogenic pathway of NTDs in babies born to obese mothers.

9.8 Low pregnancy weight gain

9.8.1 Maternal health

Low pregnancy weight gains (1–14 lbs) have been found to increase the risk of delivering infants that are SGA, when compared against women gaining sufficient levels of weight during pregnancy (15–25 lbs) (Dietz *et al.*, 2009). There is also fairly strong evidence that pregnancy weight gain below original IoM guidelines increases the risk of preterm and low birth weight infants and the initiation of breastfeeding may be more difficult in these mothers (Viswanathan *et al.*, 2008). Research conducted by Tsukamoto *et al.* (2007) studied the effects of restricting pregnancy weight gain in a large (3071 sample) population. The study showed that women gaining 8 kg or less had an increased risk of delivering a low birth weight or SGA infants. As mentioned earlier, similar findings have also been observed in Japanese women with low pregnancy weight gains (less than 9 kg) (Watanabe *et al.*, 2010). It seems that when levels of pregnancy weight gain are restricted, this is a strong risk factor for SGA infants, particularly when coupled with low pre-pregnancy body weights.

9.8.2 Eating disorders

Around 5–7% of women of childbearing age have eating disorders. It is not uncommon for eating disorders to occur and/or continue into pregnancy. Two main theories have been built around the occurrence of eating disorders in pregnancy. One theory is that eating behaviours should improve in pregnancy, mainly because of concern for the well-being of the developing child. The other is that body changes and weight gain in pregnancy can rekindle concerns leading to the development of eating disorders in pregnancy and after birth (Micali *et al.*, 2007). The Norwegin mother and child cohort study (MoBa) has assessed women's attitudes towards pregnancy weight gain and has observed the effects of eating disorders on pregnancy outcomes. The findings from this research are discussed in the next research highlight.

Research Highlight   Attitudes towards pregnancy weight gain and effect on infant health

The MoBa study is a large follow-through study comprising 35,929 Norwegian pregnant women. Given the large sample size of this study, scientists have been able to draw some important conclusions relating to women's attitudes towards pregnancy weight gain and whether disordered eating in pregnancy can affect birth outcomes.

The study found that women with a history of eating disorders worry most about pregnancy-related weight gain (Swann *et al.*, 2009). Levels of pregnancy weight gain also seem to vary according to the type of eating disorder women have had; those with a history of binge eating disorders are most likely to experience high pregnancy weight gains and deliver large-for-gestational-age (LGA) by c-section (Bulik *et al.*, 2009). Overall, supporting women in early pregnancy and educating them about what constitutes a healthy level of pregnant weight gain could help to alleviate and moderate the concerns of these women.

9.8.3   Folate levels

In addition, attempts to lose weight, fasting diets, or self-reported eating disorders and low folate intakes in early pregnancy may be associated with an increased risk of spina bifida (Takimoto and Tamura, 2006) and NTDs (Carmichael *et al.*, 2003). Such dieting behaviours appear to be most strongly associated with NTDs in the first 3 months of pregnancy when foetal organogenesis is taking place (Carmichael *et al.*, 2003). It has also been demonstrated that weight gain and dietary behaviours in the second trimester of pregnancy could affect birth weight and length (Sekiya *et al.*, 2007). One the whole, scientific evidence implies that dietary restriction early in pregnancy and low levels of weight gain could affect the health short term and long term health of the offspring (Table 9.7).

Table 9.7   Implications of inadequate maternal weight gain.

Maternal health – increased risk of
Maternal micronutrient deficiencies
Perineal tears
Preterm labour
Shortened gestation

Infant health – increased risk of
Low birth weight
Neural tube defects
Prematurity
Spina bifida
Spontaneous abortion

Poor adult health – increased risk of
Hypertension
Diabetes
Obesity
Coronary artery disease

Table 9.8   Revised weight gain guidelines for singleton pregnancies.

| Pre-pregnancy BMI | BMI category | Total weight gain | |
		Range in kg	Range in lb
<18.5 kg/m^2	Underweight	12.5–18	28—40
18.5–24.9 kg/m^2	Normal weight	11.5–16	25—35
25.0–29.9 kg/m^2	Overweight	7–11.5	15—25
≥30.0 kg/m^2	Obese	5–9	11—20

Source: Adapted from Rasmussen and Yaktine (2009), with permission.

9.8.4   Infant health

A spectrum of research has investigated links between maternal nutrition, infant birth weight and adult health status (Table 9.8). As discussed previously, the 'foetal origins' hypothesis has been derived from such research; a theory proposing that inadequate maternal nutrition and a low infant birth weight can predispose the child towards chronic diseases such as hypertension, diabetes, obesity and coronary artery disease later in life (Thompson, 2007). Now, scientists need to further investigate the role on maternal overnutrition and foetal programming. It is thought that the maternal diet and rise in body mass may play a role in foetal fat cell and of the central appetite regulatory systems. It is possible that maternal overnutrition could even contribute to a cycle of intergenerational obesity (McMillen *et al.*, 2008).

9.9   Weight gain guidelines

Since the Institute of Medicine pregnancy weight gain guidelines were compiled in 1990, a lot of changes have taken place. The population now comprises a higher proportion of racial/ethnic groups and both pre-pregnancy body mass index and levels of pregnancy weight gain have increased in westernised regions (and is also rising in less developed regions). Also, it appears that rates of maternal overweight and obesity are highest amongst 'at risk' population groups, for example adolescents and low income mothers.

Weight gain recommendations are displayed in Table 9.9. As can been seen from the data, for each BMI category, weight gain guidelines are based on the notion that good pregnancy outcomes can be achieved within a range of weight gains. As emphasised earlier, it is when weight gain is at the top or bottom end of these scales that this poses at risk to the health of mother and child. It is, however, important

Table 9.9   Weight gain guidelines for multiple foetuses.

| Pre-pregnancy BMI | BMI category | Total weight gain | |
		Range in kg	Range in lbs
18.5–24.9 kg/m^2	Normal weight	17–25	37–54
25.0–29.9 kg/m^2	Overweight	14–23	31–50
≥30.0 kg/m^2	Obese	11–19	25–42

Source: Rasmussen and Yaktine (2009).

to consider that these guidelines are mainly for use in developed countries. They are not intended for use in populations that may be shorter or thinner than the average Westernised woman.

9.10   Multiple foetuses

Increasingly, more women are conceiving through assisted reproductive technologies, which has increased rates of multi-foetal pregnancies in the United Kingdom and worldwide. Several studies have investigated levels of weight gain in mothers expecting twin pregnancies and related this to pregnancy outcome. A recent US study measured the proportion of weight gained in over 6000 mothers who delivered twins. Over one-third of mothers expecting twins gained more than 20 kg (45 lbs). Women with a lower BMI before pregnancy were more likely to gain more weight while obese women with high levels of weight gain (over 30 kg or 65 lbs) delivered infants with a high birth weight (Chu and D'Angelo, 2009). Although, only a few studies have monitored levels of weight gain in women expecting multiple foetuses, the IoM have developed guidelines based on what evidence is available (Table 9.8). Unfortunately, not enough data is currently available to compile guidelines for underweight mothers expecting multiples.

9.11   Weight retention

For some women, pregnancy can put them over the healthy BMI threshold after giving birth. Many women will lose the weight that they gained during pregnancy, but for some, pregnancy acts as a trigger for developing overweight and obesity. A Swedish investigation, the Stockholm Pregnancy and Women's Nutrition Study, also known as the SPAWN study, investigated the relationship between pre-pregnancy BMI, maternal weight gain and weight retention one year and 15 years after giving birth. Of the 563 women who completed the study, 56% of the participants were categorised as high weight gainers (>15.6 kg) during pregnancy. These participants retained high levels of weight 15 years later (gaining 9.9 ± 8.3 kg) when followed up (Linné et al., 2004). In terms of susceptibility towards maternal obesity, white, black and Hispanic women may be up to 4.5 times more likely to become obese after pregnancy when compared with Asian mothers (Gunderson et al., 2000).

Adolescents have also been found to retain a proportion of their pregnancy weight when followed up one year after birth (particularly those with high levels of GWG). Consequently, pregnancy may further contribute to overweight and obesity in adolescent populations (Oken et al., 2008). Even more recently, in a mother–daughter cohort study (part of the American Nurses' Health Study), a high BMI before pregnancy and excess pregnancy weight gain were associated with higher rates of obesity amongst adolescent and adult daughters. Authors concluded that pre-pregnancy weight and GWG may be modifiable foetal origins of overweight and obesity in women (Stuebe et al., 2009).

Overall, it seems apparent that high levels of GWG in pregnancy may contribute to long-term obesity (in the mother and her offspring). By promoting the importance of attaining a healthy pre-pregnancy body weight and appropriate level of GWG, this may help to prevent overweight and obesity in the next generation.

> **Research Highlight**   Weight gain in pregnancy and children's body composition – is there a link?
>
> As described previously in Chapter 2, the Southampton Women's Survey is one of the largest, most well-designed studies assessing the dietary, lifestyle and body composition of women and their children.
>
> Levels of women's pregnancy weight gain were assessed at 34 weeks into pregnancy and categorised using the latest Institute of Medicine guidelines and the body composition of the offspring ($n = 948$) assessed at birth and at 4 and 6 years of age using DEXA measurements. Just under half (49%) of children were born to women who gained excess weight in pregnancy. Higher levels of pregnancy weight gain were associated with higher levels of fat mass after birth and weakly associated at 6 years or age (but not at 4 years) (Crozier *et al.*, 2010). Nonetheless, appropriate levels of pregnancy weight gain may help to reduce the risk of adiposity in the offspring but more remains to be understood about the effects on the long-term body composition.

9.12   Weight loss interventions

Although weight control interventions may be used once pregnancy has been confirmed; ideally, pregnancies should be planned so that women's body weight falls within recommended reference ranges before conception takes place. With regard to pregnancy weight gain, a more effective approach seems to be to guide women to gain the right proportions of extra body weight when pregnant rather than trying to reverse the effects and intervene after birth. In one study, providing nutritional advice to pregnant women helped to improve dietary quality, but levels of physical activity and GWG were unaffected (Guelinckx *et al.*, 2010). Scientists have also found that lack of time and motivation and need for support all act as individual challenges to weight loss after birth (Montgomery *et al.*, 2010). Equally, more evidence is needed to test the safety and efficacy of dieting and exercising (or both) when mothers are breastfeeding after birth to prevent long-term weight retention.

9.13   What about physical activity?

The American College of Obstetricians and Gynaecologists (ACOG) recommend that in the absence of medical or obstetric complications, women may exercise for 5 minutes per day, building this up gradually to 30 minutes per day (moderate exercise only) (ACOG, 2003). As can be seen in Table 9.10, the ACOG have established

Table 9.10   Exercise and pregnancy.

ACOG (2003) exercise guidelines for pregnancy
1. After the first trimester, avoid doing any exercises on your back.
2. Avoid brisk exercise in hot, humid weather conditions.
3. Wear comfortable clothing that will help you to keep cool.
4. Drink plenty of water to prevent overheating and dehydration.
5. Make sure the energy that you expend is in balance with your energy intake.

Table 9.11 When to stop exercising.

Stop exercise and seek advice from a doctor if any of the following symptoms are observed:
Vaginal bleeding
Dizziness or feeling faint
Increased shortness of breath
Chest pain
Headache
Muscle weakness
Calf pain or swelling
Uterine contractions
Decreased foetal movement
Fluid leaking from the vagina

Source: ACOG (2003).

a set of useful exercise guidelines for pregnant women. Equally, if women experience any of the symptoms or signs as listed in Table 9.11, women need to stop exercising immediately and seek medical advice. Leading an active lifestyle is safe during pregnancy, providing that this is undertaken in moderation and the right activities are chosen, i.e. gentle walking. As a rule of thumb, women should slow their pace of exercise immediately once they become out of breath and stop immediately if any of the symptoms shown in Table 9.11 arise.

9.14   A note on weight management

To date, much attention has been focused of the importance of folic acid in the periconceptional period, although these messages generally seem to be getting through to women too late, i.e. when they are already pregnant and the neural tube has already formed. Consequently, it is important that women are guided about these factors – getting body weight into healthy ranges and the importance of folic acid when they come into contact with health practitioners before becoming pregnant, i.e. when guided about smoking and alcohol consumption. In addition, weight loss programmes are best completed and should be recommended before women become pregnant. Women who become pregnant when either obese or dieting should also be counselled about the risks of NTDs and other birth defects.

9.15   Application in practice

Unfortunately, because a substantial proportion of pregnancies are unplanned, it is difficult to recommend that women achieve a healthy body weight before conceiving. However, for mothers planning their pregnancies, it should be advised that a healthy body weight should be attained before falling pregnant. Health professionals can play a key role in helping women to attain a healthy body weight in their childbearing years by weighing them regularly, i.e. at visits to the general practitioners. Equally, once pregnant, women should be weighed at antenatal appointments and guided about recommended weight ranges and how to stay within these; this is currently not standard or is a common practice in all hospitals. From a more general sense, women should also be advised to improve their diet quality and continue to take part in some physical activities, i.e. gentle walking (also see Table 9.12), although some

Table 9.12 Pregnancy weight gain: application in practice.

1. Women planning to conceive should aim to achieve a healthy body weight (BMI between 19.8 and 26.0).
2. Expectant mothers should be advised to gain between 11.5 and 16 kg (1.8–2.5 stones) from conception to before delivery (Rasmussen and Yaktine, 2009)
3. Women who are obese before pregnancy (pre-pregnancy BMI 30 kg/m^2) only need to gain small amounts of weight in pregnancy – 5–9 kg (Rasmussen *et al.*, 2010).
4. Women who are obese before pregnancy (BMI >35 kg/m^2) should increase their intakes of folate-rich foods and take a daily supplement containing multivitamins and 5 mg folic acid from 3 weeks before conception until 10–12 weeks (Wilson *et al.*, 2007).
5. Pregnant teenagers should be closely monitored by midwives, nutritionists or dieticians to ensure that they are eating a balanced diet and gaining adequate amount of weight.
6. Moderate levels of physical activity (around 30 min each day) are recommended throughout pregnancy (excluding impact sports such as tennis).
7. Women should be encouraged to enjoy their pregnancies and to not worry about weight loss until after birth but equally try not to gain 'excess' weight when pregnant.

women may need reassurance that certain activities are safe. Government agencies, healthcare providers and some voluntary organisations can also play a key role in helping to communicate and steer women to gain weight within the new guidelines.

9.16 Conclusion

From the evidence, it is distressing to see that pregnant women often fail to gain weight within the recommended ranges. Women should be encouraged by governments and health practitioners to obtain a healthy bodyweight 'before' becoming pregnant. Equally, once pregnant, women should be guided in terms of what constitutes an appropriate level of weight gain during pregnancy. This seems to be an area for which advice is not always given.

Overall, improving the number of women meeting weight guidelines (before and during pregnancy) could significantly help to reduce health care costs whilst improving the health of both mothers and their children. Regulation of maternal body weight may also play a key role in preventing the onset of childhood obesity. Emphasis should also be put on the importance of a balanced, good quality diet and encouraging women to maintain their energy expenditure during pregnancy through the inclusion of light activities. Although exercise interventions may be one way to regulate body weight and level of pregnancy weight gain, emphasis needs to be placed on the importance of these before pregnancy, rather than relying upon interventions during and after pregnancy.

Key Messages

- Women need to be aware of the effects body weight can have on reproductive health.
- Women should be encouraged to strive to gain weight within the revised Institute of Medicine recommended ranges – around 11.5–16 kilograms (1^1/$_2$–2^1/$_2$ stones) (Rasmussen and Yaktine, 2009).
- For women who are obese, pregnancy weight gain only need to range between 5 and 9 kg (11–20 lbs) (Bodnar *et al.*, 2010).

- It is imperative that new weight gain guidelines are imparted to both expectant mothers and women planning a pregnancy. Nurses and midwives can play a key role in helping women achieve these by regular weighing when women attend their antenatal clinics.
- Multidisciplinary management of dietary and lifestyle advice is needed to encourage young women to achieve their ideal body weight before they reach their childbearing years.
- Regulation of body weight may play a pivotal role in improving birth outcomes, preventing SGA deliveries (low weight gains) and the onset of childhood obesity (high weight gains).

Recommended reading

Hytten FE and Chamberlain G (1991) *Clinical Physiology in Obstetrics*. Blackwell Scientific Publications: Oxford.

Rasmussen KM and Yaktine AL (2009) *Weight Gain During Pregnancy: Re-examining the Guidelines*. The National Academies Press: Washington, DC.

Royal College of Obstetricians & Gynaecologists (RCOG); Centre for maternal and Child Enquiries (CEMACE) (2010) *The Management of Women with Obesity in Pregnancy*. RCOG: London.

Wilson RD, Désilets V, Wyatt P *et al.* (2007) Pre-conception vitamin/folic acid supplementation 2007: the use of folic acid in combination with a multivitamin supplement for the prevention of neural tube defects and other congenital anomalies. *Journal of Obstetrics & Gynaecology Canada* 138, 1003–13.

References

ACOG (American College of Obstetricians and Gynaecologists) (2003) *Exercise During Pregnancy*. ACOG: Washington, DC.

Amorim AR, Linne Y, Kac G and Lourenco PM (2008) Assessment of weight changes during and after pregnancy: practical approaches. *Maternal & Child Nutrition* 4(1), 1–13.

Arendas K, Qiu Q and Gruslin A (2008) Obesity in pregnancy: pre-conceptional to postpartum consequences. *Journal of Obstetrics & Gynaecology Canada* 30(6), 477–88.

Berends AL, Zillikens MC, de Groot CJ *et al.* (2009) Body composition by dual-energy X-ray absorptiometry in women with previous pre-eclampsia or small-for-gestational age offspring. *British Journal of Obstetrics & Gynaecology* 116(3), 442–51.

Beyerlein A, Lack N and von Kries R (2010) Within-population average compared with Institute of Medicine recommendations for gestational weight gain. *Obstetrics & Gynaecology* 116(5), 111–18.

Bodnar LM, Siega-Riz AM, Simhan HN, Himes KP and Abrams B (2010) Severe obesity, gestational weight gain, and adverse birth outcomes. *American Journal of Clinical Nutrition* 91(6), 1642–8.

Bulik CM, Von Holle A, Siega-Riz AM *et al.* (2009) Birth outcomes in women with eating disorders in the Norwegian Mother and Child cohort study (MoBa). *International Journal of Eating Disorders* 42(1), 9–18.

Carmichael SL, Shaw GM, Schaffer DM, Laurent C and Selvin S (2003) Dieting behaviours and the risk of neural tube defects. *American Journal of Epidemiology* 158, 1127–31.

Catalano PM, Presley L, Minium J and Hauguel-de Mouzon S (2009) Fetuses of obese mothers develop insulin resistance in utero. *Diabetes Care* 32(6), 1076–80.

Chu SY and D'Angelo DV (2009) Gestational weight gain among US women who deliver twins, 2001–2006. *American Journal of Obstetrics & Gynaecology* 200(4), 390.e1–6.

Collado MC, Isolauri E, Laitinen K and Salminen S (2008) Distinct composition of gut microbiota during pregnancy in overweight and normal-weight women. *American Journal of Clinical Nutrition* 88(4), 894–9.

Collado MC, Isolauri E, Laitinen K and Salminen S (2010) Effect of mother's weight on infant's microbiota acquisition, composition, and activity during early infancy: a prospective follow-up study initiated in early pregnancy. *American Journal of Clinical Nutrition* **92**(5), 1023–30.

Crane JM, White J, Murphy P, Burrage L and Hutchens D (2009) The effect of gestational weight gain by body mass index on maternal and neonatal outcomes. *Journal of Obstetrics & Gynaecology Canada* **31**(1), 28–35.

Crozier SR, Inskip HM, Godfrey KM *et al.*; Southampton Women's Survey Study Group (2010) Weight gain in pregnancy and childhood body composition: findings from the Southampton Women's Survey. *American Journal of Clinical Nutrition* **91**(6), 1745–51.

Dietz PM, Callaghan WM and Sharma AJ (2009) High pregnancy weight gain and risk of excessive fetal growth. *American Journal of Obstetrics & Gynaecology* **201**(1), 51.e1–6.

Gale CG, Javaid MK, Robinson SM, Law CM, Godfrey KM and Cooper C (2007) Maternal size in pregnancy and body composition in children. *The Journal of Clinical Endocrinology & Metabolism* **92**(10), 3904–11.

Groth SW and Kearney MH (2009) Diverse women's beliefs about weight gain in pregnancy. *Journal of Midwifery & Women's Health* **54**(6), 452–7.

Guelinckx I, Devlieger R, Mullie P and Vansant G (2010) Effect of lifestyle intervention on dietary habits, physical activity, and gestational weight gain in obese pregnant women: a randomized controlled trial. *American Journal of Clinical Nutrition* **91**, 373–80.

Gunderson EP, Abrams B and Selvin S (2000) The relative importance of gestational gain and maternal characteristics associated with the risk of becoming overweight after pregnancy. *International Journal of Obesity and Related Metabolic Disorders.* **24**(12), 1660–8.

Gunderson EP, Striegel-Moore R, Schreiber G *et al.* (2009) Longitudinal study of growth and adiposity in parous compared with nulligravid adolescents. *Archives of Paediatrics & Adolescent Medicine* **163**(4), 349–56.

Henriksen T (2008) The macrosomic fetus: a challenge in current obstetrics. *Acta Obstetricia et Gynecologica Scandinavica* **87**(2), 134–45.

Herring SJ, Oken E, Rifas-Shiman SL *et al.* (2009) Weight gain in pregnancy and risk of maternal hyperglycemia. *American Journal of Obstetrics & Gynaecology* **201**(1), 61.e1–7.

Hytten FE and Chamberlain G (1991) *Clinical Physiology in Obstetrics*. Blackwell Scientific Publications: Oxford.

Hytten FE and Leith I (1971) *The Physiology of Human Pregnancy*. Blackwells Scientific Publications: Oxford.

Institute of Medicine (IoM) (1990) *Nutrition During Pregnancy: Part 1: Weight Gain, Part II: Nutrient Supplements*. National Academy Press, Washington, DC.

Jones RL, Cederberg HMS, Wheeler SJ *et al.* (2010) Relationship between maternal growth, infant birth weight and nutrient partitioning in teenage pregnancies. *British Journal of Obstetrics & Gynaecology* **117**, 200–11.

Knight M, Kurinczuk JJ, Spark P, Brocklehurst P; UK Obstetric Surveillance System (2010) Extreme obesity in pregnancy in the United Kingdom. *Obstetrics & Gynaecology* **115**(5), 989–97.

Levario-Carrillo M, Avitia M, Tufiño-Olivares E, Trevizo E, Corral-Terrazas M and Reza-López S (2006) Body composition of patients with hypertensive complications during pregnancy. *Hypertension in Pregnancy* **25**(3), 259–69.

Linné Y, Dye L, Barkeling B and Rössner S (2004) Long-term weight development in women: a 15-year follow-up of the effects of pregnancy. *Obesity Research* **12**(7), 1166–78.

Mantakas A and Farrell T (2010) The influence of increasing BMI in nulliparous women on pregnancy outcome. *European Journal of Obstetrics & Gynaecology* **153**, 43–6.

McCarthy EA, Strauss BJ, Walker SP and Permezel M (2004) Determination of maternal body composition in pregnancy and its relevance to perinatal outcomes. *Obstetrical & Gynecological Survey* **59**(10), 731–42.

McMillen IC, MacLaughlin SM, Muhlhausler BS, Gentili S, Duffield JL and Morrison JL (2008) Developmental origins of adult health and disease: the role of periconceptional and foetal nutrition. *Basic & Clinical Pharmacology & Toxicology* **102**(2), 82–9.

Micali N, Treasure J and Simonoff E (2007) Eating disorders symptoms in pregnancy: a longitudinal study of women with recent and past eating disorders and obesity. *Journal of Psychosomatic Research* **63**(3), 297–303.

Mills JL, Troendle J, Conley MR, Carter T and Druschel CM (2010) Maternal obesity and congenital heart defects: a population-based study. *American Journal of Clinical Nutrition* **91**(6), 1543–9.

MoHLW (Ministry of Health, Labour and Welfare) (2008) *Dietary Reference Intakes for Japanese*. Dai-ichi Shuppan: Tokyo.

Montgomery KS, Bushee TD, Phillips JD *et al.* (2010) Women's challenges with postpartum weight loss. *Maternal & Child Health Journal* [Epub ahead of print]

Moreno Martinez S, Tufiño Olivares E *et al.* (2009) Body composition in women with gestational diabetes mellitus. *Ginecologia y Obstetricia de Mexico* 77(6), 270–6.

O'Brien TE, Ray JG and Chan WS (2003) Maternal body mass index and the risk of pre-eclampsia: a systemic overview. *Epidemiology* 14(3), 368–74.

Oken E, Rifas-Shiman SL, Field AE, Frazier AL and Gillman MW (2008) Maternal gestational weight gain and offspring weight in adolescence. *Obstetrics & Gynaecology* 112(5), 999–1006.

Prentice AM (2006) The emerging epidemic of obesity in developing countries. *International Journal of Epidemiology* 35, 93–9.

Rankin J, Tennant PW, Stothard KJ, Bythell M, Summerbell CD and Bell R (2010) Maternal body mass index and congenital anomaly risk: a cohort study. *International Journal of Obesity (London)* 34(9), 1371–80.

Rasmussen KM, Abrams B, Bodnar LM, Butte NF, Catalano PM and Maria Siega-Riz A (2010) Recommendations for weight gain during pregnancy in the context of the obesity epidemic. *Obstetrics and Gynaecology* 116(5), 1191–5.

Rasmussen SA, Chu SY, Kim SY, Schmid CH and Lau J (2008) Maternal obesity and risk of neural tube defects: a meta-analysis. *American Journal of Obstetrics and Gynaecology* 198(6), 611–9.

Rasmussen KM and Yaktine AL (2009) *Weight Gain During Pregnancy: Re-examining the Guidelines*. The National Academies Press: Washington, DC.

Retnakaran R and Shah BR (2009) Mild glucose intolerance in pregnancy and risk of cardiovascular disease: a population-based cohort study. *Canadian Medical Association Journal* 181(6–7), 371–6.

Salihu HN, Lynch O, Alio AP, Mbah AK, Kornosky JL and Marty PJ (2009b) Extreme maternal underweight and feto–infant morbidity outcomes: a population-based study. *Journal of Maternal–Fetal and Neonatal Medicine* 22(5), 428–34.

Salihu HM, Mbah AK, Alio AP, Clayton HB and Lynch O (2009a) Low pre-pregnancy body mass index and risk of medically indicated versus spontaneous preterm singleton birth. *European Journal of Obstetrics, Gynaecology & Reproductive Biology* 144(2), 119–23.

Santacruz A, Collado MC, García-Valdés L *et al.* (2010) Gut microbiota composition is associated with body weight, weight gain and biochemical parameters in pregnant women. *British Journal of Nutrition* 104(1), 83–92.

Scialli AR; Public Affairs Committee of the Teratology Society (2006) Teratology Public Affairs Committee position paper: maternal obesity and pregnancy. *Birth Defects Research Part A: Clinical & Molecular Teratology* 76(2), 73–7.

Sekiya N, Anai T, Matsubara M and Miyazaki F (2007) Maternal weight gain in the second trimester are associated with birth weight and length of gestation. *Gynaecology & Obstetric Investigation* 63(1), 45–8.

Shaw GM, Todoroff K, Schaffer DM and Selvin S (2000) Maternal height and prepregnancy body mass index as risk factors for selected congenital anomalies. *Paediatric and Perinatal Epidemiology* 14(3), 234–9.

Stotland NE, Cheng YW, Hopkins LM and Caughey AB (2006) Gestational weight gain and adverse neonatal outcome among term infants. *Obstetrics and Gynaecology* 108(3), 635–43.

Stothard KJ, Tennant PWG, Bell R and Rankin J (2009) Maternal overweight and obesity and the risk of congenital anomalies. *Journal of the American Medical Association* 301(6), 636–50

Stuebe AM, Forman MR and Michels KB (2009) Maternal-recalled gestational weight gain, pre-pregnancy body mass index, and obesity in the daughter. *International Journal of Obesity (London)* 33(7), 743–52.

Suntio K, Saarelainen H, Laitinen T *et al.* (2010) Women with hypertensive pregnancies have difficulties in regaining pre-pregnancy weight and show metabolic disturbances. *Obesity* 18(2), 282–6.

Swann RA, Von Holle A, Torgersen L, Gendall K, Reichborn-Kjennerud T and Bulik CM (2009) Attitudes toward weight gain during pregnancy: results from the Norwegian mother and child cohort study (MoBa). *International Journal of Eating Disorders* 42(5), 394–401.

Takimoto H and Tamura T (2006) Increasing trend of spina bifida and decreasing birth weight in relation to declining body-mass index of young women in Japan. *Medical Hypotheses* **67**(5), 1023–6.

Thame MM, Jackson MD, Manswell IP, Osmond C and Antoine MG (2010) Weight retention within the puerperium in adolescents: a risk factor for obesity? *Public Health Nutrition* **13**(2), 283–8.

Thame M, Trotman H, Osmond C, Fletcher H and Antoine M (2007) Body composition in pregnancies of adolescents and mature women and the relationship to birth anthropometry. *European Journal of Clinical Nutrition* **61**(1), 47–53.

Thompson JN (2007) Fetal nutrition and adult hypertension, diabetes, obesity, and coronary artery disease. *Neonatal Network* **26**(4), 235–40.

To WW and Wong MW (2009) Body fat composition and weight changes during pregnancy and 6–8 months post-partum in primiparous and multiparous women. *Australian & New Zealand Journal of Obstetrics & Gynaecology* **49**(1), 34–8.

Torloni MR, Betràn AP, Horta BL *et al.* (2008) Prepregnancy BMI and the risk of gestational diabetes: a systematic review of the literature with meta-analysis. *Obesity Reviews* **10**, 194–203.

Tsukamoto H, Fukuoka H, Koyasu M, Nagai Y and Takimoto H (2007) Risk factors for small for gestational age. *Pediatrics International* **49**(6), 985–90.

Viswanathan M, Siega-Riz AM, Moos NM *et al.* (2008) Outcomes of maternal weight gain. *Evidence Report–Technology Assessment* **168**, 1–223.

Watanabe H, Inoue K, Doi M *et al.* (2010) Risk factors for term small for gestational age infants in women with low prepregnancy body mass index. *Journal of Obstetrics & Gynaecology Research* **36**(3), 506–12.

Wilson RD, Désilets V, Wyatt P *et al.* (2007) Pre-conception vitamin/folic acid supplementation 2007: The use of folic acid in combination with a multivitamin supplement for the prevention of neural tube defects and other congenital anomalies. *Journal of Obstetrics & Gynaecology Canada* **138**, 1003–13.

Yazdy MM, Liu S, Mitchell AA and Werler MM (2010) Maternal dietary glycemic intake and the risk of neural tube defects. *American Journal of Epidemiology* **171**(4), 407–14

10 Special Cases

Summary

Nutritional needs are not necessarily the same for every expectant mother. Adolescents are an example of one group that are particularly nutritionally vulnerable should they fall pregnant. Equally, it is becoming increasingly common for women to delay conception towards the end of their childbearing years. Not only does this increase the risk of genetic and medical complications, but fecundity declines with age, a factor that means a high percentage of older mothers conceive through the use of assisted reproductive technologies. This has led to a rise in the number of multiple births, for which, the nutritional needs may vary. In addition vegetarian mothers, diabetic mothers and those with genetic disorders such as phenylketonuria are all examples of specific groups of women who may have slightly modified nutritional needs. Using available evidence, the nutritional needs of these mothers will be discussed along with other factors that may influence the nutritional status of pregnant mothers.

Learning Outcomes

- To explain why nutritional needs are not the same for every expectant mother.
- To discuss the dietary requirements of pregnant women with special nutritional needs.
- To use information in practice to help nurses, midwives, dieticians, nutritionists and other health practitioners support the nutritional needs of these mothers.

10.1 Introduction

Women need enough nutrients to support the growth of the developing foetus whilst maintaining their own nutrient stores. For some pregnant mothers, nutritional needs may surpass standard nutritional requirements, which in many instances are not specific to the needs of pregnant mothers. One example of this may be for women expecting twin or multifoetal pregnancies (MFP). Adolescents are another group when the combined effects of deprivation, growth and pregnancy mean that they have particularly high nutrient requirements that need to be accounted for. Finally, certain inherited or acquired medical conditions can also mean that women's diets need to be tailored during pregnancy.

Nutrition in the Childbearing Years, First Edition. Emma Derbyshire.
© 2011 Emma Derbyshire. Published 2011 by Blackwell Publishing Ltd.

For these reasons, it is important to consider that nutritional needs are not necessarily the same for every expectant mother. Time of conception, social status, parity, income, country of residence and medical health status are just some of the many factors that need to be contemplated when assessing the nutritional needs of these women. This chapter aims to outline some of the key factors that may influence the dietary requirements of expectant mothers. Recommendations will also be given based on the evidence that is currently available.

10.2   Pregnant adolescents

Pregnancy and adolescence are two of the most physiologically active phases of the life cycle. When combined, an adequate dietary intake is of fundamental importance to fuel both foetal and adolescent growth (Yassin *et al.*, 2004). Unfortunately, a poor diet before pregnancy means that many teenagers enter pregnancy with inadequate nutrient stores and risk of nutritional deficiencies. Rates of teenage pregnancy are generally highest in the United States when compared against other industrialised nations such as Canada and Western Europe (Guttmacher Institute, 2006). Within Europe, the United Kingdom remains to have some of the highest rates of teenage pregnancy, although there has been a small decrease over the last decade (Paranjothy *et al.*, 2009). Within less developed regions, it can be seen that rates of teenage pregnancy are particularly high in Mozambique, Bangladesh and Liberia; over 30% of teenage mothers have begun childbearing (Figure 10.1). As teenage pregnancies are often coupled with deprivation and poverty, the risk of poor health (for both mother and child) is elevated. Dieting, irregular meal patterns, consuming fast foods and body dissatisfaction are also additional factors that may impact upon diet quality during this life phase.

10.2.1   Dietary habits

As mentioned previously, young mothers are more likely to have deprived socio-economic backgrounds. Findings from key studies investigating the diets of pregnant teenagers are included in Table 10.1. Haggarty *et al.* (2009) studied the dietary habits of young, deprived mothers (*n* = 1461) living in Aberdeen, United Kingdom. Scientists found that these mothers were more likely to have low blood folate levels, diets lacking in key macronutrients and several vitamins and minerals. Blood homocysteine levels were also elevated, which was linked to higher intakes of meat, fried potatoes (chips and crisps) and snack foods. Overall, deprivation and poor diet quality were thought to increase the risk of preterm deliveries and the need for extra neonatal care amongst these women and their children.

The about teenage eating (ATE) study is another example of research that has studied the dietary habits and nutritional status of pregnant teenagers (research highlight). The study recruited nearly 500 teenagers (14–18 years) and was carried out across four hospitals in London and Manchester, United Kingdom. Scientists used highly regarded methods, which included detailed anthropometric measurements, blood analysis, multiple-pass 24-hour dietary recalls and records of pregnancy outcomes. This study was also valuable in that it collected daily solar radiation data so this could be taken into account when determining vitamin D status. As can be seen in

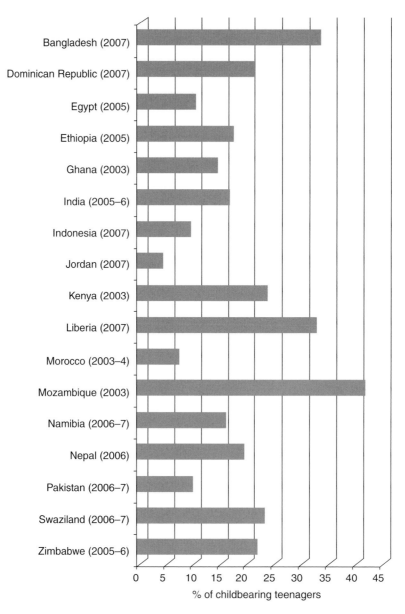

Figure 10.1 Percentage of teenagers who have begun childbearing (developing regions). (Adapted from WHOSIS 2009.)

both of these studies, dietary inadequacies in young, socially deprived mothers may ultimately contribute to social inequalities in terms of pregnancy outcome and infant health, i.e. pregnant teenagers are at high risk of delivering babies that are preterm or small for their delivery date. In addition to this, risk of infant death before and after birth may be higher and the chances of infection, lung disease, poor growth and adverse developmental outcomes may also be greater in the offspring of these mothers (Harding, 2003).

Table 10.1   Dietary habits of pregnant adolescents.

Key studies	Country	Key findings
Baker *et al.* (2009)	United Kingdom	Folate and iron intakes were lower than recommended. Low food iron intake was associated with an increased risk of SGA infants.
Haggarty *et al.* (2009)	United Kingdom	Younger mothers living in deprived areas had low blood folate levels and consumed inadequate intakes of protein, fibre, fruit, vegetables and oily fish.
Yassin *et al.* (2004)	Egypt	Poor nutritional knowledge was apparent amongst 62% pregnancy teenagers. Not all nutrient requirements were met.
Giddens *et al.* (2000)	United States	Intakes of energy, iron, zinc, calcium, magnesium, folate, and vitamins D and E were below recommended standards.
Schneck *et al.* (1990)	United States	Teens who were underweight or smoked during pregnancy had an increased likelihood of delivering LBW infants.

Table 10.2   What foods should pregnant teenagers be eating?

Nutrient	Food sources (per 100 g)
Folate	Marmite (1010 μg), wheat germ (325 μg), dark green leafy vegetables (140 μg), broccoli (130 μg), peanuts (110 μg), spinach (90 μg), kale (86 μg), whole grains (80 μg) and avocado (66 μg).
Calcium	Cheddar cheese (750 mg), sesame seeds (670 mg), almonds (230 mg), yoghurt (210 mg), horlicks and semi-skimmed milk (150 mg), low-fat cottage cheese (80 mg), pumpkin seeds (51 mg) and tofu (50 mg).
Vitamin D	Grilled herring (16.1 μg), trout (9.6 μg), steamed salmon (8.7 μg), polyunsaturated margarine (7.9 μg), egg yolk (4.9 μg) and cheddar cheese (0.3 μg).
Iron	Black pudding (20 mg), pumpkin seeds (11.2 mg), sardines (4.6 mg), raisins (3.5 mg), lean beef (2.8 mg), beans, sesame seeds (2.4 mg) and watercress (2.2 mg).
Fibre (NSP)	All-bran (24.5 g), bran flakes (13.0 g), rye crispbread (11.7 g), shredded wheat (9.8 g), dried figs (7.5 g), almonds (7.4 g), wholemeal bread (5.8 g), baked beans (3.8 g), wholemeal spaghetti (3.5 g), brown bread (3.5 g), raisins (2.0 g) and brown rice (1.9 g).

Source: FSA (2006).

Research Highlight   The ATE study – what are pregnant teenagers eating?

This study assessed the dietary habits of pregnant teenagers in their third trimester using three multiple-pass 24-hour dietary recalls, from which diet quality could be determined.

Scientists found that serum folate levels were low (<7.0 nmol/L) in 12% subjects and homocysteine levels, a marker of cardiovascular health, elevated (>10 μmol/L) in 20% of teenagers. Girls who smoked were also more likely to have depleted folate and vitamin B_{12} reserves. Over half of the pregnant girls had iron-deficiency anaemia and 30% had inadequate vitamin D status (<25 nmol/L). The scientific team also found that teenagers with low levels of red blood cell, serum folate and low intakes of iron from their diets were more likely to deliver small-for-gestational-age (SGA) babies (Baker et al., 2009).

On the whole, these findings provide a strong need to evaluate the folate, iron and vitamin D status of pregnant teenagers and encouragement to stop smoking. As fewer than half the teenagers in this study took any supplements, the need for other approaches, such as food fortification is certainly something that requires further attention.

10.2.2   Specific nutritional needs

As identified previously, pregnant adolescents are more likely to consume a diet that is lacking in certain nutrients. Providing young mothers with examples of food sources may be one way to help improve their overall diet quality (Table 10.2). In addition, it has been reported that risk of spina bifida (incomplete closure of the spinal cord) may be twice as high amongst pregnant teenagers (Noonan, 1997) although this is something that needs to be studied further.

Intakes of at least 300 μg/day have been recommended in the past (Table 10.3), but intakes of at least 400 μg/day is now the consensus for pregnant women before and in the early stages of their pregnancy (COMA, 2000; SACN, 2006). Ideally, this should be obtained from dietary sources, but supplementation with folic acid is generally needed to help women achieve adequate folate status as folate from food sources is not bioavailable.

Calcium requirements are also higher in pregnant teenage mothers. Skeletal maturity may not have been achieved by many young mothers – growth may still be ongoing. Calcium attrition can be as high as 340 mg per day during the third trimester

Table 10.3   Nutritional needs of pregnant teenagers.

Nutrient	Dietary recommendations for 15–18 year olds (with pregnancy increments; DHS, 1991)
Energy (kcal/day)	2310
Fat (% EI)	35
Protein (%EI)	15
Carbohydrate (%EI)	50
Folate (μg/day)	300*
Calcium (mg/day)	700
Iron (mg/day)	14.8
Fibre (NSP) (g/day)	18

EI, energy intake; NSP, non-starch polysaccharide.
*COMA (2000) and SACN (2006) recommends 400 μg/day.

of pregnancy, placing high demands for calcium provision upon the growing mother. As a result, maternal calcium reserves may be utilised to fuel the development of the infant's skeletal system; a process which can result in osteoporosis in later life for the adolescent young mother (Ward *et al.*, 2005). For teenagers, the adolescent growth spurt and onset of menstruation can mean that risk of developing iron deficiency-anaemia is increased if they conceive, a factor that is associated with morbidity of mothers and their infants (Lynch, 2000).

In terms of fibre intake, it has been reported that teenage girls only consume around 10 g per day (Gregory and Lowe, 2000). Higher intakes of indigestible fibre, in particular, can help to increase stool–water absorption, expand bacterial populations, form 'bulky' stools and ultimately, initiate the defecation reflex (James *et al.*, 2003). It is therefore recommended that pregnant teens eat enough fibre (an average of 18 g/day) to maintain healthy bowel function during pregnancy and prevent constipation.

Finally, it is now well documented that a diet sufficient in long-chain polyunsaturated fatty acids, particularly docosahexaenoic acid (DHA), in the third trimester can help to support foetal brain growth and visual development (Cetin *et al.*, 2009). Although intakes and health benefits have not been studied in detail in populations of pregnant teenagers, all women of reproductive age should aim to achieve a DHA intake of at least 200 mg/day (Cetin and Koletzko, 2008). Oily fish such as salmon and herring are good sources of DHA, although their consumption during pregnancy should be limited to no more than two weekly portions (SACN/CoT, 2004).

10.2.3   Application in practice

When combined with the physiological changes of both pregnancy and growth, pregnant teenagers are a particularly nutritionally vulnerable group. Although improving nutrition education in schools may be one way to improve the diet of teenage girls (and nutrient stores before pregnancy), for those that conceive, nurses, midwives and other health practitioners can play a key role in informing and educating these young women about the importance of a balanced diet during pregnancy. For most pregnant teenagers, nutritional knowledge is limited, and they are not necessarily aware of how the diet can influence their own health and the health of their child. Nutritionists and dieticians should help to support nurses and midwives deliver this important information to their patients. Future intervention studies in the form of dietary advice, support and supplement trials are also warranted.

10.3   Advanced maternal age

It is now not uncommon for childbearing to occur at a later time in a woman's life. This trend is not only apparent in the United Kingdom but also in Western Europe, Australia, New Zealand, Canada and in the United States (RCOG, 2009). As the age of childbearing rises, this means that more women are likely to enter pregnancy with medical conditions, or develop common chronic conditions such as hypertension or diabetes in pregnancy. There is increasing evidence now to indicate that this is often the case. One study carried out in Sweden studied the effect of younger (20–29 years), mature (40–44 years) and older (45+ years) maternal age on pregnancy outcome. Preterm births, gestational diabetes, and pre-eclampsia were more common amongst

Table 10.4 Advanced maternal age – medical implications.

Increased risk of
Genetic disorders
Down's syndrome
Klinefelter's syndrome
Turner's syndrome
Birth defects
Neural tube disorders (possible link)
Medical complications
Hypertension/pre-eclampsia
Gestational diabetes
Obstetric complications
Preterm labour
Premature rupture of membranes
Delivery by caesarean section
Maternal mortality
Birth outcome
Lower Apgar scores
Low birth weight infants
Multifoetal pregnancies

Source: Information from Chervenak and Kardon (1991).

women 40–44 years of age and those 45 years or older. The number of stillborn deliveries was also higher in women with these pregnancy complications, but this was not necessarily related directly to age (Jacobsson *et al.*, 2004). Another study investigated the effects of 'extremely' advanced maternal age, i.e. conception beyond 45 years on women's and infants health. Scientists found that women aged 50+ years had a higher risk of developing diabetes mellitus and pre-eclampsia in pregnancy. Risk of preterm deliveries and intensive neonatal care was also higher amongst the older mothers (Yogev *et al.*, 2010). Other medical risks associated with advanced maternal age are displayed in Table 10.4.

On the whole, more women are now waiting until later into their childbearing years to have children. This means they may be entering pregnancy with health issues or be at higher risk of developing these in pregnancy. Currently, few studies have investigated whether these mothers have different nutritional needs. For now, older mothers should continue to follow standard dietary advice for pregnancy, as recommended by government bodies and health professionals until evidence from suitable interventions becomes available.

10.4 Multifoetal pregnancies

The number of MFP (when more than one foetus develops in the womb simultaneously) is rising. Currently, worldwide, the number of MFP has risen, mainly because of increased use of assisted reproductive technologies (ART) (Rosello-Soberon *et al.*, 2005). Other factors increasing the likelihood of MFP are listed in Table 10.5.

Carrying a multiple number of foetuses can place extra physiological stress on both the mother and child. For the mother, MFP can place women at greater risk of pre-eclampsia, iron-deficiency anaemia, hyperemesis gravidarium (excessive sickness) and other medical conditions. With respect to foetal well-being, women expecting

Table 10.5 Factors increasing the possibility of a multifoetal pregnancy.

Fertility treatment
African heritage
Early age at menarche
Increased childbearing age
Maternal obesity
Parentage (particularly if the mother is a twin)
Parity

Source: Rosello-Soberon *et al.* (2005).

a multiple number of children are more likely to deliver low birth weight (LBW) (<2500 g) and preterm infants (less than 37 weeks gestation) (Brown and Carlson, 2000). Medical conditions associated with MFP are displayed in Table 10.6. Although older maternal age may increase the risk of poor pregnancy outcomes in women of lower socio-economic status expecting twins, this does not appear to be the case in women of higher socio-economic status (Zhang *et al.*, 2002).

10.4.1   Specific nutritional needs

The nutritional needs of women expecting a single child is well documented, but the requirements of women expecting multiple births is not as well known or understood. A small number of review papers have been published within this field and recommendations have generally been extrapolated using data from singleton pregnancies.

It is clear that energy requirements are higher when mothers are expecting more than one child, partly because levels of weight gain are higher. Previous studies have shown that numbers of twin pregnancies have declined in times of famine, a factor indicating that energy status is important in MFPs (Lumey and Stein, 1997). Although scientists advise that energy intakes should be higher for MFPs, there is a lack of consensus in terms of 'how much' and 'when' energy intake should be increased. Using data from weight gain studies, Brown and Carlson (2000) calculated that women expecting twins require 35,000 kcal more than women expecting a single

Table 10.6 Medical conditions associated with multifoetal pregnancies.

Maternal health	Foetal health
Caesarean section	Foetal resorption
Hyperemesis gravidarium	Foetal loss
Iron deficiency anaemia	Neonatal death
Kidney problems	Congenital abnormalities
Placenta previa	Respiratory distress
Pre-eclampsia	Intraventricular haemorrhage
Preterm delivery	Retinopathy of prematurity
	Sepsis
	Asphyxia
	Cerebral palsy

Source: Brown and Carlson (2000).
Also refer to Glossary of Terms for definitions.

foetus. This equates to an extra 150 kcal/day, on top of current energy requirements for pregnancy.

With respect to carbohydrate requirements, both blood glucose and glycogen stores are depleted more rapidly in MFPs, a factor that may result in ketonuria and increase the risk of preterm delivery (Rosello-Soberon *et al.*, 2005). It has been reported that a diet comprising 40% low glycaemic index carbohydrate, 20% protein and fat may help to regulate blood sugar levels in women expecting more than one child (Luke, 2004).

Dietary intakes of calcium, vitamin D and essential fatty acids intakes should be increased in women expecting more than one child (Brown and Carlson, 2000). Essential fatty acids (linoleic and linolenic acid) may help to support the development of the embryonic nervous systems. Sunflower, safflower, corn and soybean oil are good sources of linoleic acid whilst egg yolk, oily fish, canola and soybean oil are abundant in linoleic acid (USDA nutrient database, 2010).

10.4.2   Are supplements needed?

The Institute of Medicine (1990) recommended that women expecting more than one child take a multivitamin and mineral supplement containing 2 mg copper, 250 mg calcium, 15 mg zinc, 2 mg vitamin B_6, 300 µg folate, 50 mg vitamin C, 5 µ vitamin D and 30 mg iron after the 12th week of pregnancy (Table 10.7). These recommendations appear to be best practice at present, but will need to be updated as new evidence emerges.

Future studies, namely supplementation trials, would help to establish whether the consumption of individual or multiple vitamins and minerals would help to improve maternal and pregnancy outcome (and the levels to which these are required) in women expecting more than one child. Until this research has been completed, the compilation of recommended levels for specific micronutrients for twin/multiple pregnancies will be arduous.

10.4.3   Application in practice

Although literature on the nutritional needs of multifoetal mothers is limited, several conclusions can be drawn. Women should continue to follow standard guidelines in terms of what constitutes a healthy balanced diet. Some modifications may be needed

Table 10.7   Levels of supplementation that may support a multiple pregnancy.

IoM (1990) recommended levels of supplementation for MFP
Iron (30 mg)
Zinc (15 mg)
Copper (2 mg)
Calcium (250 mg)
Vitamin B_6 (2 mg)
Folate (300 µg)
Vitamin C (50 mg)
Vitamin D (5 µg)

Source: Institute of Medicine (1990)

in terms of adapting energy intakes, although these requirements are very subtle and do not involve the need to overconsume excess calories. In particular, intakes of key nutrients should continue to be monitored, which includes calcium, vitamin D, folic acid and the essential fatty acids. Although women should try and obtain these from their diets, achieving optimal levels of intake is not always easy. Therefore, taking a daily vitamin and mineral supplement, e.g. as a multivitamin (noting vitamin A dose; see Section 6.2.2) or pregnancy formulation, may help women to achieve desirable levels of intake.

To date, scientists from the Society of Maternal–Foetal medicine have some of the most succinct nutrition recommendations for women expecting twin pregnancies (Goodnight and Newman, 2009; Appendix 6). These may be of help to midwives, nurses and other health professionals when coming into contact with women expecting multiple births. As of yet, no specific guidelines are available for women carrying more than two children, and guidelines for MFP are yet to be integrated within standard dietary guidelines.

Can Folic Acid Increase the Likelihood of Twins?

It is well known that folic acid is needed for DNA synthesis and cell division. In theory, mothers expecting twin births should have higher folic acid requirements, but this has not been thoroughly determined. There is, however, some evidence (although controversial) suggesting that folic acid may have the opposite effect, i.e. women with higher folic acid intakes may be more likely to have twin births. This seems logical, as folic acid does help with cell replication, but scientists believe that findings from these studies may be flawed as fertility treatments and maternal age have not been adequately accounted for (Levy and Blickstein, 2006). Even though this is an interesting theory women should not be discouraged from taking folic acid supplements to avoid twin or multiple births.

10.5 Maternal obesity

Maternal obesity is associated with a spectrum of health complications and the degree of obesity is generally proportional to the severity of such problems. This has been discussed previously in Chapter 9, but, in brief, maternal obesity may increase the risk of miscarriage (Metwally *et al.*, 2008), neural tube defect (NTD) affected pregnancies (Rasmussen and Yaktine, 2009), stillborn deliveries (Chu *et al.*, 2007a) and the development of medical conditions such as pre-eclampsia and gestational diabetes (Smith *et al.*, 2009). In terms of delivery complications, obese mothers are more likely to have elective surgery, haemorrhage, develop infections and have longer recovery times (Heslehurst *et al.*, 2008).

Research also shows that, on average, obese women spend about an extra 4.8 days in hospital and the costs of antenatal care are fivefold higher than women with a healthy body weight (Galtier-Dereure *et al.*, 2000). Evidence now shows that the child of an obese mother may be exposed to a sub-optimal in-utero environment and that these early life exposures may affect adult health (Poston *et al.*, 2010). The causes behind this need to be established, but one theory is that an obese intrauterine environment could influence appetite and metabolic pathways of the developing child (Oken, 2009).

10.5.1   Specific nutritional needs

Women need to be weighed at regular intervals during their pregnancies to ensure they are gaining appropriate levels of weight gain, but ideally a healthy body weight should be achieved prior to pregnancy. It is also strongly advised that women who are overweight before or early in pregnancy meet folate dietary requirements. Women with a body mass index (BMI) of 29 kg/m² or over are reported to have a twofold risk or greater of delivering a child with NTDs compared to mothers with a pregravid BMI of >29 kg/m² (Shaw *et al.*, 2000). Although all women of childbearing age should consume a 400 µg supplement before conception and for the first 12 weeks of pregnancy, the American National Health and Nutrition Examination Survey (NHANES) estimated that women with a BMI of 30 kg/m² or more may need an additional 350 µg/day folate to achieve serum folate levels when compared to women with a BMI of <20 kg/m² (Mojtabai, 2004). As mentioned in Chapter 9, this has been reflected in Canadian guidelines with the Society of Obstetricians and Gynaecologists of Canada advising that women with a BMI >35 kg/m² take 5 mg folic 3 months before and 10–12 weeks after conception (Wilson *et al.*, 2007). Equally, findings from recent studies have shown that women with features of metabolic syndrome (diabetes prior to pregnancy, high body weight, non-white ethnicity and sensitive to C-reactive protein) had a twofold and sixfold higher risk of NTD in the presence of metabolic syndrome when one or two features were present, respectively (Ray *et al.*, 2007). Overall, the findings from this study indicate that the risk of NTDs is even higher when features of metabolic syndrome are present. It is not yet firmly established why this may be the case or whether high levels of C-reactive protein may be a possible contributory factor.

10.5.2   Application in practice

Ideally, women planning a pregnancy should aim to achieve a healthy body weight before conception. When this is not possible, women should monitor their level of weight gain, aiming to stay within latest Rasmussen & Yakine (2009) guidelines; 7–11.5 kg (15–25 lb) for women who are overweight and 5–9 kg (11–20 lb) for women who are obese before pregnancy. Once again, the importance of folic acid should be communicated to women before they become pregnant. Overweight and obese expectant mothers should at the very least meet basic guidelines (400 µg/day), although 5 mg/day before and in early pregnancy has been recommended by Canadian obstetricians (Wilson *et al.*, 2007). Women over the healthy weight threshold may also be encouraged to undertake moderate levels of physical activity starting with 5 minutes per day, building this up gradually to 30 minutes per day to help maintain a state of energy balance in pregnancy.

10.6   Diabetic mothers

In developed regions, gestational diabetes mellitus (GDM) occurs in around 5–9% of pregnancies and is increasing in prevalence (Serlin and Lash, 2009). GDM is

Table 10.8   Risk factors for gestational diabetes.

Elevated fasting plasma glucose (>7 mmol/L)

First-degree relative with diabetes

Gestational diabetes, large-for-gestational-age or unexplained stillbirth baby from a previous pregnancy

Hispanic, Black, Native American, South-East Asian, Pacific Islander or indigenous Australian ethnicity

Obesity (>120% ideal body weight)

Polycystic ovarian syndrome

Source: Hanna and Peters (2002).

a common disorder that usually develops in the third trimester when insulin resistance occurs and blood glucose levels become elevated (Cheung, 2009). Overweight or obese mothers have an increased risk of developing GDM (Chu *et al.*, 2007b). Women with a family history of gestational diabetes or Asian/Latina/Native America race are also more likely to develop insulin resistance (Cheng and Caughey, 2008). Additional risk factors for gestational diabetes are shown in Table 10.8.

Women with GDM are more likely to deliver infants with macrosomia or that are large-for-gestational age. In turn, infants born to mothers with GDM are more likely to suffer from low blood sugar levels, have high bilirubin levels, which may become toxic, and have higher proportions of red blood cells (polycythemia) (Biri *et al.*, 2009). Pregnancy GDM may also increase the risk of the mother developing type 2 diabetes or metabolic syndrome in early adulthood (Yogev and Visser, 2009).

10.6.1   Specific nutritional needs

In terms of dietary practices, the American Dietetic Association recommends that obese mothers reduce their calorie intake by 30–33% or consume around 25 kcal per kilogram of bodyweight per day. It is also advised that carbohydrate intake is limited to 35–40% calories (particularly simple carbohydrates) (Reader *et al.*, 2006). Although some non-caloric sweeteners may be used, it is recommended that saccharin is not used as this may cross the placenta.

Pregnant women with diabetes should be encouraged to test fasting and 1-hour postprandial (after eating) blood glucose levels after every meal. Women should aim for a fasting blood glucose between 3.5 and 5.9 mmol/L and 1-hour postprandial blood glucose below 7.8 mmol/L (NICE, 2008). Mothers with GDM should always seek guidance from a specialist dietician to help them achieve normal blood sugar levels.

There is emerging evidence to suggest that probiotics may have a role to play in the regulation of blood glucose levels in pregnancy. Rates of gestational diabetes were just 13% amongst women receiving dietary counselling and taking probiotics from the first trimester of pregnancy compared with rates of 36% in those receiving dietary advice and taking a placebo and 34% in controls (Luoto *et al.*, 2010). Further research is now needed to look at the effects of probiotics alone, as it is possible that dietary counselling contributed largely to these findings.

Pre-conception Care for Diabetic Mothers

Maternal diabetes during pregnancy is a well-known teratogen that increases the risk of certain birth defects, such as NTDs. There is now a wealth of information on consistent information from various bodies recommending that women with diabetes who are wishing to become pregnant take 5 mg/day folic acid from pre-conception and for the first 3 months of pregnancy. These recommendations now advised by the Scientific Advisory Committee on Nutrition (2006), National Institute of Clinical Excellence (2008) and Canadian Society of Obstetricians (Wilson *et al.*, 2007).

Most importantly, the importance of avoiding an unplanned pregnancy needs to become an essential component of diabetes education for adolescents and women with diabetes. Once women wish to have a baby, additional pre-conception advice and care should be provided before contraception is discontinued.

10.6.2   Physical activity

There is ample evidence to suggest that regular physical activity may help to improve glucose control, insulin sensitivity and regulate weight gain. Higher levels of physical activity prior to pregnancy or in early pregnancy have been associated with a significantly lower risk of developing GDM (Tobias *et al.*, 2010). Equally, some scientists have found that physical activity in pregnancy can help to reduce the risk of GDM, even if women are inactive before becoming pregnant (Liu *et al.*, 2008). Scientists have identified that simple leisure activities such a walking can help to protect against the development of GDM and then 30 minutes of daily physical activity may be beneficial to health pregnancy (Hegaard *et al.*, 2007).

10.6.3   Application in practice

Providing that the diabetes in pregnancy is adequately managed, good pregnancy outcomes may be achieved. Simple dietary practices that help to establish good glycaemic control before and continuing this throughout pregnancy will help to reduce the risk of miscarriage, birth defects, stillbirth and neonatal death. Equally, taking 5 mg/day folic acid 3 months before and after conception will also help to reduce the risk of birth defects (NICE, 2008). As recommended previously for overweight and obese mothers, moderate levels of physical activity should be encouraged and levels of weight gain monitored throughout pregnancy.

10.7   Phenylketonuria (PKU) in pregnancy

10.7.1   Maternal PKU

Maternal PKU occurs when high levels of phenylalanine (Phe) accumulate in the blood. Phe gathers in the bloodstream when individuals do not have enough of the phenylalanine hydroxylase enzyme (the enzyme that breaks downs phenylalanine). During pregnancy, the most critical time period of foetal development is during early pregnancy (the first 3 months) when embryogenesis takes place and organ systems form. Accumulation of Phe can have a teratogenic effect on the foetus and may cause facial malformalities, microcephaly (poor head growth), learning difficulties and congenital heart disease (Levy, 2003).

10.7.2   Specific nutritional needs

It is fundamentally important that Phe concentrations throughout pregnancy are well regulated, to prevent the development of birth defects. Pregnant women with PKU require a diet that contains some Phe but lower levels than normal (100–250 μmol/L) (MRC working party, 1993). Generally, high protein foods such as meat, fish, eggs, cheese and beans should be avoided and cereals, starches, fruits and vegetables should be consumed. Milk and protein supplements may also be used as protein supplements although there has been some controversy over the efficacy and cost of these (Yi and Singh, 2008).

Research undertaken by Acosta *et al.* (2001) found that when protein intakes (from medicinal food products) met or just exceeded the recommended daily intake for protein, Phe concentrations were better regulated. Consuming adequate levels of energy and fat also helped to reduce Phe levels whilst improving pregnancy outcome. Brown *et al.* (2002) identified barriers most likely to affect Phe regulation in pregnancy. Only 33% women with PKU adapted their diet before conception and just 55% regulated their Phe levels within the recommended threshold during pregnancy. Young maternal age and the high cost of specialist foods were also some of the greatest barriers to Phe regulation.

10.7.3   Application in practice

Expectant mothers with PKU should ensure that their blood Phe concentrations remain within the recommended range for pregnancy, 100–250 μmol/L. Phe levels should be monitored before and throughout gestation, particularly in mothers expecting their second or third child. Consuming a diet sufficient in energy, fat and protein (non-meat sources) may also help to regulate Phe levels (MRC working party, 1993). As research has shown that folate metabolism is altered in patients with PKU (Lucock *et al.*, 2002) and accumulation of Phe may be teratogenic, further work is needed to determine whether folic acid requirements are higher in these women.

10.8   Vegetarian mothers

There are many different definitions in terms of what constitutes a vegetarian diet. In general, a vegetarian diet may be defined as one that does not contain meat, poultry or fish, although there are some variations of vegetarian diet. A lacto–ovo vegetarian diet includes dairy and eggs whilst vegan diets exclude both dairy and animal-derived products. Macrobiotic diets mainly comprised grains, legumes, vegetables and fruits, seeds and nuts (to a lesser extent) (Penney and Miller, 2008).

Table 10.9 Vegetarian diets as a source of nutrients.

Rich in	Deficient in
Complex carbohydrates	Protein
Dietary fibre	Iron
Magnesium	Zinc
Folate	Calcium
Vitamin C	Vitamin A
Vitamin E	Vitamin B_{12} (cyanocobalamin)
Carotenoids	n-3 fatty acids
Phytochemicals	Iodine

Source: Leitzmann (2005).

10.8.1   Specific nutritional needs

It is important that vegetarian mothers plan their diets to ensure that they are nutritionally balanced. Vegetarian diets are a good source of fibre and folate but may be lacking in protein, vitamins and minerals and omega-3 fatty acids (Table 10.9). When vegetarian or ovo–lacto vegetarian diets are deficient in vitamin B_{12}, this may cause plasma homocysteine levels to rise, increasing the risk of both NTDs and pre-eclampsia (Selhub, 2008). Vitamin B_{12} is needed for the enzyme methionine synthase to function, an enzyme that facilitates the conversion of homocysteine to methionine (a less potent amino acid). It has been suggested that eating a folate-rich diet may help to improve the function of the methionine synthase enzyme and regulate homocysteine levels in vegetarian women (Resfum, 2001).

It has also been suggested that vegetarian diets may play a key role in type 2 diabetes management. Clinical trials have shown that vegetarian diets help to improve glycaemic control and promote weight loss (Barnard *et al.*, 2009). Although studies to date have not studied this specifically in pregnancy, it seems reasonable to suggest that vegetarian diets may play a key role in the management of GDM.

10.8.2   Application in practice

Vegetarian diets must be planned carefully but have the potential to be nutritionally balanced. When optimal nutrient intakes are achieved, vegetarian diets may be beneficial to both maternal and infant health (Craig and Mangels, 2009). Vegetarians need to be guided about which food sources can help to provide adequate levels of key nutrients and how the daily diet may be modified to meet their nutritional needs (Table 10.10). An example of a vegetarian case study is included in appendices.

10.9   Alternative dietary practices

10.9.1   Pica

During pregnancy, some women crave for unusual food substances, a condition known as 'pica'. This is not a new condition; the works of both Hippocrates and Aristotle have both documented concerns about immoderate consumption of cold

Table 10.10   Helping vegetarian women to achieve sufficient nutrient intakes.

Common nutrient deficiencies	Alternative food sources
Protein	Chickpeas, baked beans, tofu, boiled lentils, muesli, hard cheese and hummus
Iron	Chickpeas, spinach, bran flakes, liquorice, black treacle, baked beans and dried apricots
Zinc	Green vegetables, cheese, sesame and pumpkin seeds and wholegrain cereals
Calcium	Tofu, cheddar cheese, spinach, dried figs, raw cabbage and broccoli
Vitamin A	Carrots, tomatoes and sweet potato
Vitamin B_{12} (cyanocobalamin)	Wheat germ, pulses, green vegetables and eggs
Omega-3 fatty acids	Flaxseeds, pumpkin seeds, walnut, soy and rapeseed (canola) oils
Iodine	Milk, seaweed, vegetables and grains

water, ice and snow (pagophagia) in the context of disordered eating (Parry-Jones, 1992). The prevalence of this condition is reported to range between 8% and 65% but causes largely remain undocumented, possibly because of a lack of understanding within this area and women may be embarrassed to talk about it (Lopez *et al.*, 2004). There are three main forms of pica, each named according to the substances that are frequently ingested.

1. Pagophagia – ingestion of ice
2. Geophagia – ingestion of soil or clay
3. Amylophagia – ingestion of laundry or corn starch

Other rare cases have included ingestion of glue, hair, buttons, paper, toothpaste and oyster shells (Nicoletti, 2003). When individuals have a tendency to ingest more than one non-nutritive substance, this is known as 'polypica' (Corbett *et al.*, 2003). Women who practice pica may also exhibit other medical conditions such as anaemia and lead poisoning.

10.9.2   Theories of pica

Several theories have been proposed to explain this unusual condition (Table 10.11). In some instances, pica may have cultural causes. For example, within the area of Kilifi (a town on the Kenyan coast), prevalence of geophagia has been found to be particularly high. The study comprising 52 pregnant mothers identified that 73% ate soil regularly (mainly from the walls of houses) and daily ingestion of soil was on average 41.5 g/day! This is one example of pica with a cultural aetiology; soil eating to them had strong relations to fertility and reproduction. Women in this study also reported that they liked the taste of soil, reporting it to be 'sweet and tasty' (Geissler *et al.*, 1999). Similarly, in the Georgia Piedmont region (on the edge of the Appalachian mountains in America), kaolin (white dirt, chalk or clay) eating has been reported, which has been attributed to cultural beliefs (Grigsby *et al.*, 1999).

Table 10.11   Theories of pica.

Cultural	Some cultural beliefs may result in the consumption of non-nutritive items
Nutritional	Nutrient deficiencies such as iron and zinc may play a role in the aetiology of pica
Physiological (sensory)	Individuals may like the taste, smell of texture of the substance that they are ingesting
Psychological	Pica may be a response to stress, a habit or disorder, or manifestation of an oral fixation

Source: Mills (2007), with permission.

Iron and zinc deficiencies are also common amongst women with pica. It is, however, unclear whether this is a cause or consequence of pica (Mills, 2007). Interestingly, it has been shown that symptoms of pica were resolved after patients who had undergone gastric bypass surgery were treated with iron supplements (Kushner and Shanta Retelny, 2005). Finally, it has been suggested that in some cases, pica may be a form of obsessive-compulsive spectrum disorder (OCSD) and assessment may be required when patients are resistant to iron treatment (Herguner, 2007).

10.9.3   Application in practice

Pica is often a condition that goes undetected, as many patients do not volunteer information about their condition. Treatment generally depends on the type and cause of pica, with iron supplementation proving to be beneficial in some instances. In cases of geophagia, patients may need to be treated for intestinal helminthic (worm) infestations. When this is ineffective, counselling may be required by some individuals. Approaches should always be non-judgemental because, as mentioned, pica may be practised for cultural reasons in some instances.

10.10   Nutrition and culture

Evidence studying the effect of culture on diet quality and pregnancy outcome is scant. Vitamin D deficiency appears to be a common problem in Asian mothers. Rees *et al.* (2005) found that Asian mothers that delivered LBW infants had some of the lowest vitamin D intakes. Amongst Pakistani mothers, it is possible that frequent chapatti consumption (a source of phytates; an iron absorption inhibitor) may place them at risk of iron deficiency (Brunvand *et al.*, 1995). In terms of folic acid consumption (from fortified foods), Yang *et al.* (2007) found that Hispanic and non-Hispanic black women in their childbearing years were least likely to achieve recommended levels of intake.

Overall, research within this area is rather fragmented and in need of further development. Large epidemiological studies are required to assess and make cross-comparisons between mothers of different ethnic backgrounds and cultures. Table 10.12 summates the main targets for nutrition interventions but this is based mainly on research undertaken in non-pregnant women. On a final note, it is important that ethnic foods are added to food composition databases to ensure that nutrient intake levels are reported accurately (Abu-Saad *et al.*, 2010).

Table 10.12   Targets for nutrition interventions.

South Asians	Both communities	Afro-Caribbeans
↑ vitamin D	↓Total energy	↓Salt
↑ iron	↓Total fat	↑ Fruit and vegetables
↑ folate and vitamin B_{12}	↓Obesity and weight gain	
	↑ Fibre	
	↑ Low GI foods	
	↑ Monounsaturated and polyunsaturated fats	

Source: Thomas (2002), with permission.

Research Focus   Placental size may change during Ramadan

Ramadan is the ninth month of the year in the Islamic calendar when a daily fast is carried out from sunrise to sunset. For Muslims, fasting has a number of benefits including feelings of greater appreciation for what they have as a result of feeling hunger and thirst. It allows Muslims to practice self-control and will power, which can be beneficial throughout life and provides a time for Muslims to refresh their bodies and souls. Ramadan is generally practised by all Muslims by the time they reach puberty, including pregnant women.

Scientists from King Saud University (Saudi Arabia) have now studied the birth records (birth weight, placental weight and gestational age) of over 7000 babies born over a 4-year period. Scientists found that the birth weight of babies born during this time period were similar to that of European babies. However, the weight of the placenta and ratio of placental weight to birth weight were lower in Saudi mothers. Scientists also found that the mean placental weight and ratio were lower amongst babies who were in the second or third trimester of pregnancy in Ramadan when compared to those who were not in utero during this time (Alwasel *et al.*, 2010).

These are interesting findings and indicate that lifestyle changes linked to Ramadan may slow placental growth when women are in the later stages of their pregnancy. It is already known that placental efficiency is increased in Saudi mothers, a factor related to limited nutrient supplies to help to sustain foetal growth (even though the placenta itself may be smaller). More work is now needed to establish whether reduced placental growth in these women could affect foetal programming and the health of the next generation.

10.11   Conclusion

As can be seen from this chapter, the nutrition needs of some pregnant mothers are quite different. Women should be supported and guided, ideally before they become pregnant, i.e. particularly overweight women and those with diabetes. There is now good evidence to indicate that diabetic and obese women have higher folic acid requirements. These guidelines now need to be communicated at the appropriate time phases, i.e. before women stop using contraception or plan to become pregnant. The diets of pregnant teenagers may also benefit from further guidance. On the whole, improving women's understanding about the importance of a diet adequate in the right nutrients can play a key role in helping to improve pregnancy outcomes amongst these groups with special nutrient needs.

Key Messages

- Expectant teenagers need both support and guidance from nurses on the types and quantities of foods that need to be consumed during this important time and whether supplements are needed.
- In particular, the diets of pregnant teenagers may be high in energy and fat but low in fibre, folate, iron and vitamin D.
- More women are having children later in their childbearing years, but more research is needed to study whether these women have altered nutritional needs.
- Overweight or obese mothers should be guided to take extra folic acid – 5 mg/day 3 months before and 10–12 weeks after conception for women with a pre-pregnancy BMI >35 kg/m² (Wilson *et al.*, 2007).
- Diabetic mothers should reduce their intakes of simple carbohydrate and fat. There is also some emerging evidence that consumption of probiotics may also help to regulate blood sugar levels in pregnancy.
- Several government and professional bodies now advise that women with diabetes also take 5 mg/day folic acid before and in the early stages of pregnancy.
- For women with PKU, a diet sufficient in energy, fat and protein (from medicinal foods) may help to regulate their Phe levels.
- Vegetarian mothers should ensure that they are consuming adequate levels of protein, iron, zinc, calcium, vitamin A, B_{12}, omega-3 fatty acids and iodine.
- Pica is a condition when unusual food substances are craved and ingested. There are several theories behind this, which include cultural, nutritional, physiological and psychological reasons.

Recommended reading

NICE (National Institute of Clinical Excellence) (2008) *Diabetes in Pregnancy: Management of Diabetes and its Complications from Preconception to the Postnatal Period*. RCOG: London.

SACN (Scientific Advisory Committee on Nutrition) (2006) *Folate and Disease Prevention*. The Stationary Office: London.

WHOSIS (2009) Demographic and Health Service Statistics. Available at: http://www.who.int/whosis/en/. (accessed March 2011.)

Wilson RD, Désilets V, Wyatt P *et al.* (2007) Pre-conception vitamin/folic acid supplementation 2007: the use of folic acid in combination with a multivitamin supplement for the prevention of neural tube defects and other congenital anomalies. *Journal of Obstetrics & Gynaecology Canada* **138**, 1003–13.

References

Abu-Saad K, Shahar DR, Vardi H and Fraser D (2010) Importance of ethnic foods as predictors of and contributors to nutrient intake levels in a minority population. *European Journal of Clinical Nutrition* **64**(Suppl 3), S88–94.

Acosta PB, Matalon K, Castiglioni L *et al.* (2001) Intake of major nutrients by women in the Maternal Phenylketonuria (MPKU) Study and effects on plasma phenylalanine concentrations. *American Journal of Clinical Nutrition* **73**(4), 792–6.

Alwasel SH, Abotalib Z, Aljarallah JS *et al.* (2010) Changes in placental size during Ramadan. *Placenta* **31**(7), 607–10.

Baker PN, Wheeler SJ, Sanders TA *et al.* (2009) A prospective study of micronutrient status in adolescent pregnancy. *American Journal of Clinical Nutrition* **89**(4), 1114–24.

Barnard ND, Katcher HI, Jenkins DJ, Cohen J and Turner-McGrievy G (2009) Vegetarian and vegan diets in type 2 diabetes management. *Nutrition Reviews* **67**(5), 255–63.

Biri A, Korucuoglu U, Ozcan P, Aksakal N, Turan O and Himmetoglu O (2009) Effect of different degrees of glucose intolerance on maternal and perinatal outcomes. *Journal of Maternal Fetal & Neonatal Medicine* **22**(6), 473–8.

Brown AS, Fernhoff PM, Waisbren SE *et al.* (2002) Barriers to successful dietary control among pregnant women with phenylketonuria. *Genetics in Medicine* **4**(2), 84–9.

Brown JE and Carlson M (2000) Nutrition and multifetal pregnancy. *Journal of the American Dietetic Association* **100**, 343–8.

Brunvand L, Henriksen C, Larsson M and Sandberg AS (1995) Iron deficiency among pregnant Pakistanis in Norway and the phytic content of their diet. *Acta Obstetricia et Gynecologica Scandinavica* **74**(7), 520–5.

Cetin I, Alvino G and Cardellicchio M (2009) Long chain fatty acids and dietary fats in fetal nutrition. *Journal of Physiology* **587**(14), 3441–51.

Cetin I and Koletzko B (2008) Long-chain omega-3 fatty acid supply in pregnancy and lactation. *Current Opinion in Clinical Nutrition & Metabolic Care* **11**(3), 297–302.

Cheng YW and Caughey AB (2008) Gestational diabetes: diagnosis and management. *Journal of Perinatology* **28**(10), 657–64.

Chervenak JL and Kardon NB (1991) Advancing maternal age: the actual risks. *The Female Patient* **16**, 17–24.

Cheung NW (2009) The management of gestational diabetes. *Vascular Health and Risk Management* **5**, 153–64.

Chu ST, Callaghan WM, Kim SY *et al.* (2007b) Maternal obesity and risk of gestational diabetes mellitus. *Diabetes Care* **30**(8), 2070–6.

Chu SY, Kim SY, Lau J *et al.* (2007a) Maternal obesity and risk of stillbirth: a meta analysis. *American Journal of Obstetrics & Gynaecology* **197**(3), 223–8.

COMA (Committee on Medical Aspects of Food and Nutrition Policy) (2000) *Folic Acid and the Prevention of Disease.* The Stationery Office: London.

Corbett RW, Ryan C and Weinrich SP (2003) Pica in pregnancy: does it affect pregnancy outcome? *MCN: American Journal of Maternal/Child Nursing* **28**(3), 183–9.

Craig WJ and Mangels AR (2009) Position of the American Dietetic Association: vegetarian diets. *Journal of the American Dietetic Association* **109**(7), 1266–82.

DH (Department of Health) (1991) *Dietary Reference Values for Food Energy and Nutrients for the United Kingdom,* 2nd edition. Report on Social Subjects No. 41. The Stationery Office: London.

FSA (Food Standards Agency) (2006) *McCance and Widdowson's, the Composition of Foods.* 6th Edition. Royal Society of Chemistry: London.

Galtier-Dereure F, Boegner C and Bringer J (2000) Obesity and pregnancy: complications and cost. *American Journal of Clinical Nutrition* **71**(5), 1242S–8S.

Geissler PW, Prince RJ, Levene M *et al.* (1999) Perceptions of soil-eating and anaemia among pregnant women on the Kenyan coast. *Social Science & Medicine* **48**(8), 1069–79

Giddens JB, Krug SK, Tsang RC, Guo S, Miodovnik M and Prada JA (2000) Pregnant adolescent and adult women have similar low intakes of selected nutrients. *Journal of the American Dietetic Association* **100**(11), 1334–40.

Goodnight W, Newman R; Society of Maternal-Fetal Medicine (2009) Optimal nutrition for improved twin pregnancy outcome. *Obstetrics & Gynaecology* **114**(5), 1121–34.

Gregory J and Lowe S (2000) *National Diet and Nutrition Survey: Young People Aged 4–18 Years.* The Stationery Office: London.

Grigsby RK, Thyer BA, Waller RJ and Johnston GA Jr (1999) Chalk eating in middle Georgia: a culture-bound syndrome of pica? *Southern Medical Journal* **92**(2), 190–2.

Guttmacher Institute (2006) *U.S. Teenage Pregnancy Statistics National and State Trends and Trends by Race and Ethnicity.* Guttmacher Institute: New York.

Haggarty P, Campbell DM, Duthie S *et al.* (2009) Diet and deprivation in pregnancy. *British Journal of Nutrition* **17**, 1–11.

Hanna FWF and Peters JP (2002) Screening for gestational diabetes: past, present and future. *Diabetic Medicine* **19**, 351–8.

Harding JE (2003) Nutrition and growth before birth. *Asia Pacific Journal of Clinical Nutrition* **12**, 28.

Hegaard HK, Pedersen BK, Nielsen BB and Damm P (2007) Leisure time physical activity during pregnancy and impact on gestational diabetes mellitus, pre-eclampsia, preterm delivery and birth weight: a review. *Acta Obstetrica et Gynecologica Scandanavia* **86**(11), 1290–6.

Herguner S (2007) Is pica an eating disorder or an obsessive-compulsive spectrum disorder? *Progress in Neuro-Psychopharmacology & Biological Psychiatry* **32**, 2010–11.

Heslehurst N, Simpson H, Ells LJ *et al.* (2008) The impact of maternal BMI status on pregnancy outcomes with immediate short-term obstetric resource implications: a meta-analysis. *Obesity Reviews* **9**(6), 635–83.

IoM (Institute of Medicine) (1990) *Committee on Nutrition Status During Pregnancy and Lactation.* National Academy Press: Washington, DC.

Jacobsson B, Ladfors L and Milsom I (2004) Advanced maternal age and adverse perinatal outcome. *Obstetrics & Gynaecology* **104**(4), 727–33.

James SL, Muir JG, Curtis SL and Gibson PR (2003) Dietary fibre: a roughage guide. *Internal Medicine Journal* **33**, 291–6.

Kushner RF and Shanta Retelny V (2005) Emergence of pica (ingestion of non-food substances) accompanying iron deficiency anaemia after gastric bypass surgery. *Obesity Surgery* **15**(10), 1491–5.

Leitzmann C (2005) Vegetarian diets: what are the advantages? *Forum of Nutrition* **57**, 147–56.

Levy HL (2003) Historical background for the maternal PKU syndrome. *Pediatrics* **112**, 1516–18.

Levy T and Blickstein I (2006) Does the use of folic acid increase the risk of twinning? *International Journal of Fertility Women's Medicine* **51**(3), 130–5.

Liu J, Laditka JN, Mayer-Davis EJ and Pate RR (2008) Does physical activity during pregnancy reduce the risk of gestational diabetes among previously inactive women. *Birth* **35**(3), 188–95.

Lopez LB, Ortega Soler CR and de Portela ML (2004) Pica during pregnancy: a frequently under-estimated problem. *Archivos Latinoamicanos de Nutricion* **54**(1), 17–24 [Abstract only].

Lucock M, Yates Z, Hall K *et al.* (2002) The impact of phenylketonuria on folate metabolism. *Molecular Genetics & Metabolism* **76**(4), 305–12.

Luke B (2004) Improving multiple pregnancy outcomes. *Clinical Obstetrics and Gynaecology* **47**, 146–62.

Lumey LH and Stein AD (1997) In utero exposure to famine and subsequent fertility: The Dutch Famine Birth Cohort Study. *American Journal of Public Health* **87**(12), 1962–6.

Luoto R, Laitinen K, Nermes M and Isolauri E. (2010) Impact of maternal probiotic-supplemented dietary counselling on pregnancy outcome and prenatal and postnatal growth: a double-blind, placebo-controlled study. *British Journal of Nutrition* **103**(12), 1792–9.

Lynch SR (2000) The potential impact of iron supplementation during adolescence on iron status in pregnancy. *Journal of Nutrition* **130**(2S Suppl), 448S–51S.

Metwally M, Ong KJ, Ledger WL and Li TC (2008) Does high body mass index increase the risk of miscarriage after spontaneous and assisted conception? A meta-analysis of the evidence. *Fertility & Sterility* **90**(3), 714–26.

Mills ME (2007) Craving more than food: the implications of pica in pregnancy. *Nursing for Women's Health* **11**(3), 266–73.

Mojtabai R (2004) Body mass index and serum folate in childbearing age women. *European Journal of Epidemiology* **19**(11), 1029–36.

MRC (Medical Research Council) (1993) MRC working party on phenylketonuria: Recommendations on the dietary management of phenylketonuria. *Archives of Disease in Childhood* **68**, 426–7.

NICE (National Institute of Clinical Excellence) (2008) Diabetes in Pregnancy: Management of Diabetes and its Complications from Preconception to the Postnatal Period. RCOG: London.

Nicoletti A (2003) Perspectives on pediatric and adolescent gynecology from the allied health care professional: Pica when you least expect it. *Journal of Pediatric and Adolescent Gynaecology* **16**(1), 173–4.

Noonan SS (1997) Kids having kids: the teen birth rate. *New Jersey Medical Journal* **94**(8), 43–5.

Oken E (2009) Maternal and child obesity: the causal link. *Obstetrics & Gynaecology Clinics of North America* **36**(2), 361–77.

Paranjothy S, Broughton H, Adappa R and Fone D. (2009) Teenage pregnancy: who suffers? *Archives of Disease in Childhood* **94**(3), 239–45.

Parry-Jones B (1992) Pagophagia, or compulsive ice consumption: a historical perspective. *Psycological Medicine* **22**(3), 561–71.

Penney DS and Miller KG (2008) Nutritional counselling for vegetarians during pregnancy and lactation. *Journal of Midwifery and Women's Health* **53**(1), 37–44.

Poston L, Harthoorn L, Van Der Beek EM; on behalf of Contributors to the ILSI Workshop (2010) Obesity in pregnancy; implications for the mother and lifelong health of the child. A consensus statement. *Pediatric Research*. [Epub ahead of print.]

Rasmussen KM and Yaktine AL (2009) *Weight gain during pregnancy: re-examining the guidelines*. The National Academies Press: Washington, DC.

Ray JG, Thompson MD, Vermeulen MJ *et al.* (2007) Metabolic syndrome features and risk of neural tube defects. *BMC Pregnancy Childbirth* **7**, 21.

Reader D, Splett P and Gunderson EP (2006) Impact of gestational diabetes mellitus nutritional practice guidelines implemented by registered dieticians on pregnancy outcomes. *Journal of the American Dietetic Association* **106**, 1426–33.

Rees GA, Doyle W, Srivastava A, Brooke ZM, Crawford MA and Costeloe KL (2005) The nutrient intakes of mothers of low birth weight babies – a comparison of ethnic groups in East London, UK. *Maternal and Child Nutrition* **1**, 91–9.

Resfum H (2001) Folate, vitamin B_{12} and homocysteine in relation to birth defects and pregnancy outcome. *British Journal of Nutrition* **85**(2), S109–13.

Rosello-Soberon ME, Fuentes-Chaparro L and Casanueva E (2005) Twin pregnancies: eating for three? Maternal nutrition update. *Nutrition Reviews* **63**(9), 295–302.

Royal College of Obstetricians and Gynaecologists (RCOG) (2009) RCOG statement on later maternal age. Available at: http://www.rcog.org.uk/what-we-do/campaigning-and-opinions/statement/rcog-statement-later-maternal-age. (accessed March 2011.)

SACN (Scientific Advisory Committee on Nutrition) (2006) *Folate and Disease Prevention*. The Stationery Office: London.

Schneck ME, Sideras KS, Fox RA and Dupuis L (1990) Low-income pregnant adolescents and their infants: dietary findings and health outcomes. *Journal of the American Dietetic Association* **90**(4), 555–8.

Scientific Advisory Committee on Nutrition/Committee on Nutrition/Committee on Toxicity (SACN/CoT) (2004). *Advice on Fish Consumption: Benefits and Risks*. The Stationery Office: London.

Selhub J (2008) Public health significance of elevated homocysteine. *Food & Nutrition Bulletin* **29**(2), S116–25.

Serlin DC and Lash RW (2009) Diagnosis and management of gestational diabetes mellitus. *American Family Physician* **80**(1), 57–62.

Shaw GM, Todoroff K, Schaffer DM and Selvin S (2000) Maternal height and prepregnancy body mass index as risk factors for selected congenital anomalies. *Paediatric and Perinatal Epidemiology* **14**(3), 234–9.

Smith SA, Hulsey T and Goodnight W (2009) Effects of obesity on pregnancy. *Journal of Obstetric Gynecologic and Neonatal Nursing* **37**(2), 176–84.

Thomas J (2002) Nutrition intervention in ethnic minority groups. *Proceedings of the Nutrition Society* **61**, 559–67.

Tobias DK, Zhang C, van Dam RM, Bowers K and Hu FB (2010) Physical activity before and during pregnancy and risk of gestational diabetes mellitus: a meta-analysis. *Diabetes Care* [Epub ahead of print].

(USDA) United Sates Department of Agriculture (2010) *USDA National Nutrient Database for Standard Reference*. Available at: http://www.nal.usda.gov/fnic/foodcomp/search/. (accessed March 2011.)

Ward KA, Adams JE and Mughal MZ (2005) Bone status during adolescence, pregnancy and lactation. *Current Opinions in Obstetrics & Gynaecology* **17**(4), 435–9.

Wilson RD, Désilets V, Wyatt P *et al.* (2007) Pre-conception vitamin/folic acid supplementation 2007: the use of folic acid in combination with a multivitamin supplement for the prevention of neural tube defects and other congenital anomalies. *Journal of Obstetrics & Gynaecology Canada* **138**, 1003–13.

Xiao S, Hansen DK, Horsley ET *et al.* (2005) Maternal folate deficiency results in selective up-regulation of folate receptors and heterogeneous nuclear ribonucleoprotein-E1 associated with multiple aberrations is fetal tissues. *Birth Defects Research Part A: Clinical & Molecular Teratology* **73**, 6–28.

Yang QH, Carter HK, Mulinare J, Berry RJ, Friedman JM and Erickson JD (2007) Race-ethnicity difference in folic acid intake in women of childbearing age in the United States after folic acid fortification: findings from the National Health and Nutrition Examination Survey, 2001–2002. *American Journal of Clinical Nutrition* **85**(5), 1409–16.

Yassin SA, Sobhy SI and Ebrahim W (2004) Factors affecting dietary practices among adolescent pregnant women in Alexandria. *Journal of the Egyptian Public Health Association* **79**(3–4), 179–96.

Yi SH and Singh RH (2008) Protein substitute for children and adults with phenylketonuria. *Cochrane Database of Systemic Reviews* **8**(4), CD004731

Yogev Y, Melamed N, Bardin R *et al.* (2010) Pregnancy outcome at extremely advanced maternal age. *American Journal of Obstetrics & Gynaecology* [Epub ahead of print].

Yogev Y and Visser GH (2009) Obesity, gestational diabetes and pregnancy outcome. *Seminars in Fetal & Neonatal Medicine* **14**(2), 77–84.

Zhang J, Meikle S, Grainger DA and Trumble A (2002) Multifetal pregnancy in older women and perinatal outcomes. *Fertility & Sterility* **78**(3), 562–8.

11 Physiological and Hormonal Changes after Birth

Summary

Once a woman has given birth, a series of hormonal and physiological changes take place to help the body return to its pre-pregnant state. Although these processes may be facilitated by breastfeeding, a large proportion of women do not return to their original weight before pregnancy, for reasons that will be discussed. In turn, failure to lose excess weight after birth is contributing to rising obesity figures, more so in developed regions. This section aims to outline the key hormonal and physiological changes that take place after birth to help the body return to normal. Mood changes, bowel habit and breast changes may all be experienced to some degree after birth, largely caused by the decline in pregnancy hormones. The physiology of breastfeeding, patterns of weight loss and evidence of some effective dietary and physical activity interventions that may help to support appropriate levels of weight loss after birth will also be described in this chapter.

Learning Outcomes

- To describe the hormonal and physiological changes that occur in the transition period after birth to help the body return to normal.
- To outline the key hormonal and physiological processes involved when breast-feeding.
- To make sense of evidence studying the relationship between breastfeeding and weight loss/body composition changes.
- To consider (and provide examples of) certain dietary and lifestyle interventions that may help women return to lose weight retained after birth.

11.1 Introduction

The physiological changes that take place in both pregnancy and after birth are vast and best described in separate texts such as Stables and Rankin (2006). However, it is important that some of the key changes are explained in the course of this text, to understand how and why nutrition requirements may change after birth

Nutrition in the Childbearing Years, First Edition. Emma Derbyshire.
© 2011 Emma Derbyshire. Published 2011 by Blackwell Publishing Ltd.

(Chapter 12). The body is remarkable in that after birth physiological mechanisms are bought into play that benefit not only the child but also the mother. Equally, having a new baby is an exciting time but can also be daunting as emotional, psychological and social changes also take place, in addition to the body's physical adaptations. If women know what to expect and are prepared for parenthood, this may help to support them during this busy time. This chapter will start by defining the postpartum period, outlining some of the key physiological changes that occur (the main change being lactation) and then go on to explain the processes and health benefits linked to breastfeeding in more detail.

11.2   When is 'postpartum'?

Defining the postpartum period can be difficult. Typically, medical dictionaries define postpartum period as the length of time it takes for the mother's reproductive organs and tissues to return to normal, which is usually around six to eight weeks. There is some literature suggesting that ancient societies considered this time period to be 'unclean', a time when women could not show themselves to their husbands until around 40 days after birth (Hytten, 1995). Although times have obviously changed, it is interesting to see that some definitions of the postpartum period (6 weeks or 42 days) still coincide with these older definitions. Today, after birth, the postpartum period may also be referred to as the puerperium or '4th trimester' and is considered to be complete once ovulation begins and menstruation returns to normal.

11.3   Changes after birth

11.3.1   Hormone changes

Delivery of the placenta means that levels of hormones secreted by the placenta during pregnancy are reduced. This may not be immediate as this depends on their half-life (rate at which they break down/are removed by the body) but includes a reduction in progesterone, oestrogen, human placental lactogen (hPL) and human chorionic gonadotrophin (hCG) levels. Oestrogen levels return to pre-pregnancy levels around 7 days after birth whilst progesterone concentrations return to those present in the luteal phase (second half) of the menstrual cycle around 24–48 hours after delivery and follicular phase (first half of the menstrual cycle) by 7 days (Stables and Rankin, 2006); progesterone levels are generally higher in the luteal phase of the menstrual cycle.

11.3.2   Hair thickness after birth

Sometimes, women may find that they are losing more hair than normal after birth. This is nothing to worry about and is generally caused by changes in hormone levels. During pregnancy, women have higher oestrogen levels, which may prolong the hair's growth phases. There is good evidence that oestrogen hormones can alter hair follicle growth by binding to oestrogen receptors (Ohnemus *et al.*, 2006). After birth, when oestrogen levels fall, it is the excess hair that is shed (hair generally becomes thicker during pregnancy) and hair returns to the thickness it was before birth.

11.3.3   Blood volume changes

The blood volume is highest at the end of pregnancy. This increase is needed for extra blood flow to the uterus, kidneys and for the metabolic needs of the foetus. Although some blood is lost during the delivery process (around 500–600 mL for vaginal and 1000 mL with a caesarean section), the remainder needs to be dispersed of in other ways. Blood loss after birth, also often referred to as 'lochia' (blood and tissue from the lining of the uterus) and is a normal process that helps the uterus to shrink back to its normal size. This may take place from just 10 days up to six weeks after birth and it is normally red/brown in colour (Marchant *et al.*, 1999). Some women may not be aware that they will experience blood loss for several weeks after birth and should be guided that this will occur.

11.3.4   Involution of the uterus

After delivery of the baby, some key changes take place to the lining and muscle layers of the uterus to help it return to its shape and size before pregnancy. As mentioned previously, the lining of the uterus is shed mainly as lochia, but three other key processes also take place – ischaemia, autolysis and phogocytsis. Ischaemia is when uterine muscles contract, the blood vessels constrict and blood circulation to the uterus is reduced, helping it to shrink back and return to normal. Autolysis is when excess muscle fibres are removed by body enzymes and macrophages (a type of white blood cell) and phagocytosis is a similar process where some of the excess fibrous and elastic tissue is removed (Stables and Rankin, 2006). These changes go a long way towards helping the uterus turn back to its original state, but a degree of elastic tissue always remains.

11.3.5   Urine production

The extra water that cells retained during pregnancy and fluid from the rise in blood volume will be looking for an escape route after birth. As a result, new mothers generally produce more urine than usual the few days after giving birth, although levels excreted vary between women. Rates of perspiration may also be slightly higher than usual during this time. Urinary tract infections (UTIs) are also common after giving birth with ethnicity, unmarried status, renal disease, pre-eclampsia and length of hospital stay all being associated with increased risk of infection (Schwartz *et al.*, 1999). Some studies have also shown that women with a high body mass index (BMI) are more likely to suffer from UTIs after birth (Sebire *et al.*, 2001; Usha Kiran *et al.*, 2005).

Equally, because during labour the bladder moves up into the abdomen and the urethra is stretched, micturition can be difficult after birth. This is sometimes known as 'postpartum urinary retention' and means that women have difficulty urinating.

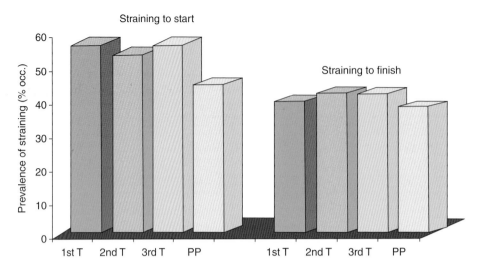

Figure 11.1 Prevalence of straining to start and finish. 1st T, first trimester; 2nd T, second trimester; 3rd T, third trimester; PP, postpartum. Changes in Bowel Function: Pregnancy and the Puerperium. (Reproduced from Derbyshire E *et al.* (2006) Digestive Diseases and Sciences, with permission from Springer.)

This can be a frustrating condition that may occur in 1.7–17.9% of women – sometimes, a warm bath can help but sometimes catheterisation may be necessary in some cases (Saultz *et al.*, 1991).

11.3.6   Constipation

Some older studies have shown that the mode of delivery, i.e. use of forceps, increased duration of second stage delivery and high infant birth weight, may all lead to anal sphincter damage (Corman, 1985; Sultan *et al.*, 1993). Research has shown that just under 20% of first-time mothers experience symptoms of constipation after birth with 44% experiencing straining to start and 37% experiencing straining to finish when defecating (Figure 11.1). As it can be seen from the Figure 11.1, bowel habits often improve after birth because the levels of pregnancy hormones that have previously relaxed the bowel and contributed to these symptoms, i.e. progesterone, have declined.

Bowel habits may also vary between lactating and non-lactating mothers with symptoms of urgency being significantly higher amongst women who are not breastfeeding (Derbyshire *et al.*, 2007). Once again, this may be because of hormonal differences, but studies are needed to confirm these. Different dietary habits/fluid intakes may lead to some bowel habit differences between lactating and non-lactating women.

11.3.7   Mood changes

Women have an increased risk of depression from early adolescence until their mid-50s and their lifetime rate of major depression 1.7–2.7 times greater than that for men (Burt and Stein, 2002). There is good evidence that hormonal fluctuations can predispose women to depressive mood states at certain phases of the female

Table 11.1 Hormones that may influence postpartum mood.

Hormone	Possible action	Source(s)
Oestrogen	Oestrogen can affect levels of neurotransmitters and neural proteins, possibly linked to depression	Wise *et al.* (2008) Zou *et al.* (2009)
Progesterone	Withdrawal of progesterone has been linked to depressive symptoms after birth	Zou *et al.* (2009)
Testosterone	Testosterone levels have been found to correlate with feelings of anger and depression scores early after birth	Hohlagschwandtner *et al.* (2001)
Prolactin	Higher prolactin levels in breastfeeding mothers have been linked to lower anxiety levels	Asher *et al.* (1995)
Oxytocin	There is preliminary evidence linking elevated oxytocin levels to feelings of emotional distress and major depression	Parker *et al.* (2010)
Cortisol	Elevated cortisol levels in pregnancy and after birth have been linked to increased feelings of anxiety	Fan *et al.* (2009) Zou *et al.* (2009) Nierop *et al.* (2006)
Other factors (hormone precursors)		
Cholesterol	Cholesterol levels can rise by as much as 43% in pregnancy and then decline after birth has been correlated with depressive symptoms	Troisi *et al.* (2002) Nasta *et al.* (2002)
Fatty acids	Low levels of omega-3 fatty acids may be linked with depressive symptoms after birth. These fatty acids may help to produce the feel good hormone 'serotonin'	Borja-Hart and Marino (2010)

Women experiencing heightened sensitivity to hormone fluctuations may be at risk of depression. Testing levels of maternal hormones after birth may be a useful diagnostic tool for evaluating psychological stress and risk of postnatal depression.

reproductive lifecycle, including after birth when hormone levels are in a dynamic state of change.

Relating this specifically to the childbearing years in pregnancy, estradiol levels in the third trimester of pregnancy are 50 times and progesterone 10 times higher than peak levels in the menstrual cycle (Zonana and Gorman, 2005). Consequently, women may be at increased risk of low mood when levels of these hormones, amongst others, change (Table 11.1). When coupled with lack of sleep, caring demands of the new baby and the emotional adjustment of motherhood, it is no wonder that women experience mood changes after birth. It is, however, important not to confuse mood disturbances linked to hormones changes with postpartum depression (discussed in Chapter 12). This is a more serious problem that often requires appropriate medical treatment. More research is needed to study hormonal effects on mood changes after birth and whether breastfeeding can protect against depression after birth. Some meta-analysis papers within this area would also be useful.

11.3.8 Postpartum fatigue

After women have experienced the extreme physiological changes of pregnancy and delivery, it is no wonder that they may be feeling tired after birth. Fatigue can be an unrelenting condition that is heightened in women with depression but can also be a cause of this condition. It has implications for everyday activities, motivation and social interactions and can be particularly challenging after birth when new mothers have additional tasks to undertake (Corwin and Arbour, 2007). There is some evidence that home-based cardiovascular exercises, i.e. 60–120 minutes per week of aerobic exercises within target heart ranges (60–85% of maximal heart rate) may help to reduce feelings of mental and physical tiredness after birth, particular amongst women with higher depression scores after birth (Dritsa et al., 2009). This research needs to be repeated using larger samples of women, but exercise interventions could be targeted at particular groups of women who are most likely to benefit.

Research Highlight   Postpartum fatigue or iron deficiency?

There is no doubt that the causes of feelings of tiredness and fatigue after birth are multi-faceted, but iron deficiency may be another contributing factor. New mothers are at risk of developing anaemia as iron levels are often at their lowest levels after giving birth. Data from American surveys has shown that twice as many women develop anaemia after giving birth (12.7%) when compared with rates amongst women who have not had children (6.5%), especially women with low incomes (Bodnar et al., 2002).

Common signs and symptoms include feelings of breathlessness, tiredness, heart palpitations and increased susceptibility to infections. Treatment strategies in the past has included high-dose iron supplements, intravenous and subcutaneous administration of iron and erythropoietin or blood transfusions, but more work is needed to examine the effects of iron-rich diets as interventions (Dodd et al., 2004). Prevention is also always better than cure, so the importance of consuming a bio-available iron-rich diet before and throughout pregnancy should also be communicated to women of childbearing age and pregnant mothers. One final note, findings from other studies have also shown that women with low iron status after birth may also be prone to depression, stress and may not bond as well with their children after birth (Beard et al., 2005).

11.3.9 Breast changes

Although mammary glands are present from birth, they require the hormones of pregnancy to become fully functional for milk production. In the early stages of pregnancy, 'mammogenesis' takes place, which is when the mammary gland adapts, so it is fully able to produce milk after birth. During this phase, women's breasts may feel increasingly tender as subcutaneous veins enlarge and the areola becomes darker. Within the breasts, the networks of ducts proliferate and alveoli expand in size and shape (Jones and Spencer, 2007). Once the mammary glands have adapted to produce milk, the secretory mechanisms facilitating milk production and ejection starts to take place, also known as 'lactogenesis'. The processes of lactogenesis can be broken down into several distinct phases, which are discussed in the next few sections.

11.4   Lactogenesis

11.4.1   Lactogenesis I

Lactogenesis I may be defined as the stage in which the mammary glands develop the ability to produce milk. During this phase, some, but not all, of the genes involved in the secretion of milk start to become expressed. This normally occurs during the second half of pregnancy and although breast milk is produced, it is not removed. This is largely because the hormone progesterone prevents the secretion of milk in pregnancy. This means that certain breast milk components are reabsorbed back into the body, including lactose, which can be detected in blood samples (Arthur et al., 1991). After birth, when progesterone levels decline, this is one important factor that facilitates the production of breast milk.

11.4.2   Lactogenesis II

Lactogenesis II is when the secretion of colostrum, followed by breast milk, commences after birth. In this phase, there is a further increase in the expression of genes that facilitate the production of milk, particularly once the suckling process begins.

The levels of immunoglobulins and other protective substances (Table 11.2) are also transferred to the colostrums and later breast milk. One particularly important

Table 11.2   Anti-infective properties found in human breast milk.

What is it?	What does it do?
Anti-secretory factor	A protein with anti-inflammatory properties that can help to prevent mastitis in the mother and diarrhoea in the offspring.
Carbohydrate components	These include oligosaccharides, glycoproteins and glycolipids. These are produced in the mammary glands and can help to prevent potentially harmful microbes binding to the gut wall.
Cytokines	Small proteins that can alter the behaviour of cells (by stimulating the release of other factors), triggering inflammation and helping the body respond to infections.
Immunoglobulin A (IgA)	One of the main human antibodies. It prevents bacteria and viruses from reaching mucosal membranes so they cannot cause infections.
Lactoferrin	An important milk protein present in the highest levels when milk is first secreted as colostrum. This protein binds iron, preventing microorganisms using it for the growth and development.
Lysozymes	Enzymes with mild antiseptic properties that are able to destroy the cell walls of bacteria.
α-Lactalbumin	Albumin found in milk that may be lethal to tumour cells. More work is needed to establish whether breastfeeding can reduce breast cancer and childhood leukaemia risk.

Source: Points extracted from Hanson (2007).

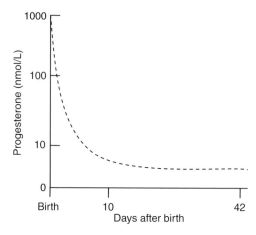

Figure 11.2 Reduction in progesterone levels after birth. (Adapted from Neville *et al.* (2002), with permission from Springer.)

phase in lactogenesis II is the withdrawal of progesterone. This hormone declines rapidly after birth once the baby and placenta have been delivered (Figure 11.2). The abrupt withdrawal of progesterone and high levels of prolactin secreted from the anterior pituitary gland mean that milk secretion can take place (Neville *et al.*, 2001), although several other key hormones are also involved. This process is usually known as the 'let down reflex'.

The Let Down Reflex

A few days after delivery, breasts can start to feel swollen, hard and tender, otherwise known as 'engorgement'. Starting to breastfeed the child can help to relieve some of these feelings. When milk is removed from the breasts, several key hormones are involved, including prolactin and oxytocin.

Prolactin, secreted from the anterior pituitary glands, helps to stimulate milk production whilst oxytocin causes the milk sacs and ducts to contact, promoting the ejection of milk. Once the infant is attached to the nipple, nerve signals transmit signals to the central nervous system where oxytocin is released from the posterior pituitary gland. The hormone oxytocin is then carried to the mammary gland via the bloodstream where it then acts with receptors on myoepithelial cells.

Myoepithelial cells have a particularly important function because they can contract, helping to expel milk from the alveoli (sacs that store the milk) into the breast ducts. Contraction of the myoepithelial cells helps the ducts to shorten and widen, propelling the milk towards the nipple (Mennella, 2001). This process is often referred to as the milk ejection or 'let down reflex' (Figure 11.3)

When women are breastfeeding, they may also experience abdominal cramping; this is because the hormone oxytocin causes uterine contractions, helping it to return to its original size.

If women decide not to breastfeed, feelings of engorgement will continue until eventually the milk supply dries up. Eventually, mammary involution will occur and the gland will lose its ability to produce milk. This process can take several weeks and can be uncomfortable at times.

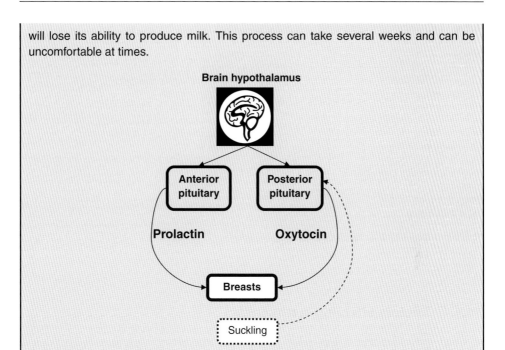

Figure 11.3   The hormonal control of the 'let down reflex'. Prolactin stimulates milk production whilst oxytocin helps milk to be removed from the breasts.

11.4.3   Lactogenesis III

After delivery, continuous removal of milk is important for synthesis to continue. This phase of lactation may be referred to as 'lactogenesis III' or 'galactopoiesis'. This process will continue as long as milk is removed on a regular basis (Jones and Spencer, 2007).

Table 11.3   How can obesity delay lactogenesis?

Reason	Explanation
Anatomical	High levels of adipose tissue can mean that progesterone levels are higher in overweight/obese women inhibiting lactation. Breast size may also lead to feeding difficulties.
Medical conditions	Diabetes, PCOS and rates of caesarean deliveries are generally higher, which have all been linked to delayed lactogenesis.
Socio-cultural	Women who are obese are more likely to belong to social groups who do not breastfeed. Large breasts may mean that it is more difficult to breastfeed discretely.
Psychological	Obese women tend to have greater body image dissatisfaction and lower levels of self-esteem.

Source: Points extracted from Amir and Donath (2007).
PCOS, polycystic ovary syndrome.

Table 11.4   Other factors that can affect breastfeeding.

Mother	Child
Caesarean section	Birth by vacuum extraction
Calorie restriction	Hyperbilirubinaemia
First-time mother	Hypoglycaemia
Inverted and/or sore nipples	Irritable infant, restless, sleepy, refusing to feed
Multiple births	Poor attachment and positioning
Overweight/obesity	Tongue tie
Prior breast surgery	Use of supplemental formula and dummies
Prior breastfeeding problems	
Smoking	
Stressful, long labour	
Type 1 diabetes	

Source: Jones and Spencer (2007), with permission.

11.4.4   Factors affecting lactogenesis

A host of factors can affect milk production after birth, but one factor that is making breastfeeding increasingly problematic is the rise in overweight and obesity. For women, being overweight or obese can lead to a range of physiological, socio-cultural and psychological factors that may affect their ability or drive to breast feed.

In particular, it is coming to light that mothers who are obese may be less likely to breastfeed because lactogenesis II may be delayed. Studies show that black women in the United States, with the highest rates of obesity, have the lowest rates and shortest duration of breastfeeding when compared with Hispanic and Caucasian mothers (Jevitt *et al.*, 2007). Research shows that prolonged labours, stress and higher rates of surgical deliveries can all delay lactogenesis II (Chen *et al.*, 1998), many of which are experienced more frequently amongst heavier mothers. There is also some evidence to suggest that overweight/obese women may have a lower prolactin response to suckling. This means their milk will not be easily produced and mothers are more likely to stop breastfeeding (Rasmussen and Kjolhede, 2004). Other factors that can also affect breastfeeding from a more general perspective are included in Table 11.4.

Research Highlight   Obesity and delayed lactogenesis

Delayed lactogenesis, i.e. failure to secrete milk, or adequate levels of milk after birth, can lead to weight loss, formula supplementation and early weaning in newborns. A new study has now studied factors associated with delayed lactogenesis, i.e. when milk production is not produced within 72 hours after delivery.

Researchers interviewed 431 women after delivery and again 3 and 7 days after birth, asking them about their lifestyle, delivery experiences and infant feeding practices. For most women, lactogenesis occurred around 68.9 hours after birth whilst 44% of women experienced delayed lactogenesis.

Risk factors for delayed onset of lactogenesis included older maternal age (≥30 years), overweight or obese BMI and an infant birth weight of >3600 g, amongst other factors (Nommsen-Rivers *et al.*, 2010).

This study shows that older maternal age and higher rates of overweight and obesity amongst women may affect their ability to breastfeed after birth. This is another important reason why women should try to get into healthy body weight ranges before becoming pregnant and gain weight within recommended ranges during pregnancy.

11.5   A note on colostrum

Colostrum is the thick fluid that is first secreted by the breasts after birth before mature milk is produced. Colostrum is a rich source of both nutritional and immunologically important components. An analysis of 505 milk samples from 115 healthy Iranian women showed that colostrum is a good source of antioxidants (Zarban *et al.*, 2009), whilst other studies have found that colostrum is also a rich source of essential fatty acids – although this very much depends on the geographic location and dietary composition of mothers, i.e. Australian mothers with diets abundant in fish have been found to secrete colostrum containing some of the highest levels of the essential fatty acids eicosapentaenoic acid (EPA) and docosahexaenoic acid (DHA) (Fidler and Koletzko, 2000).

11.6   What is transitional milk?

Transitional milk is normally produced by the breast between 2–5 days after birth. This term is used to describe the milk that is produced after colostrum has been secreted but before the breasts produce mature milk. Recently, it has been shown that a hormone named ghrelin is secreted in breast milk. Levels of this appetite-regulating hormone increase as the milk transforms from colostrum, to transitional and then to mature milk. In a small sample of 17 lactating women, ghrelin levels were found to be 70.3 pg/mL in colostrum, 83.8 pg/mL in transitional milk and 97.3 pg/mL in mature milk (Aydin *et al.*, 2006). It is possible that ghrelin may have a role to play in regulating the appetite of the infant.

11.7   Nutritional composition of milk

Neville *et al.* (1988) were some of the first scientists to measure the nutrient composition of milk during the first 8 days after birth (Figure 11.4) and have continued their research since. It can be seen that lipid levels increase in the 8 days after birth, whilst proportions of other nutrients, i.e. potassium, magnesium and calcium, level out. It is important to consider that the nutritional composition of breast milk is highly variable and depends on a host of factors. One recent study identified that sodium levels (for the first week), carbohydrate, fat and energy content of milk secreted by mothers who had delivered prematurely was significantly higher than levels present in milk secreted by mothers at term (Bauer and Gerss, 2010). Other studies clearly show that different dietary habits and the quality of the mothers' diet can affect the nutrient composition of breast milk (Peng *et al.*, 2009 and research highlight).

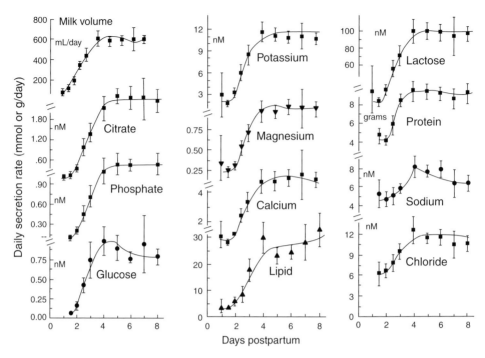

Figure 11.4   Macronutrient content of breast milk in the 8 days after birth. (Neville and Morton (2001), with permission from the American Society of Nutrition.)

Research Highlight   Ramadan may affect breast milk composition

A study carried out on a sample on 21 mothers aged 17–38 years who fasted during the month of Ramadan volunteered to give milk samples, which were then analysed by scientists. Scientists found that mothers' diets fell below dietary requirements for energy and most nutrients (except protein, vitamin A and C) and the zinc, magnesium and potassium content of breast milk declined during this period (Rakicioğlu *et al.*, 2006). Although the growth of infants appeared to be unaffected, largely because energy requirements were still met, the micronutrient content of milk was reduced, which could have implications for foetal health. More work is needed to develop this research further to establish whether lactating women and their infants may benefit from being excused from fasting during Ramadan.

11.8   Milk synthesis – use it or lose it

Earlier research by Steven Daly from the University of Western Australia has yielded several important findings. Firstly, after studying patterns of milk removal and synthesis over a 24-hour period using computerised breast measurement systems, he found that the amount of milk stored in the breast related directly to infant demand, i.e. when infants suckled and removed more milk from the breast, larger volumes of milk could then be stored in the breast (Daly *et al.*, 1993a). He also found that the degree of breast emptying affected the fat content of the milk, i.e. emptier breasts lead to higher fat levels in the hind milk (Daly *et al.*, 1993b). This was important research showing that infant demand plays a key role in regulating synthesis and storage capacity of breast milk, as well as its fat content.

When relating this work to different women, those with smaller breasts may need to feed more frequently, to prevent the breasts from becoming too full as this could switch-off milk production. Women with larger breasts may go longer between feeds but should be encouraged to feed their infant for as long as they are hungry, to help empty the breast and the synthesis of new milk.

11.9   Milk volume

Milk volume generally increases over time, providing that milk synthesis continues. Once women have given birth, just 60 minutes later they will begin to secrete colostrum (around 0–50 mL). In the first 24 hours after birth, research has shown that healthy newborn infants generally ingest around 15 mL ($\pm$11) colostrum over the course of about 3–4 feeds (Santoro *et al.*, 2010).

Volume of milk ingested by infants aged between 1 and 6 months of age has been studied by Kent *et al.* (2006). The volume of milk consumed by infants was determined by test-weighing infants before and after every breastfeeding session. Infants were exclusively breastfed and received an average of 11 feeds, providing around 76 mL milk (range 0–240 mL). The volume of milk ingested by infants largely depended on which breast was suckled, i.e. whether it was the more productive/most frequently suckled breast (most frequently used breast = greater volume of milk). Authors also concluded that night feeds made an important contribution to total milk intake and recommended that breastfed infants should be encouraged feed on demand, rather than conforming to an average number of feeds that may be appropriate to all mothers.

Research Highlight   Leptin in breast milk may help to regulate body weight in the next generation

Rates of obesity in women of childbearing age are rising, particularly within developed regions. This has implications for the offspring as these women may be more likely to use artificial feeds, possibly because of physiological difficulties with milk production. Some evidence suggests that the introduction of formulas can promote rapid weight gain in newborns, which may in turn increase their risk of obesity later in life (Stettler *et al.*, 2005).

For women who are breastfeeding, research has shown that the hormone leptin (a weight regulatory hormone) may help to regulate the body weight of newborns, as this also seems to be secreted in the breast milk. A study of 15 mothers and their newborns identified that the leptin content of milk was negatively correlated with the offspring's BMI (Doneray *et al.*, 2009). These are interesting results, but more research is needed to reinforce these initial findings.

11.10   Breastfeeding as contraception

It is well known that breastfeeding can offer a degree of protection against pregnancy, but this can depend on infant feeding patterns and maternal nutritional status to some extent. It is thought that lactation suppresses ovarian activity by disrupting the pulsatile pattern of luteinising hormone secretion (Glasier and McNeilly, 1990). This has very important implications from a public health perspective. In developing regions, lactational amenorrhea is one of the most successful contraceptive methods, especially as other forms of contraception are unavailable. Frequent and prolonged breastfeeding can help to increase birth intervals, reducing both infant and maternal morbidity and mortality (Saadeh and Benbouzid, 1990). Midwives, nurses and health care planners can play an important role in encouraging mothers to feed their infants over extended time periods. Although this cannot be relied upon fully as a contraceptive method, it can play an important role in developing regions to help women to space and recover from their pregnancies.

11.11   Breast cancer risk

Epidemiology studies have shown that risk of breast cancer is generally lower in areas where breastfeeding is practiced over prolonged time periods. These trends, however, are more difficult to try and explain. Some theories include the following:

- Breastfeeding may change hormone levels, i.e. reduced levels of estrogens
- Lead to the excretion of potentially toxic carcinogens
- Lead to physical changes in cells of the breast tissue.

Unfortunately, breastfeeding is not always practical for women living in Western societies, particularly in the case of prolonged feeding. The choice to breastfeed is mainly driven by socio-economic factors and concerns for the health of the child. Currently, there is not enough evidence to suggest that breastfeeding can protect against breast cancer. In a recent systematic review of 27 studies comparing rates of breast cancer amongst women who had breast fed against those who have never breastfed, only 11 found significant protection against breast cancer (Yang and Jacobsen, 2008). Consequently, there is not enough evidence to use protection against breast cancer as a public health recommendation to help encourage breastfeeding practices (Lipworth *et al.*, 2000).

11.12   Body weight after birth

For many women, pregnancy acts as a trigger for developing overweight and obesity. More than 30% women gain levels of weight in pregnancy that exceeds guidelines, which contributes largely to this problem (NRC/IoM, 2007). It is, however, important to consider that the relationship between pregnancy and women's weight is intertwined within a complex of other factors, which include a change in lifestyle, eating behaviours, patterns of physical activity, smoking cessation and breastfeeding habits that accompany pregnancy and birth (Linné *et al.*, 2002). Consequently, although some large studies such as the SPAWN (Stockholm Pregnancy and Women's Nutrition) study have studied changes in women's weight over the childbearing years, more research controlling carefully for as many of these factors as possible is needed. Also, more work needs to study the effects of weight retention of women's long-term health, although some new evidence is emerging (see highlight on the reset hypothesis).

11.12.1 Defining postpartum weight retention (PPWT)

There is not yet a consensus definition defining the term PPWT. It is clear that this refers to levels of body weight retained after birth, but there is currently no consistent definition that relates this to levels or weight retained or at what time period after birth. In one study, Pedersen *et al.* (2011) defined PPWR as ≥ 5 kg pre-pregnancy body weight retained at 6 and 18 months after birth. Siega-Riz *et al.* (2010) studied factors affecting levels of moderate (defined as 1–10 lbs) and high (defined as >10 lbs) levels of PPWT again using pre-pregnancy body weight as a baseline marker, but this time body weight was assessed at 3 and 12 months after birth. These are useful studies, but pre-pregnancy weight measurements should ideally not be self-reported and consistent definitions in terms of what constitutes PPWT and when weight measurements are best taken after birth would aid future comparisons between studies.

11.13 Breastfeeding and body weight

It is well documented that breastfeeding can assist in helping women to lose weight after birth. As discussed in Chapter 12, this is mainly because the production and synthesis of breast milk drives up energy expenditure to levels that are even higher than for pregnancy. There is now good evidence that for women gaining around 12 kg weight in pregnancy, breastfeeding exclusively for 6 months can help to eliminate any weight retained and also help to reduce the risk of major weight gain i.e. (>5 kg) amongst heavier women (Baker *et al.*, 2008). In developing regions, exclusive breastfeeding has been linked to weight losses of around 4.1 kg compared with an average weight loss of 1.1 kg in controls (Okechukwu *et al.*, 2009).

Key Theory – The 'Reset Hypothesis'

There is emerging evidence that breastfeeding and the length of time over which women feed their children can reduce the risk of certain metabolic diseases in the mothers. This theory also parallels findings from animal studies, which indicate that lactation can cause favourable changes in metabolism, reducing the chronic disease risk in the longer term.

During pregnancy, levels of body fat increase, triglyceride levels rise and insulin resistance occurs. These changes appear to reverse more quickly, and more completely, amongst women who breast feed their infants. The theory, now referred to as the 'reset hypothesis' suggests that regular breastfeeding may help the mother's metabolic profile return to normal (Stuebe and Rich-Edwards, 2009). This is an important theory that requires further investigation so findings can be communicated to mothers after birth. It seems that low breastfeeding rates may not only be associated with weight retention after birth but also permanent changes in women's metabolic profile, which may affect her long-term health.

11.14   Body composition changes

Earlier evidence has clearly shown that breastfeeding can help to promote weight loss (around 0.32 kg/month) and reduce levels of body fat (AbuSabha and Greene, 1998). The loss of weight retained during pregnancy may be enhanced by longer periods of more intensive breastfeeding. Equally, increased food intakes and decreased physical activity levels can dampen the weight-loss benefits of breastfeeding (Winkvist and Rasmussen, 1999). There is further evidence to now suggest that pregnant teenagers may be one group that is susceptible to weight retention and long-term weight gain (Thame et al., 2010). When coupled with low breastfeeding rates, this problem may be exacerbated further. Although all women need advice and ongoing support about the benefits of breastfeeding, this particularly applies to younger mothers (Spear, 2006). Interestingly, one recent American study found that from a sample of 688 women, 89% did not receive any weight loss advice and 77% received no advice about physical activity after birth (Ferrari et al., 2010). Clearly, the benefits these can bring need to be better communicated to mothers after birth.

11.15   Exercise and breastfeeding

Cardiovascular health, lipid levels and insulin response can all improve in breastfeeding mothers that choose to exercise. Research now shows that diet and exercise together appear to be more effective than diet alone at helping women to lose weight after childbirth. This is because the exercise helps to improve maternal cardiorespiratory fitness level and preserves fat-free mass, while diet alone reduces fat-free mass (Amorim et al., 2007)

After birth, women should start exercise slowly beginning with 15 minutes and building up to around 150 minutes a week (aerobic activity). In terms of exercise intensity, women aged 20–29 years should aim to reach a target heart rate of 110–131 beats per minute and women aged 30–39 years 108–124 beats per minute (Mottola, 2009). The 'talk test' is a good indicator as to whether full exercise capacity has been reached, i.e. if women are breathless and cannot talk, it is time to have a rest. Unfortunately, exercise alone without some degree of calorie restriction does not always promote weight loss. Lovelady (2004) has reported that once breastfeeding is well established, overweight women may reduce their daily energy intake by 500 kcal/day without affecting infant growth. This could help to promote a weight loss of 0.5 kg/week. However, women should always seek the advice of a dietician or other health professionals to find out what is best for them as an individual.

New Mothers' Views on Weight and Exercise

Women do appear to be concerned about their weight after birth, although levels of concern seem to vary according to race with Caucasian women placing a greater emphasis on weight while new black and Hispanic mothers were more focused on the how exercise could help improve levels of self-esteem. The most commonly reported barriers to exercise appear to be time constraints and health problems. Walking was seen to be the most appealing form of exercise and many women reported that having a walking partner help to integrate walking within their new daily lifestyles (Groth and David, 2008). Nurses may play an important role in helping to promote the benefits of light activity such as walking and encourage new mothers to look for walking partners.

11.16   Weight loss interventions

Having less time to exercise after birth, low motivation levels and need for extra advice and support can all affect a women's ability to lose pregnancy weight after birth (Montgomery *et al.*, 2010). A handful of studies have tested the efficacy of dietary and physical activity interventions with mixed findings. One study carried out in Taiwan found that individualised dietary and physical activity education plans helped to reduce levels of retention when women were given advice from 16 weeks into pregnancy and support until 6 weeks after birth (Huang *et al.*, 2009). Another intervention trial carried out on a sample of 450 obese women enrolled 6 weeks after birth found that a series of healthy eating and physical activity classes and telephone counselling over a 9-month period had no significant effect on levels of weight loss (Østbye *et al.*, 2009). It was concluded that asking new busy mothers to attend classes may not be feasible and postal, telephone and/or internet/e-mail approaches may be a better way forward. Overall, considerably more work is needed in this area to help establish weight management programmes that are realistic, fun to achieve and lead to results without making women feel pressured.

11.17   Conclusion

Overall, after birth is an extremely busy time physiologically as well having the day-to-day demands of looking after a new baby. The body adapts remarkably well in order to return to its pre-pregnancy state. However, high levels of pregnancy weight and failure to lose this in the busy period after birth can lead to weight retention in the longer term, which could have implications for women's health. Undoubtedly, further work is needed in terms of determining the best weight loss approaches after birth. Certainly, breastfeeding and complying with this for as long as possible is a good way forward. It does, however, seem that certain groups who are particularly susceptible to weight retention, i.e. teenagers who have been pregnant, need a much greater degree of help and support with this.

Key Messages

- Changes in hormone levels after birth can lead to low mood, bowel habit changes and a range of other symptoms after birth.
- After birth, women's bodies adapt remarkably well, helping to revert the body to its pre-pregnancy state.
- The decline in progesterone, rise in prolactin and establishment of the 'let down' reflex all play a key role in the production and secretion of breast milk after birth.
- There is now good evidence that overweight/obese women may experience more difficulties when breastfeeding, leading to lower compliance rates.
- High weight gains in pregnancy coupled with failure to lose excess weight after birth can shift women into the next BMI category, contributing to higher rates of overweight/obesity. This may have implications for women's long-term health.
- The 'reset hypothesis' proposes that breastfeeding can help revert a woman's metabolic profile to normal (otherwise, triglyceride levels and other metabolic markers may remain elevated).
- It is clear that some women may benefit from weight management programmes after birth, but more work is needed to improve the efficacy of these.

Recommended reading

Blackburn ST (2003) *Maternal, Fetal and Neonatal Physiology: A Clinical Perspective*, 2nd edition. WB Saunders: Philadelphia.

Hytten F (1995) *The Clinical Physiology of the Puerperium*. Farrand Press: London.

Stables D and Rankin J (2006) *Physiology in Childbearing*. Elsevier: London.

References

AbuSabha R and Greene G (1998) Body weight, body composition, and energy intake changes in breastfeeding mothers. *Journal of Human Lactation* 14(2), 119–24.

Amir LH and Donath S (2007) A systematic review of maternal obesity and breastfeeding intention, initiation and duration. *BMC Pregnancy Childbirth* 7, 9.

Amorim AR, Linne YM and Lourenco PM (2007) Diet or exercise, or both, for weight reduction in women after childbirth. *Cochrane Database of Systematic Reviews* 3, CD005627

Arthur PG, Kent JC, Potter JM and Hartmann PE (1991) Lactose in blood in nonpregnant, pregnant and lactating women. *Journal of Pediatric Gastroenterology & Nutrition* 13, 254–9.

Asher I, Kaplan B, Modai I, Neri A, Valevski A and Weizman A (1995) Mood and hormonal changes during late pregnancy and puerperium. *Clinical & Experimental Obstetrics & Gynecology* 22(4), 321–5.

Aydin S, Aydin S, Ozkan Y and Kumru S (2006) Ghrelin is present in human colostrum, transitional and mature milk. *Peptides* 27(4), 878–82.

Baker JL, Gamborg M, Heitmann BL, Lissner L, Sørensen TI and Rasmussen KM (2008) Breastfeeding reduces postpartum weight retention. *American Journal of Clinical Nutrition* 88(6), 1543–51.

Bauer J and Gerss J (2010) Longitudinal analysis of macronutrients and minerals in human milk produced by mothers of preterm infants. *Clinical Nutrition* [Epub ahead of print].

Beard JL, Hendricks MK, Perez EM *et al.* (2005) Maternal iron deficiency anemia affects postpartum emotions and cognition. *Journal of Nutrition* 135(2), 267–72.

Bodnar LM, Cogswell ME and Scanlon KS (2002) Low income postpartum women are at risk of iron deficiency. *Journal of Nutrition* 132(8), 2298–302.

Borja-Hart NL and Marino J (2010) Role of omega-3 fatty acids for prevention or treatment of perinatal depression. *Pharmacotherapy* 30(2), 210–6.

Burt VK and Stein K (2002) Epidemiology of depression throughout the female life cycle. *Journal of Clinical Psychiatry*. 63 Suppl 7, 9–15.

Chen DC, Nommsen-Rivers L, Dewey KG and Lönnerdal B (1998) Stress during labor and delivery and early lactation performance. *American Journal of Clinical Nutrition* 68(2), 335–44.

Corman ML (1985) Anal incontinence following obstetrical injury. *Diseases of the Colon and Rectum* 28, 86–9.

Corwin EJ, Arbour M (2007) Postpartum fatigue and evidence-based interventions. *MCN American Journal of Maternal/Child Nursing* 32(4), 215–20.

Daly SE, Di Rosso A, Owens RA and Hartmann PE (1993b) Degree of breast emptying explains changes in the fat content, but not fatty acid composition, of human milk. *Experimental Physiology* 78(6), 741–55.

Daly SE, Owens RA and Hartmann PE (1993a) The short-term synthesis and infant-regulated removal of milk in lactating women. *Experimental Physiology* 78(2), 209–20.

Derbyshire EJ, Davies J and Dettmar P (2007) Changes in bowel function: pregnancy and the puerperium. *Digestive Diseases & Sciences* 52, 324–8.

Dodd J, Dare MR and Middleton P (2004) Treatment for women with postpartum iron deficiency anaemia. *Cochrane Database of Systematic Reviews* 4, CD004222.

Doneray H, Orbak Z and Yildiz L (2009) The relationship between breast milk leptin and neonatal weight gain. *Acta Paediatrics* 98(4), 643–7.

Dritsa M, Da Costa D, Dupuis G, Lowensteyn I and Khalifé S (2009) Effects of a home-based exercise intervention on fatigue in postpartum depressed women: results of a randomized controlled trial. *Annals of Behavioural Medicine* 35(2), 179–87.

Fan F, Zou Y, Ma A, Yue Y, Mao W and Ma X (2009) Hormonal changes and somatopsychologic manifestations in the first trimester of pregnancy and postpartum. *International Journal of Gynaecology & Obstetrics* 105, 46–9.

Ferrari RM, Siega-Riz AM, Evenson KR, Moos MK, Melvin CL and Herring AH (2010) Provider advice about weight loss and physical activity in the postpartum period. *Journal of Women's Health (Larchmt)* **19**(3), 397–406.

Fidler N and Koletzko B (2000) The fatty acid composition of human colostrum. *European Journal of Nutrition* **39**(1), 31–7.

Glasier A and McNeilly AS (1990) Physiology of lactation. *Bailliere's Clinical Endocrinology & Metabolism* **4**(2), 379–95.

Groth SW and David T (2008) New mothers' views of weight and exercise. *MCN American Journal of Maternal/Child Nursing* **33**(6), 364–70.

Hanson LA (2007) Session 1: feeding and infant development breast-feeding and immune function. *Proceedings of the Nutrition Society* **66**, 384–96.

Hohlagschwandtner M, Husslein P, Klier C and Ulm B (2001) Correlation between serum testosterone levels and peripartal mood states. *Acta Obstetricia et Gynecologica Scandinavica* **80**(4), 326–30.

Huang TT, Yeh CY and Tsai YC (2009) A diet and physical activity intervention for preventing weight retention among Taiwanese childbearing women: a randomised controlled trial. *Midwifery* [Epub ahead of print].

Hytten F (1995) *The Clinical Physiology of the Puerperium*. Farrand Press: London.

Jevitt C, Hernandez I and Groër M (2007) Lactation complicated by overweight and obesity: supporting the mother and newborn. *Journal of Midwifery Women's Health* **52**(6), 606–13.

Jones E and Spencer SA (2007) The physiology of lactation. *Pediatrics and Child Health* **17**(6), 244–8.

Kent JC, Mitoulas LR, Cregan MD, Ramsay DT, Doherty DA and Hartmann PE (2006) Volume and frequency of breastfeeding and fat content of breast milk throughout the day. *Pediatrics* **117**(3), e387–95.

Linné Y, Barkeling B and Rössner S (2002) Long-term weight development after pregnancy. *Obesity Reviews* **3**(2), 75–83.

Lipworth L, Bailey LR and Trichopoulos D (2000) History of breast-feeding in relation to breast cancer risk: a review of the epidemiologic literature. *Journal of the National Cancer Institute* **92**(4), 302–12.

Lovelady CA (2004) The impact of energy restriction and exercise in lactating women. *Advances in Experimental Medicine & Biology* **554**, 115–20.

Marchant S, Alexander J, Garcia J, Ashurst H, Alderdice F and Keene J (1999) A survey of women's experiences of vaginal loss from 24 hours to three months after childbirth (the BLiPP study). *Midwifery* **15**(2), 72–81.

Mennella J (2001) Alcohol's effect on lactation. *Alcohol Research & Health* **25**(3), 230–4.

Montgomery KS, Bushee TD, Phillips JD *et al.* (2010) Women's challenges with postpartum weight loss. *Maternal & Child Health Journal* [Epub ahead of print].

Mottola MF (2009) Exercise prescription for overweight and obese women: pregnancy and postpartum. *Obstetrics & Gynaecology Clinics of North America* **36**(2), 301–16.

Nasta MT, Grussu P, Quataro RM, Cerutti R and Grella PV (2002) Cholesterol and mood states at 3 days after delivery. *Journal of Psychosomatic Research* **52**(2), 61–3.

NRC/IoM (National Research Council and the Institute of Medicine) (2007) *Influence of Pregnancy Weight on Maternal and Child Health. Workshop Report. Committee on the Impact of Pregnancy Weight on Maternal and Child Health. Board on Children, Youth, and Families, Division of Behavioural and Social Sciences and Education and Food and Nutrition Board.* The National Academies Press: Washington, DC.

Neville MC, Keller R, Seacat J *et al.* (1988) Studies in human lactation: milk volumes in lactating women during the onset of lactation and full lactation. *American Journal of Clinical Nutrition* **48**(6), 1375–86.

Neville MC, McFadden TB and Forsyth I (2002) Hormonal regulation of mammary differentiation and milk secretion. *Journal of Mammary Gland Biology and Neoplasia.* **7**(1), 49–66.

Neville MC and Morton J (2001) Physiology and endocrine changes underlying human lactogenesis II. *Journal of Nutrition* **131**(11), 3005S–8S.

Neville MC, Morton J and Umemura S (2001) Lactogenesis. The transition from pregnancy to lactation. *Pediatric Clinics of North America* **48**(1), 35–52.

Nierop A, Bratsikas A, Zimmermann R and Ehlert U (2006) Are stress-induced cortisol changes during pregnancy associated with postpartum depressive symptoms? *Psychosomatic Medicine* 68(6), 931–7.

Nommsen-Rivers LA, Chantry CJ, Peerson JM, Cohen RJ and Dewey KG (2010) Delayed onset of lactogenesis among first-time mothers is related to maternal obesity and factors associated with ineffective breastfeeding. *American Journal of Clinical Nutrition* 92(3), 574–84.

Ohnemus U, Uenalan M, Inzunza J, Gustafsson JA and Paus R (2006) The hair follicle as an estrogen target and source. *Endocrine Reviews* 27(6), 677–706.

Okechukwu AA, Okpe EC and Okolo AA (2009) Exclusive breastfeeding and postnatal changes in maternal anthropometry. *Nigerian Journal of Clinical Practice* 12(4), 383–8.

Østbye T, Krause KM, Lovelady CA et al. (2009) Active mothers postpartum: a randomized controlled weight-loss intervention trial. *American Journal of Preventative Medicine* 37 173–80.

Parker KJ, Kenna HA, Zeitzer JM et al. (2010) Preliminary evidence that plasma oxytocin levels are elevated in major depression. *Psychiatry Research* 178(2), 359–62.

Pedersen P, Baker JL, Henriksen TB, Lissner L, Heitmann BL, Sørensen TI and Nohr EA (2011) Influence of psychosocial factors on postpartum weight retention. *Obesity (Silver Spring).* 19(3), 639–46.

Peng Y, Zhou T, Wang Q et al. (2009) Fatty acid composition of diet, cord blood and breast milk in Chinese mothers with different dietary habits. *Prostaglandins Leukotrines Fatty Acids* 81(5–6), 325–30.

Rakicioğlu N, Samur G, Topçu A and Topçu AA (2006) The effect of Ramadan on maternal nutrition and composition of breast milk. *Pediatrics International* 48(3), 278–83.

Rasmussen, Kjolhede 2004 Rasmussen KM and Kjolhede CL (2004) Prepregnant overweight and obesity diminish the prolactin response to suckling in the first week postpartum. *Pediatrics* 113(5), e465–71.

Saadeh R and Benbouzid D (1990) Breast-feeding and child-spacing: importance of information collection for public health policy. *Bulletin of the World Health Organisation* 68(5), 625–31.

Santoro W Jr, Martinez FE, Ricco RG and Jorge SM (2010) Colostrum ingested during the first day of life by exclusively breastfed healthy newborn infants. *Journal of Pediatrics* 156(1), 29–32.

Saultz JW, Toffler WL and Shackles JY (1991) Postpartum urinary retention. *Journal of the American Board of Family Practice* 4(5), 341–4.

Schwartz MA, Wang CC, Eckert LO and Critchlow CW (1999) Risk factors for urinary tract infection in the postpartum period. *American Journal of Obstetrics & Gynaecology* 181(3), 547–53.

Sebire NJ, Jolly M, Harris JP et al. (2001) Maternal obesity and pregnancy outcome: a study of 287,213 pregnancies in London. *International Journal of Obesity Related Metabolic Disorders* 25(8), 1175–82.

Siega-Riz AM, Herring AH, Carrier K, Evenson KR, Dole N and Deierlein A (2010) Sociodemographic, perinatal, behavioral, and psychosocial predictors of weight retention at 3 and 12 months postpartum. *Obesity (Silver Spring)* 18(10), 1996–2003.

Spear HJ (2006) Breastfeeding behaviors and experiences of adolescent mothers. *MCN American Journal of Maternal/Child Nursing* 31(2), 106–13.

Stables D and Rankin J (2006) *Physiology in Childbearing*. Elsevier: London.

Stettler N, Stallings VA, Troxel AB et al. (2005) Weight gain in the first week of life and overweight in adulthood: a cohort study of European American subjects fed infant formula. *Circulation* 111(15), 1897–903.

Stuebe AM and Rich-Edwards JW (2009) The reset hypothesis: lactation and maternal metabolism. *American Journal of Perinatology* 26(1), 81–8.

Sultan AH, Kamm MA, Hudson CN, Thomas JM and Batram CI (1993) Anal sphincter disruption during vaginal delivery. *New England Journal of Medicine* 329, 1905–11.

Thame MM, Jackson MD, Manswell IP, Osmond C and Antoine MG (2010) Weight retention within the puerperium in adolescents: a risk factor for obesity? *Public Health Nutrition* 13(2), 283–8.

Troisi A, Moles A, Panepuccia L, Lo Russo D, Palla G and Scucchi S (2002) Serum cholesterol levels and mood symptoms in the postpartum period. *Psychiatry Research* 109(3), 213–9.

Usha Kiran TS, Hemmadi S, Bethel J and Evans J (2005) Outcome of pregnancy in a woman with an increased body mass index. *British Journal of Obstetrics & Gynaecology* 112(6), 768–72.

Winkvist A and Rasmussen KM (1999) Impact of lactation on maternal body weight and body composition. *Journal of Mammary Gland Biology & Neoplasia* 4(3), 309–18.

Wise DD, Felker A and Stahl SM (2008) Tailoring treatment of depression for women across the reproductive lifecycle: the importance of pregnancy, vasomotor symptoms, and other estrogen-related events in psychopharmacology. *CNS Spectrums* 13(8), 647–62.

Yang L and Jacobsen KH (2008) A systematic review of the association between breastfeeding and breast cancer. *Journal of Women's Health (Larchmt)* 17(10), 1635–45.

Zarban A, Taheri F, Chahkandi T, Sharifzadeh G and Khorashadizadeh M (2009) Antioxidant and radical scavenging activity of human colostrum, transitional and mature milk. *Journal of Clinical Biochemistry & Nutrition* 45(2), 150–4.

Zonana J and Gorman JM (2005) The neurobiology of postpartum depression. *CNS Spectrums* 10(10), 792–9, 805.

Zou Y, Fan F, Ma A, Yue Y, Mao W and Ma X (2009) Hormonal changes and somatopsychologic manifestations in the first trimester of pregnancy and post partum. *International Journal of Gynaecology & Obstetrics* 105(1), 46–9.

12 Nutrition after Birth

Summary

Getting the diet right after birth is just as important as before or during pregnancy. A diet adequate in the right nutrients can help to replenish nutrition stores, optimise the nutrition quality of breast milk and support the health of both mother and child. Women need to be supported and guided about how to maintain a balanced, nutritious diet at such a busy and important life phase, especially as healthy eating practices can be embedded in children during the early years. Breastfeeding should be encouraged and the full health benefits (for both mother and child) should continue to be promoted. Many women may breastfeed initially, but rates decline rapidly after birth, particularly in Western mothers. Ideally, women should try to feed their infants 'exclusively', i.e. with breast milk alone for 6 months before weaning should take place. New foods should then be introduced to infants diets gradually alongside breastfeeding. Ongoing support strategies and health campaigns are needed to help support women with breastfeeding during this important time of life.

Learning Outcomes

- To express the importance of breastfeeding and describe why many new mothers discontinue this before 6 months.
- To explain which nutrients are particularly important after birth and how dietary targets can be achieved.
- To describe the link between maternal diet/nutrition status and risk of postnatal depression (PND) after birth.
- To demonstrate that encouraging healthy eating practices in early life help to improve food choices in the next generation.

12.1 Introduction

Some of the key dietary changes that should be made during pregnancy i.e. to increase folic acid intake may be practised by some mothers but the importance of tailoring the diet after birth is not an area that is as well communicated or understood. For example, one study of full-time working mothers found that although 39% reported drinking more fluids after birth, other dietary changes were largely unfounded. Twenty-five percent of mothers ate more sweet foods to help increase milk production and 29% avoided dried legumes and grains as these were thought to be linked to colic (Kulakca *et al.*, 2006). This is a good example of how health messages can easily become confused and although some dietary changes appear to be being made, these are not necessarily the right ones.

Similar confusion seems to be apparent when it comes to breastfeeding guidelines. Findings from the latest Infant Feeding Survey showed that new mothers seem to understand that breastfeeding has health benefits but a large proportion (about 75%) of women stop feeding before the 6 months (Bolling *et al.*, 2007). This is an area that is discussed in detail in later sections but is certainly an area that warrants further attention from a public health perspective.

Taken together, the aims of this chapter are to provide evidence-based guidance about how women may benefit from adapting their diets after birth. Areas of possible confusion will hopefully become clearer and guidelines provided where appropriate. This chapter also addresses some of the health problems that can arise after birth, such as PND and discusses the nutrition evidence related to this medical condition.

12.2   Is breast best?

Breast is best because as well as having economic advantages, i.e. it is free, there is good evidence that it benefits both maternal and infant health (Table 12.1). For the women living in developed regions, breastfeeding has been associated with reduced diabetes, breast and ovarian cancer risk. For infants, the consumption of breast milk may help to protect against infections, asthma, obesity and diabetes development, amongst other medical conditions (Ip *et al.*, 2007). There is also good evidence from review papers showing that infants from developing regions who are not breastfed have mortality rates that are up to ten times higher than that of breastfed infants (Bahl *et al.*, 2005). The risk of both diarrhoea and lower respiratory tract infections have both been found to be significantly lower in infants who are breastfed when compared to those receiving artificial feeds (Quigley *et al.*, 2009).

Table 12.1   Why is breast best?

Mother	Infant
Reduced risk of	
Premenopausal breast cancer	Morbidity
Ovarian cancer	Childhood obesity
Retained pregnancy weight gain	Type 1 and 2 diabetes
Type 2 diabetes	Leukaemia
Myocardial infarction	Sudden infant death syndrome
Metabolic syndrome	

Source: Points extracted from Stuebe (2009).

Table 12.2   Average nutrient content of milk.

Per 100 mL of milk	Human milk	Cow's milk	Formula milk
Energy (kcal)	70	61	78
Fat (g)	4.4	3.3	4.2
Protein (g)	1.0	3.2	2.1
Carbohydrate (g)	6.9	4.8	7.8
Calcium (mg)	32	113	163
Vitamin D (μg)	0.1	0.1	2.9
Iron (mg)	0.03	0.03	0.3
Folate (μg)	5	5	29

Source: USDA National Nutrient Database for Standard Reference.

The view that breastfeeding is best for the baby is supported by a number of different expert bodies including the WHO, UNICEF and Australia's NHMRC. However, for women and their children to get the full health benefits of breastfeeding, it is important this it continued after birth. This is an important notion that will be discussed in later sections within this chapter.

12.3   What's in breast milk?

Breast milk provides all the energy and nutrients that a growing baby needs, as well as important antibacterial and immune supporting agents. The composition of breast milk changes with time after birth. As can be seen in Table 12.2, breast milk is a good source of fatty acids, carbohydrate, calcium and folate but has a lower energy and protein content when compared with formula milk. The lower protein content of breast milk has been linked to the '*Early Protein Hypothesis*', a theory that proposes that the lower protein content of breast milk can help to normalise infant growth and reduce the likelihood of high weight gain in infancy. To test this theory, the European Childhood Obesity Trial Study Group recruited over 1000 infants from five European countries and randomised them to receive a high or low protein infant formula. After two years, results showed that the low protein formula helped to normalise infant growth (Koletzko *et al.*, 2009).

12.4   Breastfeeding – for how long?

In the past, the optimal duration of exclusive breastfeeding, i.e. breastfeeding alone (see Table 12.3 for definitions) has been subject to much debate. The World Health Organisation revised their guidelines in 2001 after a thorough systematic review of over 3000 scientific papers was carried out (Kramer and Kakuma, 2001). The findings of the report identified that exclusive breastfeeding for the first six months (180 days) of an infants' life should be recommended for maximum health benefits. Since then, even more research has been published, further supporting the health benefits of breastfeeding. Given the fact that there is so much strong evidence in this area, these guidelines have been supported and adopted by both the UK Scientific Advisory Committee on Nutrition and Department of Health. The Department of Health's latest recommendations on feeding infants are summarised in Table 12.4.

Table 12.3   Breastfeeding terminology.

Feeding method	Definition	Source
Exclusive breastfeeding	When an infant receives only breast milk from his/her mother or wet nurse, or expressed milk, and no other liquids or solids, not even water with the exception of vitamin mineral supplements or medicines.	WHO/UNICEF/USAID (2008)
Complementary feeding	When breast milk is no longer sufficient to meet the nutritional requirements of infants and other foods/liquids are needed along with breast milk. Ideally complementary feeding should take place between 6 to 23 months of age.	PAHO/WHO (2002)

Research Highlight   Confusion over weaning times

The World Health Organisation advises that women feed their infant exclusively for 6 months and start introducing solid foods into the infant's diet after this. This should help to give the infant a good start in life, fending off infections, protecting against the development of medical conditions and helping the mother to lose her baby weight after birth.

A new study carried out in Ireland monitored the breastfeeding habits of 401 mothers, to see if these guidelines were being followed (Tarrant *et al.,* 2010a). Just 0.2% mothers followed these 6-months recommendation whilst 23% of infants were weaned early (before 3 months). The same author also carried out similar research in Hong Kong and found that breastfeeding rates were higher with 27% and 37% of mothers feeding their infants for at least 6 and 3 months, respectively (Tarrant *et al.,* 2010b). This suggests that breastfeeding promotion programmes seem to be working in this region and may be worth using in Ireland. Women still, however, need further support and guidance when it comes to breastfeeding their infants exclusively and sustaining this for the ideal 6 months. More work may be needed to improve compliance with these important guidelines that have been established with the intention of optimising infant health.

Table 12.4   Infant feeding recommendations.

Exclusive breastfeeding is recommended for the first six months (26 weeks) of an infant's life.

Six months is the recommended age for the introduction of solid foods for infants.

Breastfeeding (and/or breast milk substitutes, if used) should continue beyond the first six months, along with appropriate types and amounts of solid foods.

Every infant is different and should be managed individually so that insufficient growth or other adverse health outcomes are not ignored and appropriate advice is provided.

Source: DH (2010).

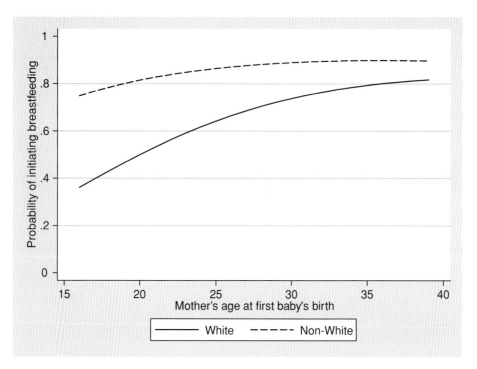

Figure 12.1 Probability of initiating breastfeeding for white and non-white mothers in England by maternal age. (Griffiths *et al.* (2005), with permission.) Graph created using logistic regression. (Griffiths *et al.* (2005), with permission.)

12.5   Who is breastfeeding?

Research conducted at the Institute of Child Health, London, studied the breastfeeding habits of 11,286 natural UK mothers 9 months after birth. Findings were similar to those from the Infant Feeding Survey. Older women with more academic qualifications were more likely to breastfeed. White mothers (Figure 12.1), those already with children, younger mothers and women in routine occupations or living in deprived areas were most likely to breastfeed their infants.

This study showed that cultural influences can have a positive impact on the rate and length of breastfeeding. Having a partner from a different ethnic group had a positive effect on breastfeeding initiation and continuation (for the first month after birth). Interestingly, lone mothers living in high ethnic minority community were also more likely to start breastfeeding (Griffiths *et al.*, 2005).

These are very important results that have wider implications. Health initiatives, training of health professionals, media campaigns and health interventions have all been found to be effective in helping to promote breastfeeding (Protheroe *et al.*, 2003). The findings from this research indicate that there may be a role for 'peer programmes' where women from multi-ethnic communities could help mentor and encourage women to breastfeed their infants. Younger mothers may equally benefit from these programmes as breastfeeding rates are lower in this generation of women also. These are certainly areas that warrant further exploration.

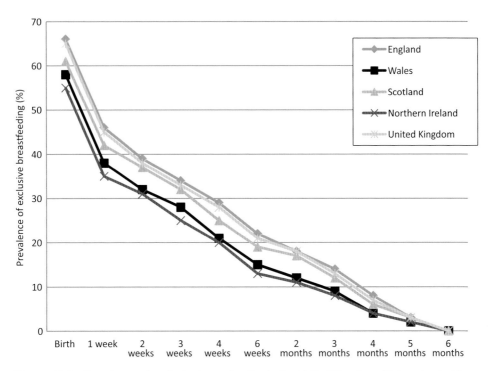

Figure 12.2 Prevalence of exclusive breastfeeding in the United Kingdom. (Data extracted from Bolling *et al.* (2007).)

12.6   Infant feeding survey

The main aim of this survey is to provide data on the incidence, prevalence and duration of both breastfeeding as well as other feeding practices after birth. The survey analyses data for all for countries in the United Kingdom as well as the United Kingdom as a whole.

Findings from the latest survey, a sample of over 9000 mothers, show that rates of breastfeeding may be high initially, but these declined rapidly after birth (Figure 12.2). Once again, older (≤30 years), working, professional mothers are more likely to breastfeed their infants. In terms of knowledge base, it was interesting to see that although 84% mothers were aware of the health benefits of breastfeeding, 75% women stopped feeding before 6 months. This is worrying considering that infants breastfed for longer were less likely to experience colic, constipation, sickness/vomiting, diarrhoea, chest infections and thrush, whilst infants formula-fed from birth had the highest rates of chest infections and thrush (Bolling *et al.*, 2007),

12.7   Why do women stop breastfeeding?

Rates of breastfeeding may be high initially but fall quickly, particularly amongst Western mothers. Recent data from Japan also showed that 95% of new mums intended to breastfeed their child after delivery, but in reality only 42% (about half of mothers) breastfed their infants one month after birth (Haku, 2007).

Table 12.5 Factors affecting breastfeeding rates.

Factors	Reason
Employment	Working mothers breastfeed for shorter periods or not at all.
Overweight/obese	Reduced prolactin response means that milk is not easily produced.
Postnatal depression	Depression inhibits the 'let down reflex', reducing milk supply.
Smoking	Smokers tend to not breastfeed or discontinue breastfeeding.
Socio-economic status	Rates of breastfeeding are positively associated with socio-economic status in most developed countries. In developing regions, higher income women may perceive breastfeeding as old fashioned and bottle-feeding may be seen as being modern and 'westernised'.
Sore nipples	A common cause of stopping of breastfeeding. Women should be guided about good feeding techniques to prevent this problem. There is some evidence that rubbing breast milk into nipples can help to promote wound healing (Mohammadzadeh et al., 2005). This is certainly worth trying if it helps women to feed longer.
Support	Support strategies through health services as well as from a partner help to encourage breastfeeding.

Source: Key points extracted from Haku (2007).

There are many reasons why women stop breastfeeding their infants early (Table 12.5). Some mothers would like to breastfeed their children for longer, but work commitments, problems producing milk, need for support strategies and painful experiences often affect compliance. This can lead to feelings of guilt, an area of common concern for physicians and medical practitioners (see Labbok, 2008, for full review). Research has shown that support from partners and family members can help to play a key role in encouraging mothers to take up and continue breastfeeding. Such support systems now need to overspill into work practices and the community (Clifford and McIntyre, 2008).

Research Highlight   Bottle-feeding experiences

Scientists from the Medical Research Council, Cambridge, evaluated findings from other 23 scientific papers to gather women's thoughts and experiences when they can do bottle-feed their infants. After evaluating the findings from the papers, it became apparent that a large portion of women felt guilty, angry, as though they were failing and were concerned about their infants' health when they stopped breastfeeding. It was also evident that very little information was available for women who chose or went on to bottle-feed their infants, which led to mistakes when preparing the feeds (Lakshman *et al.,* 2009).

Similar findings have also been observed amongst mothers taking part in the Infant Feeding Survey. Just under half of mothers did not follow guidelines, i.e. using cooled boiled water when preparing bottle-feeds and water was not always added to the bottle before the powder and around one-third of mothers did not keep pre-prepared formula chilled (Bolling *et al.,* 2007). Taking these findings as a whole, it seems that bottle-feeding mothers may need extra help and guidance when it comes to preparing infant feeds. As with breastfeeding, this will also benefit the infant in the short and longer term.

12.8   Feeding and infant growth

Understanding normal growth patterns for infants is important to both support and promote child health. It is, however, important to be aware that breastfed and formula-fed infants have very different growth patterns. Initially, breastfed infants lose more weight after birth and take longer to regain their birth weight compared with formula-fed infants. This is because breast milk has a lower energy and protein content and feed supplies can be limited. In contrast, infants receiving bottle-feeds can suckle an unlimited supply of milk from their bottle, which can lead to higher energy intakes and levels of weight gain (Nommsen-Rivers and Dewey, 2009). It is thought that these may be key factors leading to rapid weight gain after birth and increased risk of chronic disease several decades later (Stettler et al., 2005).

12.8.1   Growth charts

These differences in growth patterns between breastfed and bottle-fed infants have recently led scientists to rethink the way that infant growth charts have been compiled. Previously, growth references and standards have been based on infants receiving human milk substitutes. This is now not thought to be the best representation of infant growth and has been replaced by new standards published by the World Health Organisation in 2006. These are based on patterns of weight gain in a large sample of breastfed infants raised in environments that minimised constraints to growth, such as poor diets and infection. These standards now explicitly identify breastfeeding as the biological norm and as the new standard model for growth and development (Onis et al., 2008). It is hoped that these new growth velocity standards will be a more accurate way to monitor patterns of infant weight gain and growth, helping to prevent early excess weight gain.

12.9   Dietary requirements after birth

Women's nutrient requirements increase for several nutrients in the period after birth. It is important that women continue to eat a healthy, balanced diet as this is reflected in the quality of their breast milk. In the UK dietary guidelines for mothers after birth are in need of some revision as a wealth of new information and research has become available since these were first compiled in 1991. For now, however, these remain to act as a useful guide (Table 12.6) until the European Food Safety Authority publishes new guidelines, which are greatly awaited. Overall, a healthy, balanced diet should provide adequate levels of most nutrients, but for new mothers, the cost of purchasing the right foods, lack of knowledge about what constitutes a healthful, balanced diet and the time needed to prepare foods can mean that intakes are not what they should be.

12.9.1   Energy

It is important that new mothers consume a diet that provides enough energy to support the production of milk. Breastfeeding is an energy demanding process

Table 12.6 Dietary reference values (DRVs) for breastfeeding mothers.

Nutrient (per day)	Non-pregnant woman (19–40 years)	Lactation (0–4 months)	<4 months
Energy (kcal)	1940	+450 1st month +530 2nd month +570 3rd month	+570 if breastfeeding exclusively +480 if complementary milk are provided in addition to breastfeeding
Protein (g)	45	+11	+8
Calcium (mg)	700	+550	+550
Iodine (μg)	1.1	–	–
Copper (mg)	1.2	+0.3	+0.3
Iron (mg)	14.8	–	–
Selenium (μg)	60	+15	+15
Zinc (mg)	7.0	+6.0	+2.5
Vitamin A (μg)	600	+350	+350
Thiamine (vitamin B_1) (mg)	0.8	+0.2	+0.2
Riboflavin (vitamin B_2) (mg)	1.1	+0.5	+0.5
Niacin (vitamin B3) (mg)	13	+2.0	+2.0
Cobalamin (vitamin B_{12}) (μg)	1.5	+0.5	+0.5
Folate (μg)	200	+60	+60
Vitamin C (mg)	40	+30	+30
Vitamin D (μg)	No RNI	+10	+10

Source: DH (1991).
RNI, reference nutrient intake; (–) indicates no increment.

that can help to facilitate weight loss after birth via the mobilisation of fat stores. On average, milk production requires an extra 500 calories a day, which can be met through the diet, mobilisation of fat reserves and changes in metabolic rate (Theobald, 2007). Although this is a useful guide, this may be slightly higher or lower for certain women. For example, women exclusively breastfeeding their child will have higher energy requirements than mothers carrying out 1–2 feeds per day. Equally, women with a lower body mass index (BMI) and/or fat reserves also generally have higher calorie requirements (maternal fat stores provide around 200 calories per day towards lactation).

There is some evidence from animal studies to show that low-fat diets can improve milk production by as much as 50% in obese rats, but food restriction can lead to cessation of milk production (Rasmussen *et al.*, 2001). Although human trials are needed, women should be advised that weight loss will occur naturally if they are breastfeeding and not consuming excess calories. It should also be emphasised that diets based on food restriction are not the best way forward at this point in time, as this may restrict milk production and impact upon the nutritional quality of the breast milk.

Table 12.7 Recommendations of EPA and DHA for pregnant and lactating mothers.

	Average nutrient requirement	Upper nutrient limit
DHA	200 mg/day	1.0 g/day*
DHA + EPA	300 mg/day†	2.7 g/day*
Industrial trans fatty acids	–	As low as practical

Source: Brenna and Lapillonne (2009), with permission.
*No observed effect in RCT.
†Based on adult average nutrient requirement plus an increment for energy demands of pregnancy.

12.9.2 Omega-3 fatty acids

Omega-3 fatty acids include alpha linoleic acid (ALA), eicosapentaenoic acid (EPA) and docosahexaenoic acid (DHA). ALA, the parent fatty acid, can be converted to EPA and DHA through a series of enzymatic metabolic pathways. However, omega-6 fatty acids compete for the same enzymes. This means that diet higher in omega-6 fats (which Western diets usually are) can block and slow the metabolic production of EPA and DHA (Surette, 2008). This is of concern in pregnancy and after birth as omega-3 fats are needed to ensure optimal brain and cognitive development of the infant.

One pioneering meta-analysis of 65 studies found that breast milk only contains around 0.32% DHA although women from coastal regions eating more fish secrete higher levels (Brenna *et al.*, 2007). To achieve this level of DHA in breast milk, regression analysis has shown that women need intakes of at least 167 mg/day of DHA. On the basis of these considerations, it is advised that the average nutrient requirement for both pregnant and lactating mothers should be set at 200 mg/DHA/day, rounded for ease of use (Brenna and Lapillonne, 2009; also see Table 12.7). As can be seen from Figure 12.3, regression analysis clearly demonstrates that the dose of

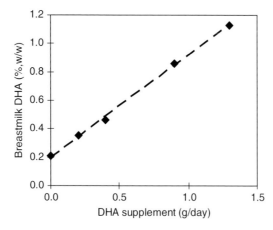

Figure 12.3 Regression analysis of breastmilk DHA (B) concentration vs. DHA intake (I). $B = (0.72 \times I) + 0.20$ ($r^2 = 0.998$). (Brenna and Lapillone, 2009.)

DHA ingested is directly proportional to the percentage of DHA in breast milk; with intakes of up to 1.5 g/day, leading to the highest concentrations.

It is also important to consider that as medical conditions such as diabetes and certain diets, i.e. vegetarian, vegan or even macrobiotic diets, may also alter the fatty acid profile of the mother's milk if they do not include seafood. Women who choose to make these dietary choices are therefore advised to monitor their omega-3 (DHA and EPA) intakes during and after pregnancy, especially if breastfeeding (Bourre, 2007).

12.9.3   Vitamin A

If breastfeeding mothers are not getting enough vitamin A from dietary sources, supplies to the newborn will also be inadequate. The American Pediatric Association claims that vitamin A is one of the most important vitamins in the breastfeeding period. This vitamin is needed for the growth and differentiation of cells and tissues and plays a key role in infant development, particularly in helping the lungs to mature (Strobel et al., 2007).

Generally, vitamin A and beta-carotene-rich foods are widely available from the diet. Orange and dark green leafy vegetables are a good source of beta-carotene, but not all women have access to such foods. This includes regions such as Pakistan, where vitamin A deficiency is prevalent. To promote infant health, the Ministry of Health in Pakistan is looking towards providing women with vitamin A supplements after birth to help replenish stores, improve the quality of women's breast milk and subsequent delivery to the infant (Siddiqi and Igbal, 2008).

12.9.4   Vitamin D

It is important that both women and infants get enough vitamin D after birth. In infancy, low vitamin D levels may lead to poor postnatal growth, hypocalcaemia and fragile bones and the development of autoimmune diseases (Mulligan et al., 2010).

Exclusive breastfeeding is recommended for the first 6 months after birth. However, it has now come to light that breast milk may not provide vitamin D in proportions needed for infant growth; infants with serum vitamin D levels below 50 nmol/L have an increased risk of rickets. This is particularly the case in countries with low latitudes (such as the United Kingdom) or where exposure to sunlight is limited for cultural reasons (Greer, 2008). The current recommended nutrient intake for pregnant and breastfeeding women is 10 µg (400 IU) vitamin D a day (DH, 1998) and for the most women, supplements will be needed to attain these levels of intake (SACN, 2007). However, NICE guidance on antenatal care recommended that, in the absence of evidence of benefit, vitamin D supplements should not be offered routinely to pregnant women (NICE, 2003).

Overall, vitamin D deficiency is not uncommon in infancy, which seems to be attributed to reduced sunlight exposures and low maternal dietary intakes. Both nationally and internationally, there is a clear need to revisit vitamin D recommendations for pregnant and lactating mothers, particularly mothers with higher levels of skin pigmentation or with limited sunlight exposure.

12.9.5   Calcium

Calcium is needed both during pregnancy but also after birth for maternal bone health. During these life phases, there is often a reduction in bone density and increased rates of bone resorption, particularly in the later stages of pregnancy and when breastfeeding. Yet, for many women, particularly teenagers and low-income mothers intakes of calcium from dietary sources do not meet dietary targets (Ruxton and Derbyshire, 2010).

Studies indicate that calcium consumption should be encouraged, to help replace maternal skeletal calcium stores that are depleted during these periods. Because the young infant through breastfeeding is dependent on mother's sources for calcium, an adequate maternal calcium intake can also have a positive effect on foetal bone health (Lowdon, 2008). Calcium can be attained through the diet by the consumption of dairy products or leafy greens (such as kale), the consumption of fortified foods, or from supplement sources (Thomas and Weisman, 2006).

Research Highlight   Drinking milk can help improve nutrient intakes in lactating mothers

Canadian researchers have compared the diet quality of mothers who drank milk or restricted their intake of milk (drank less than 250 mL/day) when breastfeeding their infants exclusively. Drinking milk helped women to meet protein requirements, as well as providing an important source of nutrients, including calcium, thiamine, riboflavin and zinc (Mannion *et al.,* 2007). Overall, women may benefit from drinking milk daily after birth, especially when breastfeeding. For those choosing not to drink milk, nutrients should be provided from other dietary sources or supplements.

12.9.6   Iron

After pregnancy, red cell mass contracts, helping iron stores return to normal, the return of the menstrual cycle is delayed and only a small amount of iron is secreted in breast milk (Food and Nutrition Board, 1990). Together, these physiologic changes should help to protect new mothers against iron deficiency, but unfortunately this is not always the enough.

Iron deficiency after birth (in mother and infant) can stem from the mother having inadequate iron stores before and during pregnancy, but also factors such as the diet providing iron that is not readily bio-available and medical complications including inflammation and infection (Lozoff *et al.,* 2006). Although further studies are needed, research carried out at Harvard Medical School found that infants with iron deficiency (defined a haemoglobin levels <110 g/L + two other abnormal markers of iron status) had signs of reduced cognitive function – objects were not recognised or retrieved as well as though with sufficient iron reserves (Carter *et al.,* 2010).

Women should be encouraged to consume foods that provide iron in a form that can be readily absorbed. Eating lean red meat and drinking orange juice with meals can help increase intestinal iron absorption. Equally, taking a multivitamin or consuming foods fortified with iron can go some way to improving iron status. Prevention is better than cure so making sure iron stores are adequate before conception and during pregnancy can help to prevent iron deficiency in infancy.

12.9.7 Zinc

Cognitive function is the way in which information is processed, which involves thinking, memory, learning and attention. Studies show that zinc is needed for brain neurons (cells) to function efficiently. Deficiencies can cause oxidative stress and affect the structure and function of brain neurons, slowing their replication and even causing cell death (Mackenzie et al., 2007). When the pool of zinc in the brain is low, this can also cause abnormal glucocorticoid secretion and interfere with the metabolism of carbohydrate, fat and protein (Takeda and Tamano, 2009).

Early animal studies have shown that the brains of zinc-deficient foetuses were smaller when maternal zinc intakes were inadequate in the third trimester (McKenzie et al., 1975) and it has been advised that premature infants receive additional zinc after delivery (Friel and Andres, 1994). Given that scientists are now starting to uncover how zinc may influence cognitive function, better-designed human studies are needed in women and their offspring. There is also some evidence linking postnatal zinc deficiencies in the mother to behavioural problems, impaired immunity and a higher risk of elevated blood pressure in the offspring (Uriu-Adams and Keen, 2010).

12.9.8 Iodine

The role of iodine is well established in pregnancy, but now there is some evidence that benefits may extend to after birth. A paper reviewing findings from 36 different studies found that the iodine content of breast milk was related directly to dietary intakes, i.e. in areas where goitre is prevalent, levels of iodine in breast milk were lowest. Studies also showed that iodine levels in breast milk were higher in areas where salt or oil had been fortified with iodine. In these areas, iodine was present in breast milk in sufficient levels (between 100 and 150 μg/dL), but parts of Europe (France, Germany, Spain, Sweden, Denmark and Belgium) had breast milk levels <100 μg/dL. Adequate levels of iodine are essential for thyroid hormone stores in the newborn and their neurological development (see Azizi and Smyth, 2009, for full review). To prevent iodine deficiency after birth and to ensure the iodine content of breast milk is sufficient for the infants' iodine requirements, the WHO/ICCIDD/UNICEF (2008) advise that the iodine intake of lactating mothers is 250 μg/day.

12.9.9 Folate

Folate and vitamin B_{12} are both important nutrients that are critical to rapid growth during early life (Obeid and Herrmann, 2005). In young children, poor folate status has been linked to respiratory infections (Strand et al., 2007). In addition, both folate and B_{12} status in the mother are a strong indicator of status in 6-month-old infants (Hay *et al.*, 2010). Studies have shown that supplements taken daily after birth for 16 weeks can help to maintain red blood cells (RBC) folate levels. Supplements containing 416 μg 5-methyl tetrahydrofolate (THF) led to significantly higher RBC folate levels (2178 nmol/L) when compared with a similar dose of folic acid (1967 nmol/L), or placebo supplements (1390 nmol/L) (Houghton *et al.*, 2006). This research shows that the natural 5-methyl THF form of folate may be more effective at maintaining women's folate status after birth and could be less likely to mask vitamin B_{12} deficiency than supplemental folic acid.

12.9.10   Water

Breast milk is about 88% water, so it is not surprising that fluid requirements are higher after birth. For women of childbearing age (19–50 years), it is advised that total water intake (from foods + beverages) should be around 2 L each day. On top of this, it is advised that lactating mothers consume extra an 700 mL water per day (as shown previously in Table 5.8). Scientifically, the reason behind this is that the average woman produces between 740 and 850 mL breast milk a day. This is about 88% water that equates to about 600–700 mL extra, until milk production slows or stops (EFSA, 2010).

Drinking additional beverages such as water, herbal teas and squash or consuming foods with a high water content, i.e. soups, stews, yoghurts, fruits and vegetables can help to meet these guidelines. On a final note, although these targets are very useful, it is important to remember that every woman's hydration needs are different. Thirst is a good signal, which should not go ignored, but signs that women may not be getting enough fluids include concentrated urine (darker, straw coloured and stronger smelling) and constipation (dark, hard stools that are difficult to expel).

12.9.11   Alcohol

Historically, it has long been thought that small amounts of alcohol can help women to relax, aiding milk release from the mammary glands. Beer drinking has been linked to higher prolactin levels and stimulation of breast milk production (Koletzko and Lehner, 2000). Although these folklores only imply that smalls amounts of alcohol could help to promote the let down reflex, in higher levels, alcohol may be counterproductive. Drinking alcohol when breastfeeding can alter hormone metabolism, changing levels of key hormones involved in milk production (i.e. reduced oxytocin) (Mennella *et al.*, 2005). So, certainly, mothers may feel more relaxed in the short term, but eventually the hormonal milieu fundamental to milk production may be disrupted, diminishing the infant's milk supply.

The National Health and Medical Research Council (2009) have recently recommended that women abstain from drinking alcohol whilst breastfeeding, rather than simply drinking minimal amounts. For women that would like to breastfeed and may feel that alcohol may help them to relax, there is some evidence that barley polysaccharides found in beer can help to facilitate prolactin secretion (rather than the alcohol itself). Therefore, some authors recommend that moderate consumption of non-alcoholic rather than alcoholic beer may help to facilitate the process of breastfeeding (Koletzko and Lehner, 2000).

12.10   Vegetarian and vegan mothers

It is well known that the quality of the mothers' diet can affect the nutrient levels present in breast milk. As vegetarian and vegan mothers are on restricted diets, they may be as risk of nutrient inadequacies, particularly vitamin B_{12} (cobalamin), iron and omega-3, which are mainly found in meat and oily fish. In particular, studies show that infants born to mothers who are vegetarian or vegan may be at risk of megoblastic anaemia (Erdeve *et al.*, 2009), cobalamin and iron deficiency (Fadyl and Inoue, 2007). Research carried out at Kings College University also found that the omega-3 content (namely, DHA) of blood samples taken from infants born to Hindu vegetarian mothers was lower than infants fed a milk formula containing butterfat or mothers who ate meat (Sanders and Reddy, 1992).

Vegetarian mothers may benefit from incorporating flaxseed oils (cold pressed) into their daily diets or algae oil-based supplements (Doughman *et al.*, 2007). Research studies have shown that consuming 2.4 or 3.6 g flax oil per day can significantly improve red blood cell levels of ALA, EPA and DHA although more research is needed on women of childbearing age (Barceló-Coblijn *et al.*, 2008). Some scientists have also reported that vitamin B_{12} supplements may be required by some pregnant vegetarian mothers, if their diets are inadequate (Weiss *et al.*, 2004).

12.11   Feeding multiples

Breastfeeding several infants can be time consuming, challenging and stressful. It can also be uncomfortable for the mother in terms of how to position the baby, particularly if the mother has delivered by caesarean section. However, with the right support and nutrition, there now seems to be good evidence that mother's can nourish more than one infant effectively.

With regard to calorie requirements, feeding more than one child can be an energy-demanding process. Women should make sure they gain the correct proportion of weight in pregnancy (Chapter 9) and correct energy intake after delivery. As a rough guide, it has been estimated that breastfeeding mothers should add an extra 500–600 kcal to her daily diet (per infant). The diet should also be balanced in carbohydrates, fat and protein (around 40% of total calories for carbohydrate and fat and 20% for protein) (Flidel-Rimon and Shinwell, 2006). Supplements can also help to top up nutrient intakes in these new, busy mothers. Goodnight and Newman (2009) advises that women expecting more than one baby take two multivitamin/mineral supplements, which could be continued after birth. As with all mothers, it can be difficult to get enough omega-3 fatty acids from the diet, so an omega-3/fish oil supplement may also be beneficial for mothers' breastfeeding multiple infants.

12.12   Allergy risk

Over the last 10 years, the relationship between infant feeding patterns and allergy risk has been one area that has been hotly debated. National recommendations have been made by some countries on how to feed infants to reduce the risk of allergy although a limited evidence base has meant that there is a lack of consensus. Although breast milk is the food of choice for infants, there is a lack of evidence supporting the theory that this can help to protect against infant allergies (Grimshaw *et al.*, 2009). Some studies have suggested that hydrolysed milk formulas may help to reduce allergy risk, but there is not enough evidence to draw firm conclusions (Zuppa *et al.*, 2005). Other authors suggest that introducing solid foods at an earlier age (around 4–6 months) may help to reduce allergy risk. This recommendation makes sense but further clarification is clearly needed (Anderson *et al.*, 2009). It is hoped that research carried out by EuroPrevall, a European multicentre research project, funded by the European Union may help to shed more light on this important area.

12.13   Postnatal depression

PND is a common medical condition occurring in 13–20% new mothers, after delivery. As this condition is frequently under-reported and not always diagnosed, the true prevalence is likely to be even higher (Mancini *et al.*, 2007). The prevalence of PND also varies globally, which may be attributed to different dietary habits and lifestyles. Rates are reported to be as low as 0.5% in Singapore and as high as 24.5% in South Africa, with a mean worldwide prevalence of around 12.4% (Hibbeln, 2002).

There are many reasons why women develop PND, some of which are summarised in Table 12.8. Symptoms may be wide-ranging and range from postpartum blues to severe depression. Postpartum blues can be defined as short-lived episodes of depressive symptoms after birth and can include feelings of anxiety, disturbed sleeping patterns, decreased appetite and irritability (Gurel and Gurel, 2000). Symptoms of PND are generally more severe and include feelings of suicide, obsessive thoughts and extreme petulance (Wisner *et al.*, 2002). Both disorders subsequently leave women

Table 12.8   Some causes of PND.

Endocrinological
Insulin reduction
Oestrogen reduction

Social
Isolation
Poor support
Unplanned/unwanted pregnancy
Financial concerns

Nutritional
Low riboflavin
Low folate
Low DHA
Low EPA
Low calcium
Low magnesium
Low zinc

Medical
Previous history of mental illness/PND
Family history of mental illness/PND
Personal history of PND
History of severe PND symptoms

Source: Derbyshire and Costarelli (2008).

feeling downhearted during a phase of the life cycle that should be enjoyed to the utmost. Although the causes of PND are undoubtedly multifaceted, this section aims to evaluate the evidence linking diet to PND.

12.13.1   Omega-3 fatty acids

A diet rich in fish, fish oils and omega-3 fatty acids may help to reduce symptoms of depression after birth. Evidence shows that these fatty acids may be involved in the synthesis and regulation of brain neurotransmitters (dopamine, monoamine and serotonin), which are thought to be reduced in patients with symptoms of depression (Sapolsky, 2000).

One report written by members of the American Omega-3 Fatty Acids Subcommittee, established by the Committee on Research on Psychiatric Treatments of the American Psychiatric Association, concluded that omega-3 fats, especially EPA and DHA appear to have a protective effect on mood disorders (Freeman et al., 2006). Recent research has shown that out of a sample of 176 pregnant women, no women were taking supplements that contained omega-3 and only 11% took a separate omega-3 supplement (Grigoriadis et al., 2010). This is concerning considering that numerous studies have linked low omega-3 levels with a higher incidence of maternal depression (Leung and Kaplan, 2009) and there are some links with PND although small patient sample sizes, short study durations and different doses of omega-3 supplements makes drawing firm conclusions difficult (Boria-Hart and Marino, 2010).

12.13.2   Dietary folate and B vitamins

In the case of the B vitamins, most research has focused on folate in the treatment of depression. Studies have shown that supplementing antidepressant medications with folic acid can enhance their therapeutic effects when treating depression both in pregnancy and after birth. This can help to reduce the side effects of antidepressant therapy because dose and period of treatment can both be reduced (Behzadi et al., 2008). One way in which folate may exert its actions is by donating methyl groups, forming S-adenosylmethionine (SAM) which in turn plays a key role in neurological function (Bottiglieri, 2005). Compared with the amount of evidence available, studying the benefits of omega-3 in preventing PND, the evidence for folate, folic acids and B vitamins is comparatively sparse. Therefore, further studies are needed in this field in order to elucidate the possible role of folate and other B vitamins in the prevention and management of PND.

12.13.3   Minerals

There is some evidence that calcium may play a role in stimulating the release of neurotransmitters from vesicles in the brain (the influx of calcium into cells acts as a trigger) (Llinas, 1977). It is also thought that low levels of magnesium ions in the hippocampus of the brain may cause brain cells to misfire and depressive symptoms (Eby and Eby, 2006). Apart from this, a clear evidence base is lacking. One study carried out on South African mothers found that women with iron deficiency after birth had reduced cognitive function and higher rates of depression when compared against those who had taken a supplement (Beard *et al.*, 2005). Many more studies are needed to elucidate how minerals may be linked to depressive symptoms, and if such a relationship exists.

12.13.4 Glycaemic index

Levels of insulin secretion are highest in the third trimester of pregnancy and fall rapidly after infant delivery. The drop in insulin levels have been linked to symptoms of PND, as insulin affects the secretion of serotonin, the 'feel good' hormone in the brain. Therefore, logically, a high-glycaemic index (GI) diet should help to stimulate the secretion of insulin and reduce symptoms of PND after birth (Chen *et al.*, 2006).

To test this theory, Japanese scientists examined the relationship between GI and GL in 865 women with postpartum depression, assessed using the EPDS. Although there was not a dose–response relationship, dietary GI in the third quartile was associated with a reduced risk of depression after birth (Murakami *et al.*, 2008). This is an interesting study but more work is needed to reconfirm findings.

The Edinburgh Postnatal Depression Scale

EPDS provides an easy way to identify women experiencing postpartum depression. The scale was first developed by the scientist John Cox in 1987. It is a 10-point scale that can be used easily in practice setting and during follow-up visits (usually between weeks 1 and 6 after birth). Generally, a score of 9 or above indicates that women may be experiencing depression, although scientists in the past have used different cutoffs.

Over the last few decades, a wealth of scientific literature has used the EPDS in their research, but unfortunately the scale may have lost its usefulness as women have become more aware of the medical condition and answer questions to avoid the diagnosis of depression. For this reason the EPDS has been used in combination with other diagnostic tools, such as the Hamilton Depression Rating Scale.

12.14 Supplement use after birth

While many women are aware that supplementation may be beneficial prior to and during the early phases of pregnancy, the evidence and possible benefits of supplementation after birth are not as well known. Equally, few detailed studies have collected data on supplement use after birth although it seems likely that usage will largely depend on demographic, sociologic and economic factors (Picciano and McGuire, 2009). It makes sense that supplements could have a role to play in replenishing pregnancy nutrient stores and improving the nutrient quality of breast milk, but more work is needed to establish what constitutes the optimal formulation (Allen, 2005). The need to continue supplementation strategies through until after birth needs to be better recognised, especially in the many situations where both mother and child could benefit.

Table 12.9 Ten simple eating habits that can be encouraged from an early age.

1. Encourage children to have plenty of opportunities to eat a range of healthy foods.
2. Encourage children to follow their natural appetite.
3. Meals should be eaten at the table with no distractions, i.e. the television.
4. Children should not rush mealtimes but be encouraged to chew their food slowly.
5. Mealtimes should be as relaxing as possible, i.e. try not to pressure children to 'finish their food' if they do not want it or 'give them a treat' if they finish their vegetables. This can send out the wrong messages and be confusing.
6. Involve children with the shopping and preparation of meals.
7. Encourage healthy snacking on nutritious foods but do not deprive children of occasional treats, i.e. crisps and biscuits.
8. Food should not be used to punish or reward children, keep it neutral.
9. Make sure children's meals outside the home are balanced, i.e. school lunches.
10. Encourage water as their beverage of choice or very dilute squash. Overconsumption of sugar-sweetened beverages has been linked with weight gain in children.

12.15   Healthy eating from an early age

Figures indicate that around 1 in 10 children is overweight, a total of about 155 million globally (IOTF, 2010). Although parents and children may genetically share the tendency to gain weight, healthy eating habits can be formed early in life. Laboratory studies of children's food acceptance show that children who are provided with the opportunity to taste a range of foods and introduced to healthy eating habits early on are less likely to become overweight or obese (Cooke, 2007). In Australia, a new study – the NOURISH randomised controlled trial – has been established to test whether early healthy eating programmes can help to encourage lifelong healthy food preferences and improve long-term health and well-being (Daniels *et al.*, 2009). In essence, it seems that healthy eating habits early in life could play a key role in helping to instill good eating habits throughout life (Table 12.9). This is something that needs to be encouraged amongst new mothers once weaning begins to take place.

12.16   Application in practice

Overall, the quality of a mother's diet is reflected in the quality of her breast milk. Women should be encouraged to breastfeed exclusively for the full 6 months and support groups may play a role in helping women to achieve this. In terms of specific nutrient requirements, 200 mg/day DHA is recommended for breastfeeding mothers to support brain and cognitive development (Koletzko *et al.*, 2007), especially if women are not regular fish-eaters (Bergmann *et al.*, 2008). The re-emergence of rickets amongst some infants, i.e. those born to British Asian mothers, has led to the question of whether 10 µg/day is enough for some pregnant and lactating mothers. However, failures for organisations to reach a consensus on these matters make practical guidelines difficult. The evidence for 250 µg/day of iodine for lactating mothers is stronger and supported by several scientific bodies (WHO, 2007). Other nutrients that are also important after birth include vitamin A, iron, zinc, folate and vitamin B_{12} (particularly for vegetarian mothers) although the evidence base for some of these is not as strong as for others.

12.17   Conclusion

A balanced diet adequate in the right proportions of nutrients not only helps to replenish depleted nutrient reserves but is reflected in the quality of breast milk secreted and infants' health. Breastfeeding is by no means as easy task and even though many women take it up to begin with, additional public health strategies are needed to help women continue this into the longer term. As evidence continues to accumulate within this field, new clear public health messages can be put forward. Certainly, the benefits of a diet adequate in omega-3 fatty acids in the later stages of pregnancy and after birth (especially when breastfeeding) are becoming increasingly apparent and need to be imparted.

Key Messages

- Women are aware that breastfeeding is important for good health, but this is not necessarily put into practice.
- Women should be encouraged not only to breastfeed their infants, but to try to continue this for the 6-month recommendation. Support groups and 'peer programmes' may be one way forward.
- Women breastfeeding multiple children may require an extra 500–600 kcal/day (per child) (Flidel-Rimon and Shinwell, 2006).
- It is advised the average nutrient requirement for both pregnant and lactating mothers should be set at 200 mg/DHA/day (Brenna and Lapillonne, 2009).
- To prevent iodine deficiency after birth and to ensure the iodine content of breast milk is sufficient, the scientific bodies advise that the iodine intake of lactating mothers is 250 µg/day (WHO, ICCIDD, UNICEF, 2008).
- On top of basic water requirements (2 L/day from food and beverage sources), lactating mothers should aim to drink an extra 700 mL water/day (EFSA, 2010).
- Certain dietary components, i.e. omega-3 fatty acids (stronger evidence) and folate (some evidence), may have a role to play in the aetiology of PND.
- Vegetarian mothers' diets may be lacking in vitamin B_{12} and omega-3. Vitamin B_{12} and algal-derived omega-3 supplements may help women to improve the nutrient profile of breast milk if these women are breastfeeding after birth.
- Body weight, dietary and lifestyle behaviours track from childhood to adulthood. Encouraging healthy eating habits from an early age may help to break this cycle. These behaviours may be more difficult to modify as children get older.
- The need to continue supplements during lactation is not recognised in many situations where maternal and infant health could benefit and is certainly worth considering.

Recommended reading

Bolling K, Grant C, Hamlyn B and Thornthon A (2007) *Infant Feeding Survey 2005*. The information Centre for health and social care and the UK Health Departments by BMRB Social Research.

WHO (2007) *Planning Guide for National Implementation of the Global Strategy for Infant and Young Child Feeding*. WHO Press: Switzerland.

WHO (2009) *Infant and Young Child Feeding. Model Chapter for Textbooks for Medical Students and Allied Health Professionals*. WHO Press: Switzerland.

References

Allen LH (2005) Multiple micronutrients in pregnancy and lactation: an overview. *American Journal of Clinical Nutrition* **81**(5), 1206S–12S.

Anderson J, Malley K and Snell R (2009) Is 6 months still the best for exclusive breastfeeding and introduction of solids? A literature review with consideration to the risk of the development of allergies. *Breastfeeding Reviews* **17**(2), 23–31.

Azizi F and Smyth P (2009) Breastfeeding and maternal and infant iodine nutrition. *Clinical Endocrinology (Oxford)* **70**(5), 803–9.

Bahl R Frost C, Kirkwood BR *et al.* (2005) Infant feeding patterns and risks of death and hospitalization in the first half of infancy: multicentre cohort study. *Bulletin of the World Health Organization* **83**, 418–26.

Barceló-Coblijn G, Murphy EJ, Othman R, Moghadasian MH, Kashour T and Friel JK (2008) Flaxseed oil and fish-oil capsule consumption alters human red blood cell n-3 fatty acid composition: a multiple-dosing trial comparing 2 sources of n-3 fatty acid. *American Journal of Clinical Nutrition* **88**(3), 801–9.

Beard JL, Hendricks MK, Perez EM, Murray-Kolb LE and Berg A (2005) Maternal iron deficiency anemia affects postpartum emotions and cognition. *Journal of Nutrition* **135**(2), 267–72.

Behzadi AH, Behbahani AS and Ostovar N (2008) Therapeutic effects of folic acid on ante partum and postpartum depression. *Medical Hypotheses* **71**(2), 313–4.

Bergmann RL, Haschke-Becher E, Klassen-Wigger P *et al.* (2008) Supplementation with 200 mg/day docosahexaenoic acid from mid-pregnancy through lactation improves the docosahexaenoic acid status of mothers with a habitually low fish intake and of their infants. *Annals of Nutrition & Metabolism* **52**(2),157–66.

Bolling K, Grant C, Hamlyn B and Thornthon A (2007) *Infant Feeding Survey 2005*. The information centre for health and social care and the UK Health Departments by BMRB Social Research.

Borja-Hart NL and Marino J (2010) Role of omega-3 fatty acids for prevention or treatment of perinatal depression. *Pharmacotherapy* **30**(2), 210–6.

Bottiglieri T (2005) Homocysteine and folate metabolism in depression. *Progress in Neuropsychopharmacology & Biological Psychiatry* **29**(7), 1103–12.

Bourre JM (2007) Dietary omega-3 fatty acids for women. *Biomedicine & Pharmacotherapy* **61**(2–3), 105–12.

Brenna JT and Lapillonne A (2009) Background paper on fat and fatty acid requirements during pregnancy and lactation. *Annals of Nutrition & Metabolism* **55**(1–3), 97–122.

Brenna JT, Varamini B, Jensen RG *et al.* (2007) Docosahexaenoic and arachidonic acid concentrations in human breast milk worldwide. *American Journal of Clinical Nutrition* **85**(6), 1457–64.

Carter RC, Jacobson JL, Burden MJ *et al.* (2010) Iron deficiency anemia and cognitive function in infancy. *Pediatrics* **126**(2), e427–34.

Chen TH, Lan TH, Yang CY and Juang KD (2006) Postpartum mood disorders may be related to a decreased insulin level after delivery. *Medical Hypotheses* **66**(4), 820–3.

Clifford J and McIntyre E (2008) Who supports breastfeeding? *Breastfeed Reviews* **16**(2), 9–19.

Cooke L (2007) The importance of exposure for healthy eating in childhood: a review. *Journal of Human Nutrition & Dietetics* **20**, 294–301.

Daniels LA, Magarey A, Battistutta D, *et al.* (2009) The NOURISH randomised control trial: positive feeding practices and food preferences in early childhood – a primary prevention programme for childhood obesity. *BMC Public Health* **9**, 387.

DH (Department of Health) (1998) *Nutrition and Bone Health: With Particular Reference to Calcium and Vitamin D*. The Stationery Office: London.

DH (Department of Health) (2010) *Infant feeding recommendation*. Available from: http://www.dh.gov.uk/prod_consum_dh/groups/dh_digitalassets/@dh/@en/documents/digitalasset/dh_4096999.pdf. (accessed March 2011.)

Doughman SD, Krupanidhi S and Sanjeevi CB (2007) Omega-3 fatty acids for nutrition and medicine: considering microalgae oil as a vegetarian source of EPA and DHA. *Current Diabetes Reviews* 3(3), 198–203.

Eby GA and Eby KL (2006) Rapid recovery from major depression using magnesium treatment. *Medical Hypotheses* 67, 362–70.

EFSA (European Food Standards Agency) (2010) Scientific Opinion on Dietary Reference Values for Water. *EFSA Journal* 8(3), 1459.

Erdeve O, Arsan S, Atasay B, Ileri T and Uysal Z (2009) A breast-fed newborn with megaloblastic anemia-treated with the vitamin B12 supplementation of the mother. *Journal of Paediatric Hematology/Oncology* 31(10), 763–5.

Fadyl H and Inoue S (2007) Combined B$_{12}$ and iron deficiency in a child breast-fed by a vegetarian mother. *Journal of Paediatric Hematology/Oncology* 29(1), 74.

Flidel-Rimon O and Shinwell ES (2006) Breast feeding twins and high multiples. *Archives of Disease in Childhood: Fetal & Neonatal Edition* 91(5), F377–80.

FNB (Food and Nutrition Board) (1990) *Institute of Medicine, Committee on Nutrition Status during Pregnancy and Lactation.* National Academy Press: Washington, DC.

Freeman MP, Hibbeln JR, Wisner KL, *et al.* (2006) Omega-3 fatty acids: evidence basis for treatment and future research in psychiatry. *Journal of Clinical Psychiatry* 67(12), 1954–67.

Friel JK and Andrews WL (1994) Zinc requirement of premature infants. *Nutrition.* 10(1), 63–5.

Goodnight W and Newman R; Society of Maternal-Fetal Medicine (2009) Optimal nutrition for improved twin pregnancy outcome. *Obstetrics & Gynaecology* 114(5), 1121–34.

Greer FR (2008) 25-Hydroxyvitamin D: functional outcomes in infants and young children. *American Journal of Clinical Nutrition* 88, 529S–33S.

Griffiths LJ, Tate AR, Dezateux C and the Millennium Cohort Study Child Health Group (2005) The contribution of parental and community ethnicity to breastfeeding practices: evidence from the Millennium Cohort Study. *International Journal of Epidemiology* 34, 1378–86.

Grigoriadis S, Barrett J, Pittini R *et al.* (2010) Omega-3 supplements in pregnancy: are we too late to identify the possible benefits? *Journal of Obstetrics & Gynaecology Canada* 32(3), 209–16.

Grimshaw KE, Allen K, Edwards CA *et al.* (2009) Infant feeding and allergy prevention: a review of current knowledge and recommendations. A EuroPrevall state of the art paper. *Allergy* 64(10), 1407–16.

Gurel S and Gurel H (2000) The evaluation of determinants of early postpartum low mood: the importance of parity and inter-pregnancy interval. *European Journal of Obstetrics & Gynaecology and Reproductive Biology* 91, 21–4.

Haku M (2007) Breastfeeding: factors associated with the continuation of breastfeeding, the current situation in Japan, and recommendations for further research. *The Journal of Medical Investigation* 54, 224–34.

Hay G, Clausen T, Whitelaw A *et al.* (2010) Maternal folate and cobalamin status predicts vitamin status in newborns and 6-month-old infants. *Journal of Nutrition* 140(3), 557–64

Hibbeln JR (2002) Seafood consumption, the DHA content of mothers' milk and prevalence rates of postpartum depression: a cross-national, ecological analysis. *Journal of Affective Disorders* 69, 15–29.

Houghton LA, Sherwood KL, Pawlosky R, Ito S and O'Connor DL (2006) [6S]-5-Methyltetrahydrofolate is at least as effective as folic acid in preventing a decline in blood folate concentrations during lactation. *American Journal of Clinical Nutrition* 83(4), 842–50.

IOTF (International Obesity Task Force) (2010) Childhood obesity. Available at: http://www.iotf.org/childhoodobesity.asp. (accessed March 2011.)

Ip S, Chung M, Raman G *et al.* (2007) Breastfeeding and maternal and infant health outcomes in developed countries. *Evidence Report – Technology Assessment (Full Rep)* 153, 1–186.

Koletzko B, Cetin I, Brenna JT and the Perinatal Lipid Intake Working Group (2007) Dietary fat intakes for pregnant and lactating women. *British Journal of Nutrition* 98(5), 873–7.

Koletzko B and Lehner F (2000) Beer and breastfeeding. *Advances in Experimental Medicine & Biology* 478, 23–8.

Koletzko B, von Kries R, Monasterolo RC, Subías JE, Scaglioni S and the European Childhood Obesity Trial Study Group (2009) Infant feeding and later obesity risk. *Advances in Experimental Medicine and Biology* 646, 15–29.

Kramer MS and Kakuma R (2001) *The Optimal Duration of Exclusive Breastfeeding: A Systematic Review.* WHO: Geneva.

Kulakac O, Oncel S, Meydanlioglu A and Muslu L (2006) The opinions of employed mothers about their own nutrition during lactation: a questionnaire survey. *International Journal of Nursing Studies* **44**(4), 589–600.

Labbok M (2008) Exploration of guilt among mothers who do not breastfeed: the physician's role. *Journal of Human Lactation* **24**(1), 80–4.

Lakshman R, Ogilvie D and Ong KK (2009) Mothers' experiences of bottle-feeding: a systematic review of qualitative and quantitative studies. *Archives of Disease in Childhood* **94**(8), 596–601.

Leung BM and Kaplan BJ (2009) Perinatal depression: prevalence, risks, and the nutrition link – a review of the literature. *Journal of the American Dietetic Association* **109**(9), 1566–75.

Llinas RR (1977) Depolarization-release coupling systems in neurons. *Neuroscience Research Programme Bulletin* **15**, 555–687.

Lowdon J (2008) Getting bone health right from the start! Pregnancy, lactation and weaning. *Journal of Family Health Care* **18**(4), 137–41.

Lozoff B, Kaciroti N and Tomás W (2006) Iron deficiency in infancy: applying a physiologic framework for prediction. *American Journal of Clinical Nutrition* **84**, 1412–21.

Mackenzie GG, Zago MP, Aimo L and Oteiza PI (2007) Zinc deficiency in neuronal biology. *IUBMB Life* **59**(4–5), 299–307.

Mancini F, Carlson C and Albers L (2007) Use of the postpartum depression screening scale in a collaborative obstetric practice. *Journal of Midwifery & Women's Health* **52**(5), 429–34.

Mannion CA, Gray-Donald K, Johnson-Down L and Koski KG (2007) Lactating women restricting milk are low on select nutrients. *Journal of the American College of Nutrition* **26**(2), 149–55.

McKenzie JM, Fosmire GJ and Sandstead HH (1975) Zinc deficiency during the latter third of pregnancy: effects on fetal rat brain, liver, and placenta. *Journal of Nutrition* **105**(11), 1466–75.

Mennella JA, Pepino MY and Teff KL (2005) Acute alcohol consumption disrupts the hormonal milieu of lactating women. *Journal of Clinical Endocrinology & Metabolism* **90**(4), 1979–85.

Mohammadzadeh A, Farhet A and Esmaeily H (2005) The effect of breast milk and lanolin on sore nipples. *Saudi Medical Journal* **26**(8), 1231–4.

Mulligan ML, Felton SK, Riek AE and Bernal-Mizrachi C (2010) Implications of vitamin D deficiency in pregnancy and lactation. *American Journal of Obstetrics & Gynaecology* **202**(5), 429 e1–9.

Murakami K, Miyake Y, Sasaki S *et al.* (2008) Dietary glycemic index and load and the risk of postpartum depression in Japan: the Osaka Maternal and Child Health Study. *Journal of Affective Disorders* **110**(1–2), 174–9.

National Health and Medical Research Council (2009) Alcohol guidelines: reducing the health risks. Available at: http://www.nhmrc.gov.au/publications/synopses/ds10syn.htm. (accessed March 2011.)

NICE (National Institute of Clinical Excellence) (2003) *Antenatal Care: Routine Care for the Healthy Pregnant Woman*. NICE: London.

Nommsen-Rivers LA and Dewey KG (2009) Growth of breastfed infants. *Breastfeeding medicine* **4**(1), S45–9.

Obeid R and Herrmann W (2005) Homocysteine, folic acid and vitamin B_{12} in relation to pre- and postnatal health aspects. *Clinical Chemistry & Laboratory Medcine* **43**, 1052–7.

Onis M, Garza C, Onyango AW *et al.* (2008) WHO growth standards for infants and young children. *Archives de Pédiatrie* **16**, 47–53.

PAHO/WHO (Pan American Health Organisation/World Health Organisation) (2002) *Guiding principles for complementary feeding of the breastfed child*. PAHO/WHO: Washington, DC.

Picciano MF and McGuire MK (2009) Use of dietary supplements by pregnant and lactating women in North America. *American Journal of Clinical Nutrition* **89**(2), 663S–7S.

Protheroe L, Dyson L, Renfrew MJ, Bull J and Mulvhill C (2003) *The Effectiveness of Interventions to Promote the Initiation of Breastfeeding*. Health Development Agency: London.

Quigley MA, Kelly YJ and Sacker A (2009) Infant feeding, solid foods and hospitalisation in the first 8 months after birth. *Archives of Diseases in Childhood* **94**(2), 148–50.

Rasmussen KM, Wallace MH and Gournis E (2001) A low-fat diet but not food restriction improves lactational performance in obese rats. *Advances in Experimental Medicine & Biology* **50**, 101–6.

Ruxton CHS and Derbyshire EJ (2010) Women's diet quality in the UK. *Nutrition Bulletin* **35**(2), 126–37.

SACN (Scientific Advisory Committee on Nutrition) (2007) *Update on Vitamin D – Position Statement by the Scientific Advisory Committee on Nutrition*. The Stationery Office: London.

Sanders TA and Reddy S (1992) The influence of a vegetarian diet on the fatty acid composition of human milk and the essential fatty acid status of the infant. *Journal of Pediatrics* **120**(4 Pt 2), S71–7.

Sapolsky RM (2000) The possibility of neurotoxicity in the hippocampus in major depression: a primer on neuron death. *Biology Psychiatry* **48**, 755–65.

Siddiqi N and Iqbal R (2008) Maternal postpartum vitamin A supplementation programme: is there a need in Pakistan? *Journal Pakistan Medical Association* **58**(5), 265–6.

Stettler N, Stallings VA, Troxel AB *et al.* (2005) Weight gain in the first week of life and overweight in adulthood: a cohort study of European American subjects fed infant formula. *Circulation* **111**(15), 1897–903.

Strand TA, Taneja S, Bhandari N *et al.* (2007) Folate, but not vitamin B-12 status, predicts respiratory morbidity in north Indian children. *American Journal of Clinical Nutrition* **86**(1), 139–44.

Strobel M, Tinz J and Biesalski HK (2007) The importance of beta-carotene as a source of vitamin A with special regard to pregnant and breastfeeding women. *European Journal of Nutrition* **46**(S1), 11–20.

Surette ME (2008) The science behind dietary omega-3 fatty acids. *Canadian Medical Association Journal* **178**(2), 177–80.

Takeda A and Tamano H (2009) Insight into zinc signaling from dietary zinc deficiency. *Brain Research Reviews* **62**(1), 33–44.

Tarrant M, Fong DY, Wu KM *et al.* (2010b) Breastfeeding and weaning practices among Hong Kong mothers: a prospective study. *BMC Pregnancy Childbirth* **10**, 27.

Tarrant RC, Younger KM, Sheridan-Pereira M, White MJ and Kearney JM (2010a) Factors associated with weaning practices in term infants: a prospective observational study in Ireland. *British Journal of Nutrition* **104**(10), 1544–54.

Theobald H (2007) Eating for pregnancy and breastfeeding. *Journal of Family Health Care* **17**(2), 45–8.

Thomas M and Weisman SM (2006) Calcium supplementation during pregnancy and lactation: effects on the mother and the fetus. *American Journal of Obstetrics & Gynaecology* **194**(4), 937–45.

Uriu-Adams JY and Keen CL (2010) Zinc and reproduction: effects of zinc deficiency on prenatal and early postnatal development. *Birth Defects Research Part B: Developmental & Reproductive Toxicology* **89**(4), 313–25.

Weiss R, Fogelman Y and Bennett M (2004) Severe vitamin B_{12} deficiency in an infant associated with a maternal deficiency and a strict vegetarian diet. *Journal of Paediatric Haematology/Oncology* **26**(4), 270–1.

WHO, UNICEF and ICCIDD (2007) *Assessment of Iodine Deficiency Disorders and Monitoring Their Elimination. A Guide for Programme Managers*, 3rd edition. World Health Organization: Geneva.

WHO/UNICEF/USAID (World Health Organisation/United Nations Children's Fund/United States Agency for International Development) (2008) *Indicators for Assessing Infant and Young Child Feeding Practices*. WHO: Geneva.

Wisner KL, Parry BL and Piontek CM (2002) Clinical practice: postpartum depression. *New England Journal of Medicine* **347**, 194–9.

Zuppa AA, Visintini F, Cota F, Maggio L, Romagnoli C and Tortorolo G (2005) Hydrolysed milk in preterm infants: an open problem. *Acta Paediatrica Supplement* **94**(449), 84–6.

APPENDICES

Appendix 1
International definitions of indices used to form dietary recommendations

Indices	Definition
Adequate intake (AI)	When there is not enough data to calculate the EAR or RDA, the AI is used. This is the amount of a nutrient that is sufficient to maintain 'satisfactory' nutritional status in a particular age and gender group.
Dietary reference value (DRV)/dietary reference intake (DRI)	An umbrella term encompassing a series of estimates used to quantify the proportion of energy and nutrients that are needed by different groups of healthy individuals.
Estimated average requirement (EAR)	The estimated daily intake level that would meet the requirement of 50% of the population of a particular gender and age group.
Lower reference nutrient intake (LRNI)	The amount of a nutrient that is only enough to meet the needs of a small number of people who have low requirements (2.5%). The majority of people need higher amounts.
Population reference intake (PRI)	Intakes that should be sufficient for most 'healthy' individuals (similar to UK RNI).
Recommended dietary allowance (RDA)/reference daily intake (RDI)	The estimated daily intake level that is considered to meet the requirements of 97–98% healthy individuals in each life-stage and sex group (similar to the UK RNI).
Reference nutrient intake (RNI)	An estimate of the amount of protein, vitamins and minerals that should meet the needs of most individuals (about 97% of people).
Tolerable upper intake level (UL)	This is the maximum level/upper limit for certain nutrients. Beyond these levels, the risk of disease development and/or toxicity symptoms may increase.

Nutrition in the Childbearing Years, First Edition. Emma Derbyshire.
© 2011 Emma Derbyshire. Published 2011 by Blackwell Publishing Ltd.

Appendix 2
Recommended nutrient intakes for women of childbearing age (19–50 years)

	UK (DoH, 1991)	Europe (EC, 1993)	USA (FNB, 2001	Australia and New Zealand (NHMRC/MoH, 2006)	Japan (Sasaki, 2008)
Macronutrients					
Energy (kcals)	1940	–	2202*	1250–1670	1700–2550†
Protein (%EI)	–	–	10–35	–	<20
Carbohydrate (%EI)	47	–	45–65	–	50–70
Fat (%EI)	33	–	20–35	–	20–30
LC *n*-3 PUFA (%EI)	0.2	0.5	0.6–1.2	–	>2.2
LC *n*-6 PUFA (%EI)	1.0	2.0	5–10	–	<10
Fibre (g/d)	18‡	–	25	25	20
Vitamins					
Vitamin A (μg)	600	600	700	700	600
Vitamin C (mg)	40	40–45	75	45	100
Vitamin D (μg)	–	–	5.0	5.0	5.0
Vitamin E (mg)	–	–	15	7.0	8.0
Vitamin K (μg)	–	–	90	60	60–65
Thiamine (mg/day)	0.8	100	1.1	1.1	1.2
Riboflavin (mg/day)	1.1	1.3	1.1	1.1	1.1
Niacin (mg/day)	14	–	14	14	12
Vitamin B_6 (μg)	1.2	–	1.3	1.3	1.2
Vitamin B_{12} (μg)	1.5	1.4	2.4	2.4	2.4
Folate (μg)	200	200	400	400	240
Biotin (μg)	–	–	30	25	45
Choline (mg)	–	–	425	425	–
Minerals					
Calcium (mg)	700–800	700–800	1000	1000	600–700
Copper (mg)	1.0	1.1	0.9	1.2	0.7
Iodine (μg)	140	130	150	150	150

Nutrition in the Childbearing Years, First Edition. Emma Derbyshire.
© 2011 Emma Derbyshire. Published 2011 by Blackwell Publishing Ltd.

	UK (DoH, 1991)	Europe (EC, 1993)	USA (FNB, 2001	Australia and New Zealand (NHMRC/MoH, 2006)	Japan (Sasaki, 2008)
Iron (mg)	14.8	20	18	18	10.5
Selenium (μg)	60	55	55	60	25
Magnesium (mg)	270	–	350–360	350–360	270–280
Zinc (mg)	7.0	7.0	8.0	8.0	7
Sodium (g)	1.6	–	1.5	0.5–0.9	0.6

*Vary for age, activity level and height; [†]depending on levels of physical activity; [‡]value for NSP; (–) not reported.

Appendix 3
Recommended nutrient intakes for pregnancy

	UK (DoH, 1991)	Europe (EC, 1993)	USA (FNB, 2001	Australia and New Zealand (NHMRC/MoH, 2006)	Japan (Sasaki, 2008)
Macronutrients					
Energy (kcals)	2140	–	–	–	1700–2550*
Protein (%EI)	–	–	10–35	–	–
Carbohydrate (%EI)	47	–	45–65	–	–
Fat (%EI)	33	–	20–35	–	20–30
LC n-3 PUFA (%EI)	0.2	0.5	0.6–1.2	–	–
LC n-6 PUFA (%EI)	1.0	2.0	5–10	–	<10
Fibre (g/day)	18†	–	28	28	–
Vitamins					
Vitamin A (μg)	950	700	770	800	670
Vitamin C (mg)	50	55	85	60	110
Vitamin D (μg)	10	–	5.0	5.0	7.5
Vitamin E (mg)	–	–	15	7.0	8.0
Vitamin K (μg)	–	–	90	60	60–65
Folate (μg)	300	400	600	600	440
Thiamine (mg/day)	0.9	–	1.4	1.4	1.2–1.5
Riboflavin (mg/day)	1.4	1.6	1.4	1.4	1.1–1.4
Niacin (mg/day)	13–14	1.6	18	18	12–15
Vitamin B_6 (μg)	1.2	–	1.9	1.9	1.3
Vitamin B_{12} (μg)	1.5	1.6	2.6	2.6	2.8
Biotin (μg)	–	–	30	30	47
Choline (mg)	–	–	450	440	–
Minerals					
Calcium (mg)	700–800	700	1000	1000	600–700
Copper (mg)	1.0–1.2	1.1	1000 (ug)	1.3	0.8
Iodine (μg)	140	130	220	220	260
Iron (mg)	14.8	‡	27	27	19.5
Magnesium (mg)	270	–	350–60	350–60	310–320
Selenium (μg)	60	55	60	65	29
Zinc (mg)	7.0	1.1	11	11	10
Sodium (g)	1.6	–	1.5	0.5–0.9	0.6

*Depending on level of physical activity +50 kcal for early pregnancy, +250 for mid pregnancy and +500 for late pregnancy; ‡ supplements recommended; (–) not reported.

Nutrition in the Childbearing Years, First Edition. Emma Derbyshire.
© 2011 Emma Derbyshire. Published 2011 by Blackwell Publishing Ltd.

Appendix 4
Recommended nutrient intakes for breastfeeding mothers

	UK (DoH, 1991)	Europe (EC, 1993)	USA (FNB, 2001)	Australia and New Zealand (NHMRC/MoH 2006)	Japan (Sasaki, 2008)
Macrominerals					
Energy (kcals)	1900*	–	–	–	1700–2550[†]
Protein (%EI)	–	–	10–35	–	–
Carbohydrate (%EI)	47	–	45–65	–	–
Fat (%EI)	33	–	20–35	–	20–30
LC n-3 PUFA (%EI)	0.2	0.5	0.6–1.2	–	<10
LC n-6 PUFA (%EI)	1.0	2.0	5–10	–	–
Fibre (g/day)	18[‡]	–	29	30	–
Vitamins					
Vitamin A (μg)	950	950	1300	1100	1020
Vitamin C (mg)	70	70	120	85	150
Vitamin D (μg)	10	–	5.0	5.0	7.5
Vitamin E (mg)	–	–	19	11	11
Vitamin K (μg)	–	–	90	60	60–65
Thiamine (mg/day)	1.0	–	1.4	1.4	1.2–1.6
Riboflavin (mg/day)	1.6	1.7	1.6	1.6	1.1–1.2
Niacin (mg/day)	15	–	17	17	14
Vitamin B_6 (μg)	1.2	–	2.0	2.0	2.0
Vitamin B_{12} (μg)	2.0	1.9	2.8	2.8	2.8
Folate (μg)	260	350	500	500	340
Biotin (μg)	–	–	35	35	49
Choline (mg)	–	–	550	550	–
Minerals					
Calcium (mg)	1250	1200	1000	1000	600–700
Copper (mg)	1.5	1.4	1300 (ug)	1.5	1.3
Iodine (μg)	140	160	290	270	340
Iron (mg)	14.8	10	9	9	9.0
Magnesium (mg)	320	–	310–320	310–320	270–280
Selenium (μg)	75	70	70	75	45
Zinc (mg)	13.0[§]	1.4	12	12	10
Sodium (g)	1.6	–	1.5	0.5–0.9	0.6

* +450–570 depending on the length of breastfeeding; [†]+450 for lactating mothers; [‡]value for NSP; [§]decreases to 9.5 mg/day after 4 months.

Nutrition in the Childbearing Years, First Edition. Emma Derbyshire.
© 2011 Emma Derbyshire. Published 2011 by Blackwell Publishing Ltd.

Appendix 5
Recommended nutrient intakes for pregnant and lactating adolescents (14–18 years)

	Pregnancy	Lactation	Source
Macronutrients			
Energy (kcals)	2310	2680*	DoH (1991)
Protein (g/day)	71	71	FNB (2002)
Carbohydrate (g/day)	175	210	FNB (2002), EFSA (2010a)
Fibre (g/day)	28	29	FNB (2002), EFSA (2010a)
LC n-3 (DHA/EPA/DPA) (mg/day)	110	140	NHMRC/MoH (2006), EFSA (2010b)
Vitamins			
Vitamin A (μg/day)	750	1200	FNB (2001)
Vitamin C (mg/day)	80	115	FNB (2000)
Vitamin D (μg/day)	5	5	FNB (1997)
Vitamin E (mg/day)	15	19	FNB (2000)
Vitamin K (μg/day)	75	75	FNB (2001)
Folate (μg/day)	600	500	FNB (1998)
Vitamin B_{12} (μg/day)	2.6	2.8	FNB (1998)
Biotin (μg/day)	30	35	FNB (1998)
Choline (mg/day)	450	550	FNB (1998)
Minerals			
Calcium (mg)	1300	1300	FNB (1997)
Copper (μg)	1000	1300	FNB (2001)
Iodine (μg)	220	290	FNB (2001)
Iron (mg)	27	10	FNB (2001)
Selenium (μg)	60	70	FNB (2000)
Zinc (mg)	12	13	FNB (2001)
Sodium (g)	1.5	1.5	FNB (2004)
Water (L/day)	2.3	2.7	EFSA (2010c)[†]

*3 months after birth (DoH, 1991); [†]from food, beverages and drinking water.

Nutrition in the Childbearing Years, First Edition. Emma Derbyshire.
© 2011 Emma Derbyshire. Published 2011 by Blackwell Publishing Ltd.

Appendix 6
Suggested nutritional recommendations for twin pregnancies

Recommendations	1st trimester	2nd trimester	3rd trimester
Calorie requirements (kcal/kg^{-1} d^{-1}) Normal BMI Overweight Underweight	40–45 42–50 30–35	Monitor weight gain and alter as necessary for weight gain goal	Monitor weight gain and alter as necessary for weight gain goal
Calcium (mg)	1500	2500	2500
Vitamin D (IU)	1000	1000	1000
Magnesium (mg)	400	800	800
Zinc (mg)	15	30	30
DHA/EPA (mg)	300–500	300–500	300–500
Folic acid (mg)	1	1	1
Vitamin C (mg)	500–1000	500–1000	500–1000
Vitamin E (IU)	400	400	400
Micronutrient supplement	1	2	2
Laboratory nutritional assessment	Haemoglobin, ferritin, screen for GDM, vitamin D status	Follow up results from 1st trimester	Haemoglobin, ferritin, GDM with or without vitamin D

Source: Goodnight and Newman (2009), with permission.
BMI, body mass index; DHA, docosahexaenoic acid; EPA, eicosapentaenoic acid; GDM, gestational diabetes mellitus.
40 IU vitamin D = 1μg.

Nutrition in the Childbearing Years, First Edition. Emma Derbyshire.
© 2011 Emma Derbyshire. Published 2011 by Blackwell Publishing Ltd.

Appendix 7
Tolerable upper intake levels (ULs) for vitamins and minerals

	UL	Population
Vitamins		
Vitamin A (μg/day)	3000	Women of childbearing age
Vitamin C (mg/day)	–	Insufficient data available
Vitamin D (μg/day)	50	Women, pregnancy and lactation
Vitamin E (mg/day)	300	Women, pregnancy and lactation
Vitamin B_{12} (μg/day)	–	Insufficient data available*
Vitamin K (mg/day)	–	Insufficient data available
Folic acid (μg/day)	1000	Women, pregnancy and lactation
Minerals		
Calcium (g/day)	2.5	Women, pregnancy and lactation
Iodine (μg/day)	600	Women, pregnancy and lactation
Iron (mg/day)	–	Insufficient data available[†]
Selenium (μg/day)	300	Women, pregnancy and lactation
Zinc (mg/day)	25	Women, pregnancy and lactation
Sodium (g/day)	–	Insufficient data available
Fluoride (mg/day)	7	Women, pregnancy and lactation

Source: EFSA (2006).
UL, upper intake level. *Intakes of up to 1000 μg/day orally for prolonged periods have been tested without adverse effects being reported; [†]50–60 mg associated with gastrointestinal symptoms, including constipation.

Nutrition in the Childbearing Years, First Edition. Emma Derbyshire.
© 2011 Emma Derbyshire. Published 2011 by Blackwell Publishing Ltd.

Appendix 8
Institute of Medicine pregnancy weight gain guidelines

| Pre-pregnancy BMI | BMI category | Recommended level of pregnancy weight gain | |
		Range in kg	Range in lbs
<18.5 kg/m²	Underweight	12.5–18	28–40
18.5–24.9 kg/m²	Normal weight	11.5–16	25–35
25.0–29.9 kg/m²	Overweight	7–11.5	15–25
≥30.0 kg/m²	Obese	5–9	11–20

Source: Rasmussen and Yaktine (2009).

Nutrition in the Childbearing Years, First Edition. Emma Derbyshire.
© 2011 Emma Derbyshire. Published 2011 by Blackwell Publishing Ltd.

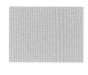

Appendix 9
Examples of common food safety concerns

Concern	Advice
Fish	
Is it safe to eat shellfish and oysters when pregnant?	Generally these should be avoided unless cooked thoroughly.
Can I eat fish?	Yes, so long as you eat no more than the recommended weekly two portions. Fish that may be a source of mercury should not be eaten, i.e. shark, swordfish and marlin (larger predatory fish).
Is it OK to eat sushi?	Yes, as long as the fish used has been frozen first or is smoked. Both methods kill parasites.
Cheese and dairy	
Can I eat goat's cheese?	Yes, as long as it is pasteurised. Avoid goat's cheese with a white rind known as Chevre.
Can I eat blue cheese?	Yes, as long as it is cooked thoroughly, which should kill any *listeria* bacteria.
Can cold meats be eaten?	Ideally, meats should be heated; cold meats may be a source of *listeria* although the risk is low.
Is it safe to eat soft boiled or 'runny' eggs in pregnancy?	Eggs may be a source of *Salmonella*, so unless hard boiled or pasteurised are best avoided. Also avoid eating homemade mayonnaise or meringue, which may also contain raw eggs.
Can I eat mayonnaise?	Homemade mayonnaise is best avoided because it may contain unpasteurised raw egg. Shop-bought mayonnaise is fine if it uses pasteurised eggs.
Other	
Can I eat honey when pregnant?	Yes, provided that it is pasteurised. Raw, unpasteurised honey may be a source of *Clostridium botulinum* bacteria.

Nutrition in the Childbearing Years, First Edition. Emma Derbyshire.
© 2011 Emma Derbyshire. Published 2011 by Blackwell Publishing Ltd.

Concern	Advice
Is it safe to eat salt in pregnancy?	Yes, this only needs to be monitored if you have a history of high blood pressure or pre-eclampsia. Moderate amounts may help to regulate fluid balance in pregnancy.
Can I use sweeteners in pregnancy?	Saccharin and cyclamates are not generally recommended during pregnancy.
Can I eat peanuts?	These are generally fine, but should be avoided if the mother, father or another sibling has a history of allergic reactions.

References

DoH (Department of Health) (1991) *Dietary Reference Values for Food Energy and Nutrients for the United Kingdom*, 2nd edition. Report on Social Subjects no. 41. The Stationery Office: London.

(EC) European Commission (1993) *Reports of the Scientific Committee for Food. Nutrition and energy Intakes for the European Community*. Commission of the European Communities: Luxembourg.

EFSA (European Food Safety Authority) (2006) *Tolerable Upper Intake Levels of Vitamins and Minerals by the Scientific Panel on Dietetic Products, Nutrition and Allergies (NDA) and Scientific Committee on Food (SCF)*. Available at: http://www.efsa.europa.eu/cs/BlobServer/Scientific_Document/upper_level_opinions_full-part33.pdf (accessed 4 January 2009).

EFSA (European Food Standards Agency) (2010a) Scientific opinion on dietary reference values for carbohydrates and dietary fibre. *EFSA Journal* 8(3), 1462.

EFSA (European Food Standards Agency) (2010b) Scientific opinion on dietary reference values for fats, including saturated fatty acids, polyunsaturated fatty acids, monounsaturated fatty acids, trans fatty acids, and cholesterol. *EFSA Journal* 8(3), 1461.

EFSA (European Food Standards Agency) (2010c) Scientific opinion on dietary reference values for water. *EFSA Journal* 8(3), 1459.

FNB (Food and Nutrition Board) Institute of Medicine (1997) *Dietary Reference Intakes for Calcium, Phosphorus, Magnesium, Vitamin D, and Fluoride*. National Academy Press: Washington, DC.

FNB (Food and Nutrition Board) Institute of Medicine (1998) *Dietary Reference Intakes for Thiamine, Riboflavin, Niacin, Vitamin B6, Folate, Vitamin B12, Pantothenic Acid, Biotin, and Choline*. National Academy Press: Washington, DC.

FNB (Food and Nutrition Board): Institute of Medicine (2000) *Dietary Reference Intakes for Vitamin C, Vitamin E, Selenium and Carotenoids*. National Academy Press: Washington, DC.

FNB (Food and Nutrition Board): Institute of Medicine (2001) *Dietary Reference Intakes for Vitamin A, Vitamin K, Arsenic, Boron, Chromium, Copper, Iodine, Iron, manganese, Molybdenum, Nickel, Silicon, Vanadium and Zinc*. National Academy Press: Washington, DC.

FNB (Food and Nutrition Board): Institute of Medicine (2002) *Dietary Reference Intakes for Energy, Carbohydrate, Fiber, Fat, Fatty Acids, Cholesterol, Protein and Amino Acids (Macronutrients)*. National Academy Press: Washington, DC.

FNB (Food and Nutrition Board): Institute of Medicine (2004) *Dietary Reference Intakes for Water, Potassium, Sodium, Chloride and Sulphate*. Panel on the dietary reference intakes for electrolytes and water. National Academy Press: Washington, DC.

Goodnight W and Newman R (2009) Optimal nutrition for improved twin pregnancy outcome. *Obstetrics and Gynaecology* 114(5): 1121–32.

NHMRC (National Health and Medical Research Council)/MoH (2006) *Nutrient Reference Values for Australia and New Zealand*. NHMRC Publications: Australia. Available at: https://www.nhmrc.gov.au (accessed 14 January 2009).

Rasmussen KM and Yaktine AL (2009) *Weight Gain During Pregnancy: Re-examining the Guidelines*. The National Academies Press: Washington DC.

Sasaki S (2008) Dietary reference intakes (DRIs) in Japan. *Asia Pacific Journal of Clinical Nutrition.* 17(S2), 420–44.

CASE STUDIES

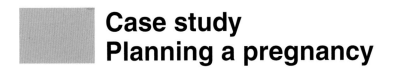

Case study
Planning a pregnancy

About the case

Alex is 32 years old and planning to have a baby. She is very busy at work, eats on the go and is a little overweight (BMI 28).

Breakfast

Fruit yoghurt pot (cereals, fruit purée and natural yoghurt)
1 large Cafe latté

Lunch

Tuna and cheese Panini
1 pack of mixed fruit salad
1 bottle mineral water
1 cup of tea and skimmed milk

Evening meal

Tomato, basil and mozzarella salad
Salmon tagliatelle (white cream sauce)
2 slices garlic bread
1 slice lemon cheesecake and a dash of cream
2 glasses red wine
2 glasses still water

Snacks

1 packet crisps
3 oaty biscuits
1 large mug hot chocolate

Simple strategies

It's good that Alex tries to select healthier food when she is out and about. However, when planning to have a baby, this is not always enough. Alcohol should ideally be avoided and Alex may also wish to monitor her caffeine intakes.

Nutrition in the Childbearing Years, First Edition. Emma Derbyshire.
© 2011 Emma Derbyshire. Published 2011 by Blackwell Publishing Ltd.

Alex should also make sure she achieves a healthy body weight 'before' she becomes pregnant. Excess body weight can lead to higher risk of pregnancy complications and long-term weight gain. Taking a daily pre-conceptual supplement will also help Alex to ensure that she is getting the right levels or vitamins, particularly folic acid, before and in the early stages of pregnancy.

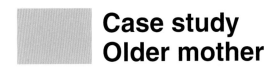

Case study
Older mother

About the case

Karen is in her mid-forties and expecting a baby. She has a healthy diet but is not sure how this could be improved further.

Breakfast

Porridge, semi-skimmed milk, raisins and a squeeze of honey
1 mug fruit herbal tea

Lunch

Tuna salad, tomato, watercress and black olives
1 oaty flapjack
1 bottle of still water

Evening meal

Lemon chicken, green kale and puy lentils
Fruit salad (apple, orange, strawberries, grapes) and crème fraiche
1 small white wine spritzer
1 large glass of water

Snacks

Small bag of mixed dried fruit
A cereal and fruit yoghurt pot
A handful sunflower seeds

Simple strategies

Although Karen generally has a healthy diet, older women are more likely to enter pregnancy with medical conditions or develop common chronic conditions such as hypertension or diabetes in pregnancy. There is also evidence that older mothers have a higher risk of delivering babies with birth defects (for a host of reasons), so folic acid supplementation is recommended before and in the early stages of pregnancy.

It is important that Karen continues eating a healthy diet, avoids drinking alcohol and has regular health checkups. Taking a pregnancy supplement would also help to ensure that Karen is getting the nutrients she needs in the right levels.

Nutrition in the Childbearing Years, First Edition. Emma Derbyshire.
© 2011 Emma Derbyshire. Published 2011 by Blackwell Publishing Ltd.

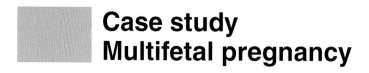

Case study
Multifetal pregnancy

About the case

Madeline is a 36-year-old mother who has undergone fertility treatment and is expecting twins. She tries to eat a healthy diet but is not sure 'how much' more food she should be eating. She is tempted to treat herself to more snacks; after all she is eating now for three.

Breakfast

Two slices wholemeal toast, butter and jam
1 bowl of Cornflakes and semi-skimmed milk
A sprinkle of sugar
1 large glass of milk

Lunch

Prawn and mayonnaise sandwich
2 blueberry muffins
1 bag of salt and vinegar crisps
1 cup of tea, semi-skimmed milk and a teaspoon of sugar

Evening meal

Lasagna, chips and a green salad
3 scoops vanilla ice cream
1 large pint glass of water

Snacks

4 chocolate digestive biscuits and a mug of hot chocolate before bed
1 chocolate cake bar in the afternoon

Simple strategies

Drinking a glass of milk each day is good practice, as calcium requirements are higher from women having more than one baby. Madeline does not need to increase her energy intake too much – two slices of wholemeal toast with marmite would be sufficient. It is important that any extra calories are nutritious and not 'empty' calories, i.e. the crisps and biscuits could be swapped for more nutritious alternatives, i.e. a bowl of cereals or some fruit.

Nutrition in the Childbearing Years, First Edition. Emma Derbyshire.
© 2011 Emma Derbyshire. Published 2011 by Blackwell Publishing Ltd.

Equally, energy intake only needs to increase in the second half of pregnancy (when the baby starts growing). Increasing this too early on may lead to unnecessary weight gain. On a final note, Madeline may consider taking a pregnancy supplement that contains suitable levels of iron, vitamin D and omega-3 fatty acids. Madeline may should also seek advice from relative health professionals.

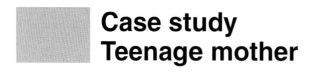

Case study
Teenage mother

About the case
Heidi is 16 years old and pregnant. She has not changed her diet much since becoming pregnant and eats much the same way as she used to. She generally eats what her mum prepares or buys snacks when hungry at school.

Breakfast
None – got up late
1 cup of tea and skimmed milk

Lunch
Chicken nuggets, ketchup and chips
1 bottle of lucozade energy from the vending machine

Evening meal
Margarita pizza (two slices)
Oven-cooked chips
2 large glasses of cola
1 cup of tea and skimmed milk before bed

Snacks
1 bottle of cola in the afternoon
Chewy sweets
2 twix sticks

Simple strategies
Heidi's diet is lacking in many essential nutrients and she is also consuming a lot of sugary beverages. These are providing extra calories and may increase the risk of developing medical conditions such as gestational diabetes in pregnancy. Heidi should swap these for healthier alternatives such as a glass of water, milk or fruit juice.

Overall, Heidi's diet is lacking in calcium, iron and essential fatty acids. This may affect her own health, i.e. bone health in the future and will not give her child the best start in life. The child may be born small and have delayed cognitive development.

Nutrition in the Childbearing Years, First Edition. Emma Derbyshire.
© 2011 Emma Derbyshire. Published 2011 by Blackwell Publishing Ltd.

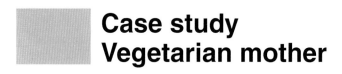

Case study
Vegetarian mother

About the case
Ruby is 29 years old and has been vegetarian for the last 15 years. She is 12 weeks pregnant and is re-evaluating her diet to make sure she is eating enough of the right foods and nutrients for her pregnancy.

Breakfast
Large bowl of muesli and soy milk
1 mug herbal tea

Lunch
Cheese and coleslaw sandwich with green rocket salad on wholemeal bread
Fruit salad
1 bottle of elderflower water

Evening meal
Tofu and noodle stir fry with soy sauce and Chinese vegetables
A strawberry organic yoghurt
2 large glasses water

Snacks
Fruit and nut cereal bar
Crackerbread and cream cheese (3 portions)
2 oat biscuits

Simple strategies
Ruby has a good diet to work with. Generally, it is balanced but a few simple changes would help to improve this further. Firstly, Ruby needs to make sure she is eating enough essential fatty acids, sprinkling sunflower seeds on her muesli or eating these as a snack may be one way to achieve this.

Nutrition in the Childbearing Years, First Edition. Emma Derbyshire.
© 2011 Emma Derbyshire. Published 2011 by Blackwell Publishing Ltd.

Equally, Ruby needs to make sure that she is eating enough foods rich in iron. A leafy green salad, with some protein and a glass of orange juice may go some way to improving her iron status. Some pregnant vegetarians may also be at risk of vitamin B_{12} deficiency, so it is worth making sure that soy milk is fortified and foods derived from yeast, i.e. marmite, are included in the diet. Supplemental vitamin preparations may be worth considering. Ideally, these should contain iron, vitamin B_{12} and omega-3 fatty acids to meet the needs of vegetarians.

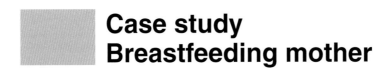

Case study
Breastfeeding mother

About the case

Sue is enjoying breastfeeding. It can be painful, but she wants to continue and make sure she is eating the right foods that will help to improve the quality of her breast milk.

Breakfast

2 slices wholemeal toast, butter and marmalade
1 large banana
1 large mug of herbal tea

Lunch

Ham sandwich, with margarine and tomato
Egg custard tart
1 cup of tea and skimmed milk

Evening meal

Steamed salmon with broccoli, carrots and potatoes
Strawberries and yoghurt
1 large glass of lemonade

Snacks

A green apple and peach
Fruit and nut chewy cereal bar
4 digestive biscuits

Simple strategies

Breast milk is about 87% water, so Sue should make sure that she is getting enough water throughout the day (about 2.7 L from food and beverage sources). It is great that Sue eats so much fresh fruit and vegetables, but it is worth making sure that these are washed thoroughly to remove any pesticide residues.

In families with a history of allergies, mothers may be advised to avoid peanuts or other allergens, i.e. cow's milk. Mothers should also be aware that some foods such as carrots may change the colour of their breast milk and alcohol should also be avoided when breastfeeding. On a final note, it is good to see that Sue is eating oily fish (a source of essential fatty acids).

Nutrition in the Childbearing Years, First Edition. Emma Derbyshire.
© 2011 Emma Derbyshire. Published 2011 by Blackwell Publishing Ltd.

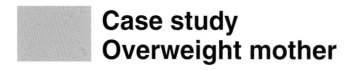

Case study
Overweight mother

About the case
Anna is 20 years old and expecting a baby. She is 5′3 and weighed 13 stone before she became pregnant (BMI 41.3). Anna is worried that she is going to deliver a big baby and is trying not to put on too much weight in her pregnancy.

Breakfast
1 bowl rice puffs, one teaspoon of sugar and semi-skimmed milk
2 slices white toast, butter and jam
A mug of tea, semi-skimmed milk and two sugars

Lunch
Fish finger sandwich on white bread, butter and tomato ketchup
1 bottle of diet cola

Evening meal
Lasagna, chips and beans
1 bottle of diet cola

Snacks
One cereal bar and some chew sweets
Another mug of tea (as before) later in the day

Simple strategies
It's great that Anna is thinking about her weight and how this may affect the size of her baby, but this is a little late. Ideally, Anna should have aimed to have been a healthier body weight 'before' she became pregnant and improved her diet quality (less refined and more fresh, nutritious foods).

Anna should aim to stay within the pregnancy weight guidelines for heavier mothers (about 5–9 kg weight gain; IoM, 2009). The importance of taking a folic acid supplement before and in the early stages of pregnancy needs to be communicated to heavier women, as their risk of having a neural tube defect affected pregnancy is higher.

Nutrition in the Childbearing Years, First Edition. Emma Derbyshire.
© 2011 Emma Derbyshire. Published 2011 by Blackwell Publishing Ltd.

Index

Note: Page numbers with italicised *f*'s and *t*'s refer to figures and tables, respectively.